GENERAL SURGICAL ONCOLOGY

GENERAL SURGICAL ONCOLOGY

GLENN STEELE, Jr., M.D.

The William V. McDermott Professor of Surgery,
Harvard Medical School;
Chairman, Department of Surgery,
New England Deaconess Hospital,
Boston, Massachusetts

BLAKE CADY, M.D.

Associate Professor of Surgery,
Harvard Medical School;
Chief, Division of Surgical Oncology,
New England Deaconess Hospital,
Boston, Massachusetts

W.B. SAUNDERS COMPANY *Philadelphia, London, Toronto, Montreal, Sydney, Tokyo*
Harcourt Brace Jovanovich, Inc.

W. B. SAUNDERS COMPANY
Harcourt Brace Jovanovich, Inc.
The Curtis Center
Independence Square West
Philadelphia, PA 19106

Library of Congress Cataloging-in-Publication Data

General surgical oncology / [editors] Glenn Steele, Jr., Blake Cady.

p. cm.

1. Cancer—Surgery.   I. Steele, Glenn.   II. Cady, Blake   [DNLM: 1. Neoplasms.   2. Neoplasms—surgery.   QZ 268 G326]

RD651.G46 1992   616.99′4059——dc20

DNLM/DLC   91–26529

ISBN 0–7216–2471–5

Production Manager: Frank Polizzano
Indexer: Susan Thomas

General Surgical Oncology   ISBN 0–7216–2471–5

Copyright © 1992 by W. B. Saunders Company

All rights reserved. No part of this publication may be reproduced or transmitted in any form or by any means, electronic or mechanical, including photocopy, recording, or any information storage and retrieval system, without permission in writing from the publisher.

Printed in MEXICO.

Last digit is the print number: 9   8   7   6   5   4   3   2   1

CONTRIBUTORS

PETER N. BENOTTI, M.D.
Associate Clinical Professor of Surgery, Harvard Medical School; New England Deaconess Hospital, Boston, Massachusetts
Management of Regional and Local Tumor Recurrence

ALBERT BOTHE, Jr., M.D.
Associate Professor of Surgery, Harvard Medical School; Associate Chairman, Department of Surgery, and Director, General Surgical Training, New England Deaconess Hospital, Boston, Massachusetts
Management of Regional and Local Tumor Recurrence

BLAKE CADY, M.D.
Associate Professor of Surgery, Harvard Medical School; Chief, Surgical Oncology, New England Deaconess Hospital, Boston, Massachusetts
Biologic Implications for Clinical Phenomena and Clinical Application of Biologic Phenomena; Influence of the Practice Setting on the Role of the Surgical Oncologist; The Surgical Oncologist as the Patient Manager; Gastric Cancer; Primary and Metastatic Cancer of the Liver; Breast Cancer; Endocrine Gland Cancers; Melanoma; Soft Tissue Sarcomas

PAUL A. CHURCH, M.D.
Clinical Instructor of Surgery, Harvard Medical School; Active Staff (Urology), New England Deaconess Hospital, Boston, Massachusetts
Urologic Carcinoma: Prostate Cancer; Testicular Cancer

F. HENRY ELLIS, Jr., M.D., Ph.D.
Clinical Professor of Surgery, Harvard Medical School; Chief Emeritus, New England Deaconess Hospital, Boston, Massachusetts
Esophageal Carcinoma

ROBERT C. EYRE, M.D.
Assistant Clinical Professor of Surgery, Harvard Medical School; Chief of Urology, New England Deaconess Hospital, Boston, Massachusetts
Urologic Carcinoma; Renal Cell Carcinoma; Transitional Cell Carcinoma of the Bladder

HOWARD M. GOODMAN, M.D.
Assistant Professor, Obstetrics, Gynecology, and Reproductive Biology, Harvard Medical School; Division of Gynecologic Oncology, Brigham and Women's Hospital, Boston, Massachusetts
Gynecologic Oncology

ROGER L. JENKINS, M.D.
Associate Professor of Surgery, Harvard Medical School; Staff Surgeon and Director of Intensive Care and Nutritional Support Service, Faulkner Hospital; Clinical Surgical Consultant, Manchester Veterans Administration Hospital; Clinical Associate in Surgery, Tuft's New England Medical Center, Children's Hospital Medical Center, and Massachusetts General Hospital; Director of Outpatient Surgery, Director of Section of Liver Transplantation, and Chief, Division of Hepatobiliary Surgery and Liver Transplantation, New England Deaconess Hospital, Boston, Massachusetts
Primary and Metastatic Cancer of the Liver

J. MILBURN JESSUP, M.D.
Associate Professor of Surgery, Harvard Medical School; New England Deaconess Hospital, Boston, Massachusetts
Rectal and Anal Carcinoma

MOHAMMED KARBASSI, M.D.
Surgical Resident, Deaconess-Harvard Surgical Service, New England Deaconess Hospital, Boston, Massachusetts
Management of Regional and Local Tumor Recurrence

SIDNEY LEVITSKY, M.D.
David W. and David Cheever Professor of Surgery, Harvard Medical School; Chief, Division of Cardiothoracic Surgery, New England Deaconess Hospital, Boston, Massachusetts
Esophageal Carcinoma: Discussion; Primary Lung Cancer: Discussion

JAMES W. LUCARINI, M.D.
Clinical Instructor in Otolaryngology, Harvard Medical School; Active Staff, New England Deaconess Hospital, Dana-Farber Cancer Institute, and Massachusetts Eye and Ear Infirmary; Courtesy Staff, The Children's Hospital, Boston, Massachusetts
Nasopharyngeal Carcinoma

WILLIAM V. McDERMOTT, Jr., M.D., F.A.C.S.
Cheever Professor of Surgery, Emeritus, Harvard Medical School; Chairman (Retired), Department of Surgery, New England Deaconess Hospital, Boston, Massachusetts
Primary and Metastatic Cancer of the Liver

DANIEL MILLER, M.D.
Clinical Professor Otolaryngology Emeritus, Harvard Medical School; New England Deaconess Hospital, Dana-Farber Cancer Institute, Massachusetts Eye and Ear Infirmary, Boston, Massachusetts
Nasopharyngeal Carcinoma

WILFORD B. NEPTUNE, M.D.
Clinical Associate Professor of Surgery, Harvard Medical School; Assistant Clinical Professor of Surgery, Tufts College of Medicine; Clinical Director, Cardiothoracic Surgery, New England Deaconess Hospital, Boston, Massachusetts
Primary Lung Cancer

JONATHAN M. NILOFF, M.D., F.A.C.S.
Associate Professor, Obstetrics, Gynecology, and Reproductive Biology, Harvard

Medical School; Director, Division of Gynecologic Oncology, Beth Israel Hospital, Boston, Massachusetts
Gynecologic Oncology

CHARLES M. NORRIS, Jr., M.D.
Assistant Professor, Otolaryngology, Harvard Medical School; Chief, Division of Otolaryngology–Head and Neck Surgery, Department of Surgery, New England Deaconess Hospital; Surgical Coordinator, Head and Neck Oncology Clinic, Dana-Farber Cancer Institute, Boston, Massachusetts
Head and Neck Cancer: Fundamentals; The Floor of the Mouth and Tongue; Larynx; Hypopharynx and Cervical Esophagus; Role of Neoadjuvant Chemotherapy in Head and Neck Cancer

T. S. RAVIKUMAR, M.D.
Associate Professor, Yale School of Medicine; Chief, Surgical Oncology Division, West Haven Veteran's Administration Hospital, and Yale–New Haven Hospital, New Haven, Connecticut
Colon Cancer; Management of Regional and Local Tumor Recurrence

GLENN STEELE, Jr., M.D.
The William V. McDermott Professor of Surgery, Harvard Medical School; Chairman, Department of Surgery, Deaconess Surgical Associates, Boston, Massachusetts
Introduction to Surgical Oncology: Surgical Oncology—Definition/Training; Biologic Implications for Clinical Phenomena and Clinical Application of Biologic Phenomena; Influence of the Practice Setting on the Role of the Surgical Oncologist; The Surgical Oncologist as the Patient Manager; Colon Cancer; Rectal and Anal Carcinoma; Primary and Metastatic Cancer of the Liver; Management of Regional and Local Tumor Recurrence

MICHAEL D. STONE, M.D.
Assistant Professor of Surgery, Harvard Medical School; Attending Surgeon, Division of Surgical Oncology, New England Deaconess Hospital, Boston, Massachusetts
Soft Tissue Sarcomas

PREFACE

The intent of *General Surgical Oncology* is to take advantage of a unique opportunity that may not last for a particularly long time. The New England Deaconess Hospital is one of the major teaching hospitals associated with Harvard Medical School and represents one of four separate general surgical training programs in the Harvard system. In contrast to the other Harvard hospitals, the Deaconess has evolved into an exclusively secondary and tertiary referral center, having personnel with particular expertise in the medical and surgical treatment of patients with solid tumors. Its collection of cancer treatment experience represents almost four generations of individuals with eminence in the surgical therapy of solid cancers. This is rare, if not unheard of, at least among the faculty of general hospitals in the United States. It occurred to us several years ago, therefore, that this collection of talent provided a reason to design a book that attempts to achieve a distinct purpose.

Perhaps others would agree with us that a major problem occurs when an author attempts to write about something with which he or she is not personally familiar (whether or not the book happens to be on a medical subject). If one scans many of the standard textbooks in general surgery and/or in surgical subspecialties, one notes that often the onerous task of writing any comprehensive review falls either to a junior faculty member or a fellow who accepts the quid pro quo of first authorship. The senior author with the more familiar name is added on for the necessary patina, credibility, name-recognition, and as a reward for recruiting the "real worker." In the attempt to present definitive, almost Talmudic, expositions, what is produced often is neither of interest nor familiar to the writer. In addition, "definitive" approaches must provide balance since on any given topic in medicine, there are at least two—and usually many more—reasonably argued views. The result is encyclopedic at best and boring at worst.

The intent of this volume has been to produce what undoubtedly will be reviewed as an idiosyncratic single-institutional view of the training of surgical oncologists and the surgical treatment of patients with the most prevalent solid cancers. Many of the authors of these chapters are well known. All have been asked to use their own patient series and data. Most refer to their own previous peer-reviewed publications; this gives their narratives a stronger background. However, the goal of this book, as originally purveyed to the individual contributors, is to present personal views in narrative style and convey the collected wisdom of experts with significant clinical knowledge who regularly interact in a single general hospital.

In some chapters, this approach has produced rather biased expositions, such that the editors have felt the need to add small commentaries to assure readers that the editors themselves recognize that what has been written may not necessarily be a customary, let alone balanced, approach.

As opposed to most textbooks that we have either read or participated in as author/editor, this effort has actually been fun. We hope that it will be enjoyable to read and, in addition, provide useful information to practicing surgeons who would like to know how things are really done at a hospital in which caregivers spend all of their time dealing with these problems.

GLENN STEELE, JR., M.D.
BLAKE CADY, M.D.

CONTENTS

1
INTRODUCTION TO SURGICAL ONCOLOGY ... 1
Surgical Oncology—Definition/Training ... 1
Glenn Steele, Jr.

Biologic Implications for Clinical Phenomena and Clinical Application of Biologic Phenomena ... 10
Glenn Steele, Jr. and Blake Cady

Influence of the Practice Setting on the Role of the Surgical Oncologist ... 14
Glenn Steele, Jr. and Blake Cady

The Surgical Oncologist as the Patient Manager ... 18
Glenn Steele, Jr. and Blake Cady

2
HEAD AND NECK CANCER ... 23
Fundamentals ... 23
Charles M. Norris, Jr.

The Floor of the Mouth and Tongue ... 41
Charles M. Norris, Jr.

Larynx ... 56
Charles M. Norris, Jr.

Hypopharynx and Cervical Esophagus ... 68
Charles M. Norris, Jr.

Role of Neoadjuvant Chemotherapy in Head and Neck Cancer ... 72
Charles M. Norris, Jr.

Nasopharyngeal Carcinoma ... 77
James W. Lucarini and Daniel Miller

3
ESOPHAGEAL CARCINOMA ... 87
F. Henry Ellis, Jr.

Discussion ... 105
Sidney Levitsky

4
PRIMARY LUNG CANCER 107
Wilford B. Neptune

Discussion 135
Sidney Levitsky

5
GASTRIC CANCER 139
Blake Cady

6
COLON CANCER 149
T. S. Ravikumar and Glenn Steele, Jr.

7
RECTAL AND ANAL CARCINOMA 171
J. Milburn Jessup and Glenn Steele, Jr.

8
PRIMARY AND METASTATIC CANCER OF THE LIVER 185
William V. McDermott, Jr., Roger L. Jenkins, Blake Cady, and Glenn Steele, Jr.

9
BREAST CANCER 195
Blake Cady

10
ENDOCRINE GLAND CANCERS 219
Blake Cady

11
MELANOMA 233
Blake Cady

12
SOFT TISSUE SARCOMAS 247
Michael D. Stone and Blake Cady

13
UROLOGIC CARCINOMA 275

Prostate Cancer 275
Paul A. Church

Renal Cell Carcinoma 285
Robert C. Eyre

Testicular Cancer 292
Paul A. Church

Transitional Cell Carcinoma of the Bladder 298
   Robert C. Eyre

14
GYNECOLOGIC ONCOLOGY 309
   Jonathan M. Niloff and Howard M. Goodman

15
MANAGEMENT OF REGIONAL AND LOCAL TUMOR RECURRENCE 341
   *Peter N. Benotti, Mohammed Karbassi, T. S. Ravikumar,
   Albert Bothe, Jr. and Glenn Steele, Jr.*

INDEX 355

1

INTRODUCTION TO SURGICAL ONCOLOGY

SURGICAL ONCOLOGY— DEFINITION/TRAINING
by Glenn Steele, Jr., M.D.

One of the opportunities (and for the reader, dangers) of a non-peer–reviewed book such as this is that the author expresses completely unsupported, biased, and somewhat colorful opinions. In designing the theme of *General Surgical Oncology*, we have asked each of our contributors to avoid encyclopedic exegesis, preferring a more personal approach to specific disease entities. Of course, in the individual chapters themselves or in the appended commentary, we have felt the need to convince readers and reviewers that we at least know what the conventionally accepted diagnostic/therapeutic approaches are. Nevertheless, our preference as editors has been to ask leaders in the field, all of whom happen to have been at a single institution at the time of writing, to speak from their personal experience, from their own series, or from their involvement in multi-institutional trials.

In a similar manner, we would like to introduce the book by presenting our own answers to many of the generic questions about surgical oncology asked when we visit other areas of the country and when we visit noncancer center practices. Here, we will try to address our unique and admittedly personal definition of what surgical oncology is, and what it will be in the future, regardless of specific decisions about certification or lack of certification by the American Board of Surgery or specialty societies such as the Society of Surgical Oncology.

First, my bias. I believe that "surgical oncology" cannot be created by fiat (i.e., certification), and certainly not at the expense of gutting the core out of general surgery. This reflects a philosophy appropriate to a chairman of a general surgery department. The argument that specialty certification alone in medicine has allowed medical oncologists to control new clinical treatment ideas, to preempt protocol design, and to manage patient flow is specious. The way to obtain credibility in conceptual or practical patient management areas of general oncologic surgery, with medical colleagues and with patients, is through performance over time, and this will most naturally follow appropriate training, not simply certification.

A surgical oncologist is essentially a function of his or her training. How then, should the surgical oncologist be trained? Another of my biases comes immediately to the fore. I believe that there should be no *one* prescribed training pathway. This does not imply that some core knowledge of the natural history of common cancers, their surgical treatment options, and the place of surgical treatment among other therapy modalities should not be clearly defined and taught to all surgical oncology trainees. The majority of this knowledge should, however, be incorporated equally well into the data base of any well-trained general surgeon. What then is the difference between the two?

First, the surgical oncologist should take extra training. Either during surgical residency or immediately after, additional significant time (two to four years, ideally) should be spent outside of the usual environment of the general surgery residency program. Numerous clinical and research opportunities exist. The selection of these will depend on the needs of the particular trainee and will largely determine the type and perhaps even the location of the subsequent post-training practice venue.

If a basic research experience is sought, precise goals must be set, but can vary from individual to individual. Many openings are now available in and outside of surgical departments in which basic science laboratories offer NIH-sponsored research training fellowships. So called "T32" surgical oncology training positions have proliferated during the past several years. They now number approximately 68 at 18 different university-associated training programs (Table 1–1; Fig. 1–1). These fellowships differ, but most offer at least one to three years of uninterrupted basic research training. If the goal is to "try out" research, then the laboratory "virgin" probably would prefer to cut his or her risk and move toward the shorter time option. Additional typical "fail-safe" planning often consists of designing a so-called "research" program either in or near the home residency institution, making arrangements to keep some footing in the clinical arena in case the laboratory experience turns out to be a bust! Such non-full-commitment options must be avoided.

Ideally, the basic research T32 positions should be quite limited in number, should be highly competed for, and should be filled only by those who have shown a considerable desire and perseverance as well as talent in getting a laboratory slot. All of these attributes will be needed (in addition to luck and an excellent basic research preceptor) if the clinical trainee is to learn "real science" in a relatively short time. Most thoughtful general surgery departmental chairmen agree that not everyone should go into the laboratory. However, I would go further in suggesting that very few should go into the laboratory. Once there, at least in our program, fellows remain for a minimum of two and, ideally, three years during their mandatory elective between the third and fourth year of the general surgery residency. An alternative laboratory time is after the surgical chief residency. In either time period, the research trainee must commit to two or three years of basic

TABLE 1–1. NIH-FUNDED SURGICAL ONCOLOGY TRAINING—FISCAL YEAR 1990–1991

Institution	Positions
Brigham and Women's Hospital	4
City of Hope	4
Johns Hopkins	2
Johns Hopkins (Pediatric)	2
New England Deaconess	4
RPMI	4
University of Alabama	2
UCLA	6
UCSF	2
University of Chicago	6
University of Florida	2
University of Illinois	2
University of Minnesota	4
University of Pennsylvania	4
University of Texas	9
University of Texas (Thoracic)	3
Virginia Commonwealth	2
Washington University	6
18 Institutions	68

laboratory work, should disconnect from all clinical duties, and should choose the best possible basic research laboratory in an area intellectually contiguous to whatever clinical interest he or she may have already developed, although this is not absolutely necessary. I insist that such clinical trainees going into our own basic research laboratories work on a moment-to-moment basis with either an M.D. or a Ph.D. whose full-time job is research. Finally, particularly in the case of research trainees who are beginning to experience some success in the laboratory, they must constantly be reminded who they are and how they differ from the basic scientists around them. This last cliché is only important if the research training is successful. More will be discussed on this later.

The phases of "self-experience" when a laboratory "neophyte" goes from the clinic to a basic research environment are predictable. First, there is euphoria. I am assuming that the trainee really wanted to learn substantive science, and wasn't just sent away to the laboratory to meet his program director's perceptions of the Residency Review Committee's requirement for overall progam credibility. This euphoric period generally lasts three to six months and does not depend on whether experiments work or whether or not the trainee is asked to think about what he or she is doing. Rather, it is a predictable response to a new environment, a new challenge (excellent surgical residents always respond well to challenge), and the resumption of a regular wake/sleep cycle. Most often, after a brief period of chaos during introduction to gels (Southerns, Westerns, Northerns, and now Southwesterns) and other basic laboratory techniques, data begin to flow.

The basic science preceptor, particularly if a Ph.D., must be made aware that surgical residents need immediate feedback. In most of the laboratory settings that I have experienced, immediate feedback is rare unless it is negative and posteuphoric depression is almost always a response to this

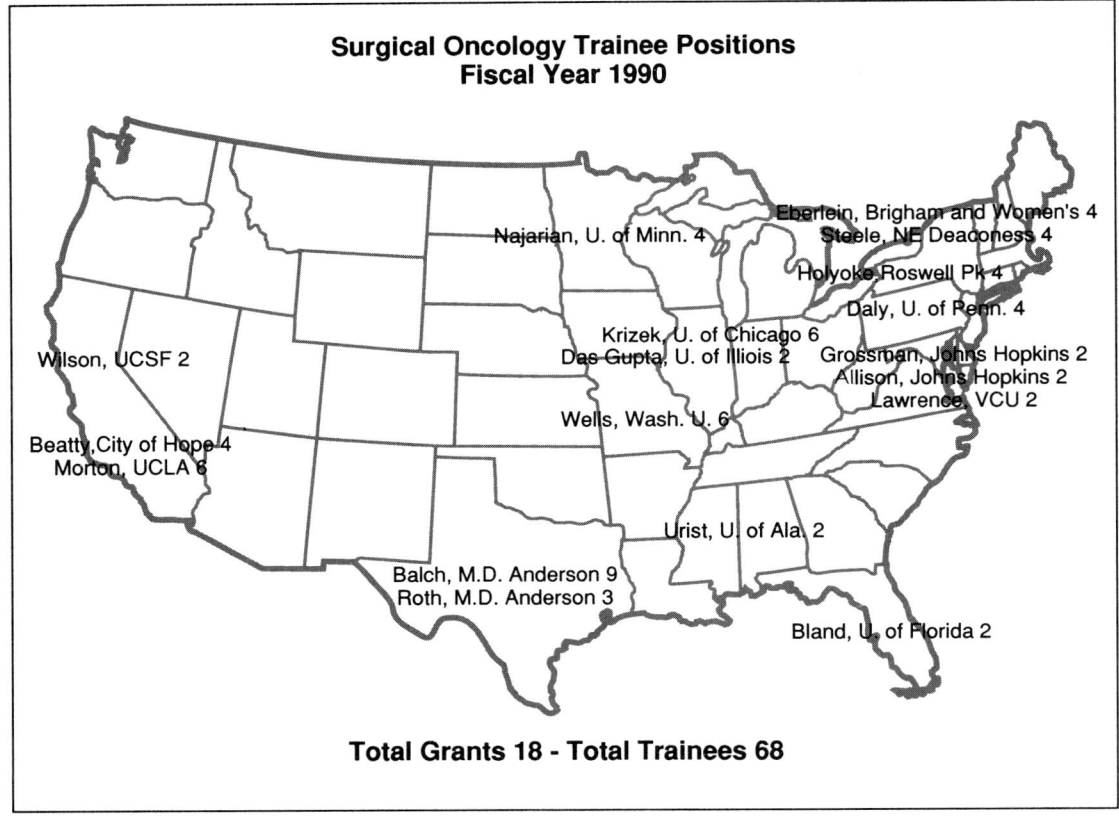

Figure 1–1. Principal investigators and location of T32 fellowships in surgical oncology.

most basic of changes in the rhythms of feedback when the resident goes from the clinic to the laboratory environment. Through all of these psychological as well as intellectual challenges, escape back to the clinic must be proscribed.

A second easy way out for many first-time research trainees is to become super technicians. Without continual prodding, particularly by the clinical department or divisional chief, the fellow and the basic research preceptor may fall into an easy pattern. The resident assumes the role of an extremely competent, but basically brainless, laboratory assistant with limited creativity defined only by solving specific experimental procedure problems. Each trainee *must* be asked again and again what his or her experimental line is.

Additional crucial questions are: "How does this experiment fit into your experimental line? What will you do when your data disprove your postulate? (This is an oblique way of proving that a postulate does, in fact, exist!) When will your data allow you to write a first draft abstract or, even better, a full manuscript?" These questions prepare the trainee for the inevitable pitfall of accumulating ever greater mounds of data without beginning the much more difficult challenge of pulling it together to finish a project. No beginning researcher has any idea of the many facets we take for granted in the progression from postulate to accepted/published and then, finally, challenged manuscript. And finally, "How will you distinguish your own unique identity in science and in clinical surgery different from your full-time basic research preceptor and equally distinct from your strictly clinical colleagues?" In our own laboratory setting, world class (i.e., they have their own grants) biologists, biochemists, immunologists, and geneticists teach surgical residents. Regardless of how effective a two- to three-year stint in a basic research laboratory may be, there is little probability that our surgical trainees will be grant-competitive if they design their experimental questions to compete directly with these basic research paradigms. Thus, it is important to ask the trainees repeatedly how what they view and what they ask as clinical scientists will be unique.

No one model exists for establishing the uniqueness of the clinician/scientist. More than likely, Francis D. Moore characterized it best when he described the position of the well-trained scientist who is also a respected surgeon as straddling two distinct cultures in a protracted and uncomfortable stance. My own summary of the integration is as follows. Questions that emanate from a thorough knowledge of various human cancers can be linked to the more artificial (the usual scientific euphemism is "elegant") but achievable goals in the defined setting of a basic science experiment. A unique ability to translate basic science results into "real" English for intelligent clinical colleagues and the ability to frame scientific postulates from clinical dilemmas is perhaps the easiest job description. As detailed below, the problem is best discussed by citing a number of specific examples that are pertinent to our own investigations of the biology and clinical treatment of colorectal cancer and thyroid neoplasms. In short, we convince our trainees that many of the most basic research questions that occur to clinicians who treat patients will not occur to basic scientists but are, nevertheless, amenable to basic science investigation.

Equally important is the ability of the clinician/scientist to take information from the laboratory to the clinic. Such "Phase I or II" experiments are the beginnings of a formal human research pathway attempting to lead to improved diagnostic and therapeutic utility in the treatment of specific human diseases. Such attempts at making a transition from basic science output to clinical medicine entail no compromise in research design or effort and, in fact, are met with much less condescension among basic scientists today than a number of years ago when, almost by definition, "applied" science was thought to be "mediocre" science. The major technical breakthroughs in bioscience (something as conceptually simple as a quantitative PCR assay, for instance) have allowed molecular biologists, biochemists, and other basic scientists to shorten the developmental lag time among studies on yeast, studies on liquid tumors in humans, and now studies on solid tumor patients.

Just as enervating in this recent upgrading of applied science in clinical medicine is the introduction of the profit motive for any new device or new idea's successful application to a majority of patients with a prevalent disease. In any case, the clinician/scientist should become the crucial determinant of appropriate experimental design for all human trials, the key to establishing ethical guidelines ensuring detachment of profit potential and experimental results, and the arbiter of what is best for the individual patient involved. The most successful surgical scientists are those who balance their commitment to scientific studies with the ultimate clinical question of what is best for the patient at hand.

The goals of our own basic science training for surgical oncology fellows are straightforward. We expect the most successful trainees to be peer-review grant–competitive, and we expect them to provide the unique set of talents summarized previously that will make them leaders in creating new knowledge.

A slightly less ideal goal is the establishment for the trainee of what "real science" is and the provision of a unique two- to three-year interaction with "real scientists." If this goal is achieved, we consider it a successful laboratory experience. If the clinical trainee does not ultimately become grant-competitive, at least he or she may provide an important link between basic researchers and clinical colleagues and clinical problems. These individuals may still help create new knowledge in various areas, but they will need assistance.

Finally, at the very least, our basic laboratory experience can convince some trainees stuck at the emotional and intellectual nadir of their research jobs (usually after the 3 to 6 months of euphoria) that relief is a return to their clinical job. The reward here is to have proved to themselves that science is not for them. The challenge for such individuals is to find one of the many nonresearch differentiation pathways into surgical oncology. These individuals should be assured that they are not failures and that their careers are not destroyed, particularly if they have worked diligently in the laboratory but to no avail. Such an outcome is quite rare if the trainee has chosen the laboratory carefully, is placed with committed basic or clinical scientist mentors, and is nurtured through at least two years of intense scientific method.

Two caveats. First, if the trainee is going into the laboratory during his general surgery residency, he or she must have a guaranteed residency training slot afterward. This should be known at the outset of the research training. All research slots should be reserved for the best of our aspiring academic surgical oncologists. No slots should be used for those who are searching for other training positions after they have been exfoliated from their original clinical program.

If the laboratory training occurs at the end of the general surgical residency, both the research preceptor and department head must assist the most successful of fellows in finding the right chairman for whom to work. For any junior staff surgeon, when peer-reviewed grant funding research is expected, protection from clinical volume-driven salary demands will be necessary for at least two to three years. Certainly no more than 25 per cent to at most 50 per cent of such an individual's time should be clinical if a start-up laboratory effort is to be instituted.

Second, is a one-year research experience ever valuable? Perhaps, but only if there are goals specified to be distinct from any subsequent expectation to compete for peer-reviewed grant funding. For most "real" research laboratories, even laboratories such as ours in a clinical department, the time and effort necessary to train a laboratory "virgin" are simply not worthwhile without a significant payback. Thus, a one-year trainee is almost always relegated to a mediocre laboratory or is used as a technician or "observer" in a good laboratory. Only if a specific and formalized exposure to clinical trials research is available and is the defined goal of a potential trainee should a one-year position be elected. Such training slots are available, but rare. As is the case with basic research trainees, preceptors who are successful clinical researchers themselves must ensure that the trainee understands the underlying foundations of clinical trial design and performance and is not simply functioning as a data manager.

In both clinical research and basic research settings, the surgical trainee needs to remember that his or her research training experience will be significantly shorter than that of competitors in basic research (three to five years obtaining a Ph.D. and another two to five years doing a postdoctoral fellowship) or academic medical oncologists who spend what amounts to a postdoctoral fellowship of three to five years protected from the demands of patient care while they begin their junior faculty careers. Such protection will generally be considerably less, even in the best of academic surgical departments. This emphasizes a need for complete immersion (i.e., no moonlighting, if possible) and intense concentration during the relatively brief research elective (even if it is three years long). As noted earlier, the surgeon must continue to ask what it is that distinguishes his or her unique view of surgical disease. And finally, perhaps even more important in clinical research (compared with the precise, elegant, but less applicable basic research setting) the surgeon must learn to condense the questions he or she asks. Only in these ways will the surgical oncologist who aspires to excellent research compete effectively with a profusion of academic medical oncology or basic research colleagues.

Although many more basic research fellowship slots are available now than several years ago, few well-defined, formalized clinical research training positions are identifiable. This is unfortunate since surgeons should be as steeped in the understanding of clinical trial design and clinical trial limitations as our medical oncology colleagues. Perhaps the appreciation of this need among all surgical trainees will become apparent only when our major surgical societies (American Surgical Association, Society of Surgical Oncology, and various regional surgical societies) accept a preponderance of papers for presentation containing obvious postulates to be tested and report identifiable clinical trials from which data are shown to support or refute well-defined conclusions. The objection by anachronistic surgical role models that prospective appropriately controlled clinical trials invade the unique personal relationship that exists between surgeon and patient is simply not true. As most clinicians now know, if the surgeon or the internist believes in a particular trial or the general worth of prospective clinical trial design as the best way to answer many human disease questions, patients will sense this and will readily agree to participate in a given trial without diluting the patient-surgeon relationship. In many areas of the country, including the Northeast, patients are often insistent that their primary surgeon review with them all available treatment protocols (conventional and experimental). Only if the surgeon objects or is unresponsive to such requests will the patient seek alternative care.

A question frequently asked by potential surgical oncologists is, "What should I do to prepare myself for a career in academic cancer surgery?" The answer is simple. Do either what is of greatest importance and interest to the individual or focus on an area felt to be a weakness. Particularly if this is a clinical area not prominent in most general surgical training programs (e.g., head and neck oncology), extra clinical training should be considered.

And remember, any surgeon who aspires to a leadership role in cancer care must learn not only the technical repertoire necessary to diagnose and treat all common solid tumors (and nonsolid tumors where surgery has a role) but, just as important, needs to understand the biology of the diseases for which surgery is contemplated.

For strictly clinical preparation, surgical oncology programs presently approved by the Society of Surgical Oncology (SSO) entail excellent technical preparation as well as a good grounding in the basics of clinical trial design and application. Present fellowship slots in such SSO-approved programs are summarized in Table 1–2. Most of the SSO fellowships stress clinical preparation and some research. Almost all of the basic research fellowships (see Table 1–1) involve both basic research (usually 18 to 24 months) and a clinical oncology framework that varies a good deal from program to program. Additional opportunities in clinical surgical oncology are undoubtedly available but not listed in the two formal categories already summarized. If a candidate has a particular area needing strengthening, each non-NIH- or SSO-approved program should be looked at with the expectation that precise numbers of patients seen with a given diagnosis, numbers of patients entered into treatment protocols, and the relationship between the surgical oncology fellow and the general surgery residents be articulated. The best situation is the one with the most patients, a high rate of protocol accrual, and a relationship in which the surgical oncology fellow is performing as a junior staff person (particularly in the educational relationship to the general surgery resident). Ideally, each clinical fellow would assume responsibility for the design and initiation of at least one treatment protocol during his or her clinical research training fellowship.

Occasionally, academic aspirants phrase their career question as follows, "Tell me what would be best to get ahead in my academic career in surgical oncology." This is a subtle but telling difference in emphasis from the career preparation question paraphrased previously. I generally suggest to such individuals that if they are thinking only of their careers, and have no basic glimmer of interest in either a basic research or a clinical research area, they should probably go into something other than surgical oncology. Naturally, such individuals continue to pursue what they desire, but they are certainly off my list of potentially interesting junior staff recruits.

TABLE 1–2. SSO-APPROVED SURGICAL ONCOLOGY TRAINING PROGRAMS—FISCAL YEAR 1990

Institution	Program Director
City of Hope	J. Terz
M.D. Anderson	C. Balch
Medical College Virginia	G. Parker
Memorial Sloan-Kettering	M. Brennan
Ohio State University	W. Farrar
RPMI	E. Holyoke
Tulane	D. Carter
University of Chicago	F. Michelassi
University of Illinois	T. Das Gupta
University of Medicine and Dentistry/ New Jersey Medical School	G. Hill
University of Miami	A. Ketcham

Despite lengthy discussions between various specialty societies and the American Board of Surgery, special certificates of competence seem to be less highly proliferative at present than in the past. Even if some sort of certification in cancer surgery is offered in the future by the American Board of Surgery or the Society of Surgical Oncology, I would hope that candidates could qualify despite having progressed through a variety of differentiation or training pathways. Quite simply, the well-trained clinical oncologist should be expected to know a corpus of knowledge including the biology and clinical diagnosis and therapy possibilities of most solid tumors and nonsolid tumors in which surgeons play a role. But hopefully, a heterogeneous array of training programs and areas of particular expertise can continue to be available that will meet the varied and individual interests and needs of bright and motivated academic surgeons. More than likely, the success or failure of our attempts to influence basic biology research or the design of clinical trials in solid tumors will be more dependent on the success of our commitment to a varied set of training pathways than to the initiation of any certification process.

What happens then, after training? How is one to define "surgical oncologist" after successful completion of one or another of the training pathways? First, a heterogeneity of practice venues (academic as well as nonacademic) should allow for wide selection of job opportunities for the well-trained surgical oncologist. Exclusively clinical, clinical research, or a combination of basic research and clinical jobs is available. All of these jobs should demand at least one of the following characteristics of anyone who calls himself or herself a surgical oncologist:

1. Leadership in application and evaluation of diagnostic and therapeutic techniques involved in secondary or tertiary referral patients with extensive but common primary cancers, recurrent cancers, or rare tumors;

2. Leadership in clinical cancer research either in multimodality protocols or in establishing surgery-only treatment plans or trials;

3. Leadership in the training of general surgery residents or surgical oncology fellows in the technical and biologic aspects of solid tumor diagnosis and therapy; and

4. Leadership in the creation of new knowledge through "surgically framed" basic research questions.

What a surgical oncologist should not be is a general surgeon who has secured a franchise by the perception of special expertise (certification or not) and who is designated by the hospital administrator to be the sole performer of procedures that could and should quite confidently be performed by any well-trained general surgeon.

BIOLOGIC IMPLICATIONS FOR CLINICAL PHENOMENA AND THE CLINICAL APPLICATION OF BIOLOGIC PHENOMENA

by Glenn Steele, Jr., M.D., and
Blake Cady, M.D.

Assuming that there are numerous pathways to becoming a surgical oncologist, some basic agreed-to repertoire of surgical diagnostic and therapeutic techniques (i.e., tests and operations) should be in the grasp of every cancer surgeon. Most of the core diseases are reviewed in succeeding chapters and are organized by organ system.

Often, in a highly competitive academic or urban secondary or tertiary referral practice setting such as ours, a practicing surgical oncologist will subspecialize. Much of this subspecialization is patient- or referring internist–driven and, at least initially, independent of the neophyte surgical oncologist's talents or wishes. Thus, there is little reason that one of the authors (G.S. Jr.) would select only patients with secondary or tertiary referral gastrointestinal and hepatobiliary cancers to the exclusion of endocrine neoplasms or melanomas in my practice. Likewise, the second author (B.C.) may not choose to be treating predominantly patients with breast cancer, sarcoma, or endocrine neoplasms. Nevertheless, it is natural in this particular setting that one begins to learn more and more about less and less. Our practice patterns ultimately reflect this. It is to be hoped that in other medical venues patients and referring physicians will not demand that every breast biopsy be done by a so-called "breast surgeon"—breast surgeon being defined as a surgeon who does nothing but operate on the breast and surrounding integument.

Regardless of the breadth or narrowness of one's clinical practice pattern, the surgical oncologist should understand the place of surgical expertise within the overall biology of the cancer being treated. Knowledge of the natural history of each disease should clarify the limits of surgery. Additionally, at least in academic settings, such knowledge should allow the surgical oncologist to frame the most essential scientific questions to expedite the translation of new biology to benefit patients through better disease diagnosis or therapy.

Let us give some specific examples from our own area of interest—gastrointestinal (GI) cancer. These examples help to define how we and our colleagues attempt to interdigitate biologists' expertise in cell biology with our role as operating cancer surgeons. Each of the basic science questions investigated in our laboratory derives from a thorough clinical knowledge of the natural history of colorectal cancer and from particular diagnostic and therapeutic weaknesses perceived to be areas where the biggest clinical gains might come from application of new biologic techniques.

Thus, our laboratory's investigations of the function of CEA (carcinoembryonic antigen) emanate from clinical phenomenology. CEA is a particularly good marker for colorectal cancer metastatic to the liver or lung. Why? Specific postulates we have derived from the clinical data include studies to determine if secreted or membrane-bound CEA is an important mechanism in site-specific metastasis. Even more narrowly framed, the question becomes whether there may be specific CEA or CEA-like receptors on human Kupffer cells and/or fixed alveolar macrophages. If such receptors were defined, isolated, and related to a variety of model systems, we could test if site specificity of CEA-producing colon and rectum carcinoma could be reproducibly perturbed either by blocking receptors or specifically changing CEA-like molecules on the tumor cell membranes. Assessing any difference in the pattern of metastases after such precise manipulation is presently under way in a variety of clinically applicable metastasis models.

Similarly, the clinical phenomenon of poorly differentiated colon and rectum carcinoma that behaves significantly more aggressively than the "wild type" moderate to well-differentiated adenocarcinoma has allowed us to frame precise experimental questions. Using these rare subsets of human colorectal cancer that have predictably poor prognoses, we have asked which of a series of molecular markers might explain the observed increased aggressiveness (markers of invasion, motility, multiple distant organ seeding, angiogenesis, and the like). Any molecular mechanisms identified that are linked to one or another aspect of aggressive behavior *in vivo* among these unusual subsets of colon and rectum carcinoma (poorly differentiated, highly mucinous, or signet ring–cell tumors) might then be studied as potential prognostic markers when applied to the more heterogenous, common, and less predictable moderate or well-differentiated primary colon and rectum carcinomas. Specific biologic markers of aggressive subpopulations among the more usual moderate to well-differentiated colon and rectum carcinomas have included various laminin-binding proteins, enzymes such as sucrase isomaltase that correlate with morphologic definition of differentiation among colorectal carcinoma, and molecules that may be involved at specific steps from tumor attachment to basement membrane, invasion through the basement membrane, and reattachment to and invasion or permeation through endothelial cells leading to the most prevalent metastatic sites in liver and lung. Knowledge of the clinical behavior of colon and rectum carcinoma, and specifically the unusual behavior of subsets of colon and rectum carcinomas such as predominantly poorly differentiated, has allowed us to ask the specific cell biology questions previously summarized.

Information also must travel in the opposite direction (from the laboratory to the clinic). This is an equally important aspect of the bridging role of the surgical oncologist. Specifically, a number of monoclonal antibodies to adhesion molecules found to be more richly expressed in less-differentiated colorectal cancer (e.g., a 67 Kd laminin-binding protein) are presently being examined immunohistochemically in a multi-institution gastrointestinal therapy protocol to establish more defined prognostic criteria than are presently available by conventional morphology. Availability of the cDNA clones has recently provided multiple oligonucleotide probes that will allow us to ask even more specific questions about transcription of mRNAs postulated to control various aspects of malignant behavior in GI cancer.

Clinical awareness of a unique group of patients whose recurrent colorectal cancers do not represent profuse distant disease (i.e., those 25 to 30 per cent of patients whose isolated liver and lung metastases can be cured by surgery) has compelled us to ask why this biologic minority is different and, furthermore, how we can identify the patients who can benefit by surgery compared with the much larger group of patients who do not benefit from resection of isolated hepatic or pulmonary recurrences. As of this writing there are no clinical or morphologic criteria that can prospectively discriminate between the two groups.

Application of marker studies to a disease such as colorectal carcinoma is best exemplified by 25 years of CEA investigation. The lack of patient survival benefit by such marker studies need not dampen enthusiasm. All tumor markers will be limited in producing patient benefit until more effective systemic therapy is available.

Given the relatively ineffective systemic therapy in gastrointestinal cancers, particularly when applied at the time of widespread recurrence, numerous research areas for marker application become obvious. In addition to the functional CEA questions summarized above, numerous probes have become available enabling us to define specific members of the CEA super gene family. Thus, questions can be asked about the presence of one or another secreted or membrane-bound CEA moiety and prediction of site-specific metastatic proclivity.

CEA and non-CEA marker studies can benefit from our ability to simultaneously harvest primary colon or rectum carcinoma, lymph node metastases, and occasionally, synchronous distant metastases and contiguous normal tissue. cDNA library construction can be designed to subtract normal from tumor, or primary tumor from lymph node metastases or distant metastases to attempt to identify specific mRNAs more abundantly expressed in one or another of these tissues. Such techniques should eventually allow us to define regulatory proteins that control each step along the pathway of tumor invasion and metastasis.

Access to patients with colonic polyps and the clinical realization that adenomatous and villous polyps represent *the* premalignant GI phenotypes have stimulated a direct search for genetic markers of GI epithelial initiation. If we can develop, through allelic deletion studies such as those of Vogelstein et al.[1-3] at Johns Hopkins, a schema of stepwise genetic change leading from premalignant to malignant GI epithelium, and if a limited number of individuals are found to be at risk for "initiated" GI epithelium, then rational guidelines for routine colonoscopic surveillance and removal of polyps could preempt subsequent malignant transformation.

And finally, the surgical oncologist, more than most physicians, realizes that despite recent adjuvant therapy successes in solid tumor multimodality trials (including colon and rectum cancer), overall patient benefit is suboptimal. The drugs used are minimally effective and toxicities are often considerable. Quite simply, the patient subsets benefitted are few and not easily identifable before treatment. Until better systemic therapy becomes available for such major cancers as breast or colorectal cancer, the most rational clinical and scientific thrust should be to better define those patients who are at the highest possible risk for recurrence where aggressive adjuvant therapy can be justified, and conversely avoid treatment in the majority of patients who will not benefit. For instance, in women with breast cancer, the argument as to whether patients with $T_1N_0M_0$ or $T_2N_0M_0$ breast primaries will benefit from adjuvant systemic therapy begs the real biologic issue—that is to find a better biologic marker for patients with the most aggressive tumors. Funding of statistically powerful clinical trials (with huge numbers of patients receiving minimally effective drugs) is not the most cost-effective or rational approach.

Melanoma provides another example. The question of establishing minimal survival benefit by prophylactic elective lymph node dissection in patients with intermediate level thickness melanomas may or may not be answered by accession of an ever larger number of patients with primary melanomas to available multi-institution national protocols. The improbable expectation of defining a minor benefit in an exceedingly small subset of patients undergoing such an extension of their surgical procedures should make the clinician/biologist wonder if a more rational effort might be in defining molecular markers that could predict which intermediate level melanomas spread and which do not spread to regional lymph nodes.

If the pathway chosen for surgical oncology training is strictly clinical, the "true" surgical oncologist should still be thoughtful and perceptive of the biology of each of the major diseases treated. This should lead to an acknowledgement of when treatment is known to be effective and when it is simply dogmatic. If the latter is true (and this is often the case), each diagnostic and surgical technique applied should be questioned and, if possible, put into the context of the overall disease process. A good example is the question of what operation should be performed for thyroid cancer.

Sophisticated empiric study of thyroid carcinoma patients has led to the development of clinical criteria that are highly effective in separating patients who are at high or low risk of metastatic disease and death. The "death rate ratio" between the high-risk and low-risk patients in differentiated thyroid carcinoma is 26:1. This indicates an extremely effective set of clinical parameters that enable treatment options to be selected; more aggressive surgery and adjuvant treatment can be confined to a small group of patients. Such a clinical prognostic scoring system can be an exceedingly valuable contribution to both understanding the biology and selecting appropriate treatment in this group of surgical oncology patients.

Another example is an analysis of the recent enthusiasm for "R2" and "R3" lymph node dissections in gastric carcinoma. This enthusiasm has largely arisen from Japan where gastric carcinoma clinically presents in a much different manner than in the United States. There are far fewer cases of "diffuse" histology and most of the cases are of the lower-grade "intestinal" histology and anatomically distal in the stomach. We have shown in earlier studies that lymph node metastases in the "intestinal" histologic variety carry a considerably better prognostic implication than lymph node metastases in the "diffuse" histologic variety. Thus translating the Japanese experience to American cases is fraught with misinterpretations and misunderstandings. Furthermore, the Japanese experience of developing a new radical surgical scheme at a time when their clinical case material is being discovered at markedly earlier stages confuses the interpretation of results from the effect of change in therapy in contrast to the change in presentation. This is a classic mistake in analyzing outcome data and not only re-emphasizes the need for concurrent prospective trials to evaluate treatment changes but also indicates the level of sophistication required of the surgical oncologist in interpreting reports in the surgical literature.

While an ongoing multi-institutional and multinational trial testing the concept of radical lymphadenectomy in gastric carcinoma is currently under way, by observing differences in clinical and biologic behavior of the subsets of gastric carcinoma, one can safely predict that more radical surgery will not lead to better outcome. This would also be predicted by recognition that repeated attempts at more radical primary surgical techniques have uniformly not increased survival but have increased morbidity and operative mortality. This truism has been found in lung cancer, esophagus cancer, breast cancer, melanoma, rectal cancer, colon cancer, primary and metastatic liver cancer, and sarcomas. Thus one would not expect this general principle to be altered significantly in gastric carcinoma.

The beginning of the next section perhaps hints at the sophistication needed by individuals who would call themselves surgical oncologists in interpreting the literature, designing trials, and conducting surgical practice.

References

1. Vogelstein, B., Fearon, E.R., Hamilton, S.R., et al.: Genetic alterations during colorectal tumor development. N. Engl. J. Med. *319*:525–532, 1988.
2. Vogelstein, B., Fearon, E.R., Kern, S.E., et al.: Allelotype of colorectal carcinomas. Science *244*:207–211, 1989.
3. Fearon, E.R., and Vogelstein, B.: A genetic model for colorectal tumorigenesis. Cell *61*:759–767, 1990.

INFLUENCE OF THE PRACTICE SETTING ON THE ROLE OF THE SURGICAL ONCOLOGIST

by Glenn Steele, Jr., M.D., and Blake Cady, M.D.

Another good example of how a cancer surgeon should be attuned to the clinical biology of his patients' disease is in attempting to design appropriate follow-up. Follow-up plans must be structured according to the particular practice venue and, ideally, will be assessed on the basis of whether or not the patient benefits. Thus, in the setting of an academic secondary or tertiary referral center, or if the patient is being treated and followed after treatment as a part of a formalized clinical trial, follow-up will usually be "by-the-book," particularly if disease-free interval is an endpoint of the trial, or if patterns of failure are to be established after a particular kind of multimodality adjuvant treatment protocol. In such settings, blood tests, radiologic diagnostic studies, and office visits may be excessively frequent. If, for instance, after an R2 gastric resection is performed for a gastric cancer or if a low anterior resection is performed for a high-risk rectal cancer, patients receiving subsequent adjuvant combination radiation and chemotherapy are usually seen every two to three months for the first several years as part of a formalized follow-up procedure. Blood tests, tumor marker sampling, liver/spleen scans, CT or MRI studies, and endoscopy will be aggressively and frequently pursued in order to establish differences in time to first recurrence between treated and control patients. Additional information about overall survival will be most accurate in such a maximal follow-up setting. Even when this kind of a formalized follow-up schema is mandated, however, the primary cancer surgeon should ask how often the particular follow-up visit or study has, in fact, led to a diagnosis of recurrence, and (even more important) how often such a diagnosis of recurrence has led to a subsequent cure.

Some of the more important information from randomized prospective clinical trials has, in fact, come from careful assessment of the cost effectiveness of follow-up procedures. In the early colon cancer adjuvant therapy trials, the multi-institution assessment of serial CEA monitoring of patients who were at high risk of recurrence after primary tumor resection was such an example. This provided valuable information, despite the fact that initial programs of adjuvant therapy for colon cancer patients were shown not to be effective. Single plasma sample CEA values were confirmed to be of independent prognostic value in patients with nodal disease. Proper monitoring of serial CEA changes after primary tumor resection was confirmed to be an excellent predictor of tumor recurrence, usually preceding conventional diagnostic indication of recurrence by three to six months. Particular rates of serial CEA rise from post primary tumor resection baseline in a given patient were shown to predict specific sites where recurrence was most likely to be found. Furthermore, the liver and lung were shown to be the metastatic sites most likely associated with rapid CEA rises.

Other less optimistic tumor marker data were also apparent. As opposed to earlier single-institution CEA second-look surgery trials, failures foreshadowed by rising CEA in the multi-institutional studies were, most often, not amenable to curative re-resection.

In whatever practice setting the surgical oncologist finds himself or herself, therefore, CEA follow-up monitoring should be thought of as a paradigm for the balance between proven benefit to the patient and our search for new knowledge. At present, our own approach is determined by the availability of experimental treatment protocols for systemic colon and rectum cancer once recurrence is diagnosed, and whether there is any evidence that such treatment may be more effective if started earlier. An additional motivation to follow colon and rectum cancer patients closely after tumor resection is to facilitate the clinical introduction of better serologic tumor markers that can be compared with CEA as a standard. In the absence of either of these experimental rationales, however, the knowledge that in only two metastatic sites, liver and lung, can isolated colon and rectum carcinoma recurrences be resected for cure has largely removed our enthusiasm for CEA-initiated second-look surgery. If the patient has a serial CEA rise, we focus on the liver and lung with CT/MRI/ultrasound. Only if we define potentially curable lesions before surgery do we perform surgery. Otherwise, we await signs or symptoms of recurrence and accommodate to a palliative rather than a curative goal.

In general, if the surgical oncologist asks why a particular follow-up plan is applied, and whether the treatment of a patient's recurrence is for cure or palliation, different rules will be applied in different environments. Using the example of a patient with colorectal carcinoma, we have recommended the following variety of follow-up plans depending on practice setting and the particular intent of the diagnostic study:

Practice Setting	Follow-up Plan
A. SECONDARY/TERTIARY Patient part of protocol. Committed to new treatment of recurrence.	Table 1–3
B. PRIMARY Patient not part of protocol. Committed to treating symptomatic recurrence only.	Table 1–4

The essential requirement for a practical follow-up program is that the early detection of a recurrence can still be treated for cure. If the early detection of an asymptomatic recurrence inevitably leads to death, there is little justification for early detection since it merely increases the patient's total duration of terror, panic, and "illness" without changing the eventual outcome and probably without changing the time of the outcome. Thus, local and regional phenomena need to be looked for assiduously only in certain patients depending on their initial treatment program and the disease behavior. Thus, a melanoma treated without prophylactic node dissection requires three monthly follow-ups of these regional nodal basins for two to three years and then slightly less frequent examination through five years before reverting to annual follow-up. Indeed, an indication for prophylactic nodal dissection in a melanoma patient may be that careful follow-up cannot

TABLE 1–3. RECOMMENDED FOLLOW-UP SCHEDULE FOR SELECTED PATIENTS

Schedule	History/Physical Laboratory	Hemoccult Stool	CEA	Colonoscopy	Double Contrast/Chest X-Ray
Preoperative	X	X	X 2	X	X
Postoperative, 3–4 weeks, and every 2–3 months for 2 years	X		X 2		
3 months			X	X (if not done before)	
6 months	X	X	X		
9 months	X	X	X		
12 months	X	X	X		X
15 months	X	X	X		
18 months	X	X	X		
21 months	X	X	X		
24 months	X	X	X	X	X
Every 6 months	X	X	X		
Yearly	X	X	X		X
Every 2–3 years				X	

(From Steele, G. Jr., and Osteen, R. T. [Eds.]: Colorectal Cancer: Current Concepts in Diagnosis and Treatment. New York, Marcel Dekker, Inc., 1986.)

TABLE 1–4. BASIC FOLLOW-UP SCHEDULE

Schedule	History/Physical Laboratory	CEA	Colonoscopy or Double Contrast	Chest X-Ray
Preoperative	X	X 2		X
Postoperative, 3–4 weeks		X 2		
Every 2–3 months for 5 years		X		
3 months			X (if not done before)	
Every 2–3 years			X	

(From Steele, G. Jr., and Osteen, R. T. [Eds.]: Colorectal Cancer: Current Concepts in Diagnosis and Treatment. New York, Marcel Dekker, Inc., 1986.)

be achieved (if the patient is going overseas or is unreliable, or the like). Similarly, if conservative management with breast preservation is undertaken for carcinoma of the breast, whether DCIS or invasive, the breast should be examined at least every three months for the first two years with a mammogram at least every six months during that time to look for recurrent disease in the breast itself. This is particularly true if a high-risk situation exists in the case such as very young age or an extensive intraductal component. Since the majority of breast recurrences can lead to curative surgery by either another local excision or mastectomy, such curable recurrences need to be detected as early as possible. If axillary lymphadenectomy is not performed as part of an early breast cancer excision, then the axillary lymph nodes need to be evaluated frequently in addition. However, chest wall disease detected early after mastectomy is rarely curable and therefore should not be sought for too assiduously.

Obtaining chest x-rays after original appropriate surgical or combined treatment of a soft-part sarcoma is a crucial part of the follow-up of some sarcomas but not others. A peripheral limb sarcoma of moderate to low grade probably should be followed by chest x-rays every six months during the first several years after excision to attempt early detection of localized pulmonary metastases for potential curative pulmonary resection. However, an extremely poor-prognosis sarcoma, because of very high-grade or retroperitoneal location, hardly justifies chest x-ray since curative pulmonary metastases seldom, if ever, occur in those settings.

Detailed follow-up for patients with low-risk differentiated thyroid carcinoma is really not justified since the death rate is less than 1 per cent and recurrence largely consists of recurrent lymph node metastases in the neck in papillary carcinoma in young people. Thus, a vigorous program of detailed follow-up examinations with chest x-rays, thyroid scans, and the like can hardly be justified from a cost-effective basis in low-risk patients. On the other hand, in high-risk differentiated thyroid carcinoma, a much more intensive program may well be justified because of the high frequency of recurrence, metastases, and death that may be aided by appropriate early detection, although early detection itself is in some doubt in these situations. Thus, the early detection of incurable metastases or failure to have a pattern of metastatic disease that lends itself to cure would be an indication for minimal technical follow-up. Follow-up should relate to psychologic support for everyone. Thus, the surgical oncologist must have enough biologic sophistication and data to know which follow-up program is appropriate for which patient. Again, this judgment justifies the field of special knowledge and focal interest designated as surgical oncology.

The responsibility for design and accomplishment of follow-up in all solid tumor patients should be within the domain of the surgical oncologist. Regardless of practice setting, the tendency for a surgeon to perform a technical procedure (i.e., an operation) after the diagnosis is made by a referring internist, and then hand the patient back to the internist for continued care is not tolerable. At the very least, the surgical oncologist must be involved in designing the overall approach to primary tumor treatment, establishing the timing and role of surgery among other modalities if the patient is to receive multimodality treatment for the primary tumor, and possibly sharing in the planning and carrying out of follow-up studies after the primary tumor is treated. This does not mean that the surgeon needs to give chemotherapy if chemotherapy is to be a part of the treatment. Nor does the patient need to be scheduled for redundant follow-up visits. Often, alternating visits can be arranged among the various treating physicians, or the medical and surgical oncologist can see the patient together.

THE SURGICAL ONCOLOGIST AS THE PATIENT MANAGER
by Glenn Steele, Jr., M.D., and
Blake Cady, M.D.

There are several basic prerequisites to be met if the surgical oncologist is to remain pivotal in the care of the cancer patient. First, he or she must understand the disease process as well as if not better than medical or radiation oncology colleagues. Second, the surgical oncologist must be an acknowledged leader within a clinical or basic research area generally focused on one or another solid tumor that has particular surgical diagnostic or therapeutic import. Third, the surgical oncologist must be a teacher or a role model in some important aspect of his or her clinical repertoire—either in the excellence of clinical surgery performed or in the excellence of mixing clinical talent and the knowledge of the biologic perspective of the disease treated—and ideally in both areas. Fourth, the surgical oncologist must ask questions about the worth of what is being done, and must find the time to be involved in designing ways to assess outcome of conventional diagnostic and therapeutic approaches. In other words, the surgical oncologist should be a leader out of the operating room in the conceptual arena as much as in the operating room. At the very least, the surgical oncologist should understand why formalized clinical trials are necessary when what we are doing is quite often simply dogmatic. If not actually leading such trials, the surgical oncologist should help colleagues overcome emotional, financial, and intellectual paranoia about convincing their patients to join such trials when available.

A surgical oncologist should be a skilled technical surgeon. This skill is even more important in conducting major destructive operations since the potential for disaster is greater, the need to mobilize and coordinate numerous specialties in the operating room and postoperatively is more crucial, and the need to conduct expeditious surgery with minimum hazard to the patients and minimum morbidity and mortality from the surgical procedure is particularly important as the magnitude of the operative procedure increases.

The surgical oncologist must be thoroughly grounded in the sophisticated biologic understanding of tumor behavior. This knowledge must also be constantly updated by devotion to the surgical literature as well as the literature of associated fields such as medical oncology and radiotherapy. It is as important to understand which patients should not have a radical surgical approach to a primary cancer or a cancer recurrence and those that should. The surgical oncologist who appreciates a biologic understanding will make such decisions with a greater chance of success either if a surgical procedure is undertaken or if a more focused approach to nonsurgical treatment is elected. As an example, it is illogical to embark on hepatic resections for metastatic colorectal carcinoma when 10 or more nodules exist in the liver or a simultaneous, extrahepatic lesion occurs since the chance of success by major surgery will approach zero. On the other hand, a patient with a persistent recurrence following right colon carcinoma with a relatively slowly rising and low CEA level and a long interval from the primary resection may well justify a radical surgical approach even removing bone, retroperitoneal structures, kidney, femoral nerve, and bowel with some expectation of permanent local control in contrast to a similar situation that occurred with a high CEA and a short disease-free interval.

Since the biologic understanding of tumor behavior is constantly changing, it is essential that the surgeon keep contemporary with the literature. The dramatic changes in the appreciation of breast cancer behavior over the past 15 years have rendered some individuals who trained in surgical oncology 20 years ago totally obsolete because they adhere to a rigid pattern of treatment in contrast to others who have been willing to keep general principles in mind while adjusting their thinking with a new understanding of behavior patterns. For instance, there are still surgeons who believe that supraradical resection of lymph node drainage basins in rectal carcinoma and the no-touch technique of colon cancer generally are required procedures, failing to have recognized newer knowledge that invalidates both of those concepts. Arbitrary performance of abdominoperineal resection for lower rectal carcinomas without recognizing variations in results based on size, differentiation, and location that permit local excision therapy is yet another example of such rigidity and failure to appreciate newer trends and biologic understandings.

The surgical oncologist should be an educator of students, residents, and general surgeons who do not specialize in cancer. No greater justification of a designation of "surgical oncologist" can be made than that his or her sophistication should be enough to act as a consultant to the frontline general surgeons who have many more fields of surgical responsibility and knowledge and cannot always keep up with the latest in studies and interpretations in the cancer area. Thus, above all, the surgical oncologist should be an educator of colleagues, residents, and students.

The surgical oncologist should be adept at reoperations and radical procedures. For instance, liver surgery, major amputations such as hemipelvectomy, pelvic exenterations, node dissections, and radical retroperitoneal sarcoma resections should all be familiar and accomplishable by the well-trained surgical oncologist. Conversely, the surgical oncologist must know the appropriate conservative procedures that are available today such as rectal preservation with local excision of small rectal cancers and restricted resections of melanomas and breast carcinomas. These features illustrate why a surgical oncologist is not just a breast surgeon or a colorectal surgeon. While these skills are crucial for selected members of the surgical community, the surgical oncologist should be able to do such procedures plus many others and thus put the entire surgical spectrum of cancer in perspective so that the most appropriate procedure might be achieved. For instance, most surgeons who specialize only in breast surgery would be reluctant to undertake a chest wall resection for a recurrent and ulcerated breast carcinoma that involved the chest wall yet was still localized enough to permit radical local procedures for palliation if not for cure. Similarly, a surgical oncologist should be willing to undertake *per primam* a pelvic exenteration for an advanced rectal carcinoma without compromising the tumor margin against the bladder if that were the appropriate step in a selected patient. The average, even well-trained, general surgeon might be reluctant to undertake such a procedure and therefore compromise a surgical margin and lead to a later recurrence.

The clinical surgical oncologist must be knowledgeable about the principles of adjuvant treatments such as chemotherapy and radiotherapy. The knowledge must be sophisticated enough to know when adjuvant therapy is appropriate, which general approaches should be done, and in what sequence. For instance, the surgical oncologist must be able to discuss with the radiotherapist the suitability of radiation techniques in the particular tumor being handled. Since many radiotherapists are fixed on radical regional radiotherapy philosophy, it takes the knowledgeable and committed surgeon to convince the average radiotherapist not to perform nodal basin radiation therapy as an adjunct to breast cancer treatment knowing that no impact on survival has been shown in studies addressing that issue. Nevertheless, the vast majority of breast cancer patients today who do have radiation therapy have wide-field–nodal radiation therapy as an adjunct, which is inappropriate. No cooperative program involving surgeon and radiotherapist or surgeon and chemotherapist can be undertaken unless the surgeon has enough knowledge about the other disciplines to recognize the limitations, advantages, and disadvantages of the adjuvant being proposed.

Furthermore, the applicability of plastic surgical reconstruction is essential to enable the surgical oncologist to embark on radical procedures for palliation and cure in specialized situations where reconstruction is required. If chest wall reconstruction is required for an advanced local breast cancer, plastic surgical colleagues must be brought in for appropriate reconstruction. Similarly, radical groin dissections with recurrent disease directly over vessels might require extensive sacrifice of skin that can only be compensated for by flap reconstruction. Breast reconstruction is a common procedure done today, frequently at the time of an initial mastectomy, and such reconstructive procedures are best handled as a team with a plastic surgeon who is familiar to the surgeon and able to work cooperatively to solve difficult clinical problems.

The surgical oncologist must be adept enough at interpersonal skills to be able to discuss such difficult concepts, procedures, and complications as suggested above with the patient and the patient's family as well as the other oncology workers. This requires a humanity and empathy that go above and beyond those of the usual surgical procedure because of the life and death issues involved and the major cosmetic and functional disabilities that may result from the most appropriately designed surgical procedures for recurrent or advanced cancers. For instance, in the contemporary management of breast carcinoma, at least 45 minutes to an hour must be spent with the patient and family, sometimes on more than one occasion, to go through the myriad treatment options available to the patient today. This task best falls to the surgical oncologist who can deal with the overview of the tumor problem and coordinate the various disciplines.

The surgical oncologist should be committed to community education through involvement with the American Cancer Society, the Commission on Cancer of the American College of Surgeons, or other appropriate groups. In addition, a commitment to the education of the medical field generally, and the surgical community in particular, should be demonstrated by involvement in trials, solicitation of patients for prospective trials, and investigation of clinical problems through retrospective surveys and contributions to the surgical literature.

And finally, and most importantly, the surgical oncologist must enjoy patient contact and accept the inevitable failure of many of his or her treatment approaches in most solid tumor patients. The natural tendency to frustration and ego withdrawal that leads to abandonment of the patient that we know is going to die is not tolerable in this specialty. Part of every surgeon's psyche, whether a surgical oncologist or not, is to demand a win every time. Most of us would prefer to be heros to our patients, and probably to ourselves. Perhaps this is the major motivation for sending the tumor patient with recurrence back to the medical oncologist or radiation oncologist just as soon as we can, even when we know that what really will be offered is nothing more than 5-fluorouracil, external beam radiation, and solace, with the solace as the most cost-effective part of the treatment. Despite the enormous time and energy this demands of any busy surgeon, the responsibility for treating a solid tumor patient must be assumed from the beginning of the patient's surgical therapy until the end of his or her life. Quite often, the dying patient and the dying patient's family will be more grateful for this continued commitment by the cancer surgeon than for the particular technical brilliance of the original surgical procedure. Certainly, the credibility of the surgical oncologist as a patient manager will be most obvious in this context to his or her patients and to his or her colleagues regardless of whether or not a particular certification of special expertise is hanging on the office wall.

2

HEAD AND NECK CANCER

FUNDAMENTALS
by Charles M. Norris, Jr., M.D.

INTRODUCTION

A discussion of head and neck cancer almost exclusively centers on squamous cell (or epidermoid) carcinoma of the upper aerodigestive tract. Related aspects include its epidemiology, etiology, classification, prognosis, the clinical and diagnostic approach to the patient, and the multidisciplinary features of treatment. Because of the diverse anatomy and clinical behavior of the regions involved, only so many generalities can be made by way of introduction. Given a basic perspective, the unique features of each site require separate discussion.

Head and neck oncology increasingly and appropriately involves the participation and judgment of multiple medical disciplines, including medical oncology, radiation therapy, head and neck surgery, dentistry, maxillofacial prosthodontics, nutrition, speech therapy, social work, nursing, and hospice care. The problems faced by the patient, even when successfully treated, are often functionally and socially meaningful, and of potentially significant psychologic impact. Although comprising a relatively small portion of all cancers, those in the head and neck nevertheless represent a visible and significant threat to life and lifestyle, with multiple relevant variables that require an individualized approach to treatment decisions. Treatment and mortality parameters cannot be universally applied, as the natural history and consequent clinical expectations vary from site to site. Survival cannot be viewed only statistically but must be considered in relation to its quality as well. Consequently, rather than only imparting to the reader a series of clinical observations, facts, and numerical data, this discussion also offers some insight into a philosophy of oncologic patient management.

Squamous cell carcinoma of the upper aerodigestive tract mucosa has mainly been a disease of males in their fifth and sixth decades, comprising roughly 8.5 per cent[1] of all malignancies in this group. The proportion of females with these lesions has always been less by a factor of 2 to 4, with some dependence on the site. This disparity may be lessening, especially in laryngeal carcinoma, as more women, smoking for longer periods of time, are approaching the traditional age group of risk. Overall, there have been approximately 44,000 new cases of epidermoid head and neck cancer in the United States in 1988, accounting for some 13,000 deaths.[2] Other head and neck cancers, thyroid, salivary gland, lymphoma, paranasal sinus, and sarcomas tend to occur in younger individuals.

The etiology of head and neck cancer is multivariate, which is understandable given the number of environmental agents that can come into contact with the air and swallowing passages. Tobacco (whether inhaled or chewed), ethyl alcohol, and the combination of tobacco and alcohol together are the best established and most significant carcinogens of mucosal malignancy in the oral cavity, oropharynx, hypopharynx, and larynx. These are not invariable, however, nor exclusive in a given patient, as indicated in Table 2–1, adapted from Myer and Suen.[3] Because the effect of multiple etiologic factors can be synergistic, the elimination of even a single factor can have more than a simply subtractive influence on overall risk. Present data favor a two-stage model of carcinogenesis, in which both mutation and malignant transformation are integrated.[4]

Nutritional deficiency and suboptimal orodental health are generally implicated in a number of patients, and not infrequently as social concomitants of alcoholism. Viral and genetic observations have provided additional insight into cancer pathogenesis, as well as a substrate for research, but are not as readily eliminated as the environmental factors. It must be emphasized,

TABLE 2–1. CARCINOGENS IN HEAD AND NECK CANCER[3]

Site	Carcinogen Factors	Other Factors
Nasal cavity	Wood dust (furniture)	? Chronic sinusitis
Paranasal sinuses	Leather manufacturing Textile industry Nickel refining Thorotrast (radiochemical) Mustard gas	? Cigarette smoke
Nasopharynx	Nitrosamines	Epstein-Barr virus Genetics—Chinese
Oral cavity	Cigarettes Ethyl alcohol Snuff, Chewing tobacco Textile industry Leather manufacturing	Syphilis Vitamin deficiencies
Hypopharynx Larynx	Cigarettes Asbestos (Ship builders) Mustard gas Ethyl alcohol Wood exposure	Nutrition deficiencies
Esophagus	Ethyl alcohol Cigarettes	Nutrition deficiency Race—Eskimos, Blacks
Salivary gland	Radiation	Genetics—Eskimos

particularly to the novice clinician, that while an interest in cancer-causing variables is important from a medical research and public health standpoint (i.e., preventive and occupational), it assists relatively little in the practical diagnosis and treatment of individual patients. The lack of identifiable carcinogens does not preclude the occurrence of head and neck cancer in a given individual. And while multiple risk factors may coexist in a patient, they should not be weighed so heavily that other causes for symptoms go unconsidered.

NATURAL HISTORY

Primary Site

Squamous cell head and neck cancer generally arises on the surface of the mucosal lining of the upper aerodigestive tract. True or apparent submucosal lesions do occur when the tumor starts within epithelial invaginations, such as in the tonsils or tongue base, or within the ducts of minor salivary glands. Recurrent cancer after previous treatment is quite often submucosal and elusive, invisible to the eye, but possibly palpable. Likewise glandular (nonepidermoid) adenocarcinomas, which may arise in the same parts of the upper aerodigestive tract, appear below the surface lining within minor salivary glands as palpable mass lesions, with mucosal change (ulceration) occurring late in their course.

The so-called "typical" mucosal carcinoma will appear as an ulceration, roughening, thickening, outcropping, cauliflower-like fungation, or as combinations of these. The color of early lesions can be either red (erythroplastic) or whitish (leukoplakic). As a tumor grows, surface infection, necrosis, or bleeding may evolve. Progressive infiltration into underlying muscles will result in their dysfunction. Centripetal mucosal expansion as well as invasion along tissue planes (including perichondrium or periosteum) or nerves occurs. Direct invasion into bone is a late event, though tumors may extend into bony structures through pre-existent anatomic openings, such as a nerve canal or dental extraction site. Extension along nerves, or within lymphatics or small vessels, can facilitate the spread of malignant cells beyond the area discernible by examination techniques.

Primary site symptoms are caused by inflammation, mass or pressure effect, nerve impingement, or muscle dysfunction. Symptoms may be lacking altogether. Certain sites (tongue base, pyriform sinus, nasopharynx, paranasal sinuses) tend to become noticeable to the patient only when tumors are advanced. Symptom trends and patterns of tumor spread vary from site to site but are neither unique nor exclusive.

Lymphatic

Epidermoid cancer in the head and neck spreads both locally (at and around the primary site of origin) and regionally via lymphatic channels, through which tumor implantation into lymph nodes occurs. Enlarged cervical nodes, in the presence of a known head and neck malignancy, reflect this form of spread and may be an initial symptom or sign. In general, nodal dissemination reflects advanced primary site disease, either longstanding, large, or both. Different sites and histologic subtypes have varying propensities for occult or overt lymphatic spread. For example, nasopharyngeal carcinoma uncommonly occurs without identifiable nodal metastases, which are usually multiple, and often bilateral. Notwithstanding, in laryngeal carcinoma localized to the true vocal cord, nodal disease is rare, even with advanced primaries. Virtually any head and neck malignancy, epidermoid or other, has the capacity to infiltrate and spread via lymphatics. Adenoid cystic adenocarcinoma of the salivary glands has a greater propensity toward perineural extension and blood-borne dissemination (distant metastasis), which are both aggressive behavior patterns. Yet, lymphatic spread is considerably less likely. Progressive lymphatic spread of head and neck malignancies tends to occur in recognizable anatomic patterns as well. A lesion of the anterior floor of mouth is much more likely to seed a submandibular triangle node, even a contralateral one, than a tonsil fossa primary, which tends to seed upper or middle deep jugular nodes. The nasopharynx is the sole site in which posterior triangle cervical adenopathy is likely. The expected patterns are altered after treatment with either surgery or radiation, due to lymphatic scarring and obstruction, with shunting of the usual drainage pathways. The sequestration of persisting tumor cells can lead to elusive manifestations of tumor recurrence in spite of diligent observation.

Distant

The invasion of malignant cells into the venous circulation can allow dissemination throughout the body. As with any seed, the tendency for any tumor cell to establish itself and propagate in a distant site depends on a number of factors. These include the cancer cell's own biology, its ability to pass through the recipient tissue's capillary wall, its resistance to local and systemic immune surveillance, its resistance to any active medical therapy, and the receptiveness of the host tissue. There is also, of course, a dosage-response phenomenon, reflected in the observation that the larger the primary tumor or more extensive the nodal deposits, i.e., the more advanced the stage of disease, the greater the risk of distant dissemination.

As with site and tumor-type variations in local and regional spread, there is a difference in the incidence of distant metastasis according to the location of the primary lesion. While the nasopharynx and hypopharynx are associated with a high (23 to 28 per cent) likelihood of systemic spread, carcinoma of the vocal cord (glottic larynx) and oral cavity metastasizes via the blood stream relatively infrequently (3 to 7 per cent). As previously noted, adenoid cystic adenocarcinoma, by contrast, has an even higher chance of systemic spread (over 70 per cent). The lungs are the most common location for distant metastasis from head and neck cancer, with bone, liver, and brain sites occurring much less frequently.

The natural history of a given tumor must additionally address its recurrence after treatment. Thus, particular patterns of spread are also reflected in associated patterns of failure. To use previous examples, glottic and oral cavity lesions will tend to recur as local problems, while adenoid cystic carcinoma will tend to recur as lung metastases. Tumors that tend to spread early on into either lymphatics or the blood stream, but are themselves responsive to treatment at the primary site, will tend to recur at either the nodal or distant site, or both.

Patterns of spread of a tumor site, histology, and extent are reflected in the natural history of a given lesion and also in the course of a patient so afflicted. This somewhat predictable biologic behavior, in turn, must be considered when determining the type and extent of treatment and plans for follow-up.

CLASSIFICATION AND STAGING

Classification and staging of cancers are necessary in order to clinically compare patient groups within and among treating institutions, to communicate data in the same language, to provide guidelines for treatment, and to evaluate response to that treatment. The ideal staging system would be simple enough to use from memory and apply on a daily basis. It must be relevant to the natural history of the disease process in question and complete enough to allow a statistical inquiry into not only the most significant aspects of the disease, but moreover into those variables that are reasonably and practically evaluable on a routine basis during a patient's evaluation and course of treatment. Most importantly, a correlation should be demonstrable between the extent of disease at the time of treatment (stage), the treatment rendered, and the outcome, expressed both in quantity and quality of life. Dealing with the complex biologic systems represented by a malignancy in a human host, superimposed on the rapidly progressing and technology-weighted field of medicine, it is understandable that a perfect classification system cannot exist.

Reflecting the patterns of spread observed in head and neck cancer, a version of the TNM system of tumor classification has been developed and is periodically refined.[5] (See anatomic sections for site-specific details.) The designation "T," for tumor, classifies the primary origin of the malignancy according to several variables that vary from site to site. These include tumor size or extension into adjacent anatomic structures. Assigning a T-stage depends on accurately locating and measuring the tumor, either by inspection, palpation, endoscopic examination, or other modality such as imaging study. Mapping biopsies, by way of a circumferential tumor survey, are occasionally useful. Since tumors are three-dimensional, not always encompassed by examination techniques, and sometimes difficult to delineate, a T-stage may be only an approximation. The reconciliation of a patient's symptoms with the measurable tumor volume may allow a presumption of deep tumor infiltration, even though the deep margin of the tumor cannot be assessed (i.e., severe trismus associated with a tonsil lesion, or fixation of movement with a tongue base cancer). While for a given anatomic subdivision in the upper aerodigestive tract advancing T-stage correlates with disease severity and prognosis, a comparison between sites of like T-stages is not at all valid, because of site differences in tumor natural history. A T_2 glottic laryngeal carcinoma carries a much more favorable prognosis, even with less radical treatment, than a T_2 lesion of the hypopharynx or supraglottic larynx, for instance. Though it does have some impact on prognosis, histologic grading is not included as a parameter for T-staging in the present system.

(Other proposed classification schemes, particularly in Europe, have included this variable.)

The "N" classification, for nodal, seeks to group the number, size, and laterality of lymphatic metastases. Assigning an N-stage is generally more consistent, with good correlation between pretreatment N-stage and outcome. Clinically false positive nodes are rare. Included in other classification schemes, but absent from the present version, are provisions for nodal fixation or striation for different or multiple levels of nodal disease (location within the neck compartment). Nodal fixation, while often emphasized in describing a patient's physical findings, is extremely subjective. Implicit, but difficult to confirm without surgery, is an invasion of the nodal tumor into the carotid artery, bone, or some other conventionally unresectable structure. When present, as with any extension of tumor outside the lymph node capsule (extracapsular spread), these findings do indeed portend prognostic pessimism. Not infrequently, however, surgical exploration reveals so-called "fixed" nodes to be resectable after all. Nevertheless, fixation and extracapsular invasion correlate well with tumor size, so these variables are indirectly represented.

Given the natural history of head and neck cancer spread via lymphatics, and given the likelihood that in the presence of a clinically apparent nodal metastasis there are other occult, microscopically involved nodes, the concept of multiple nodal levels is really implicit in the experienced clinician's interpretation of the N designation.

"M," for metastasis, designates the systemic dissemination of cancer cells to other organs of the body. The term M_0 communicates only that at a point in time, usually prior to treatment, there were no identifiable distant metastases detected by the modalities employed for examination. Since it is rare, even in the presence of massive primary and nodal disease, for pulmonary or other sites of blood-borne spread to be evident, evaluation is often limited to a chest x-ray. Any suggestive symptoms outside the head and neck area are considered and evaluated accordingly. M_1, qualified by a location, designates metastasis to that location. The identification of distant metastasis may or may not influence the immediate treatment plan.

The finding of a solitary pulmonary nodule during the preliminary evaluation of a patient with head and neck cancer represents an occasional management problem.[6] Thus, while the nodule could be a metastasis from the known primary in the upper aerodigestive tract, it could also be a primary lung malignancy, toward which there is a proclivity shared by the smoking population, which evolves head and neck cancer. Investigating the pulmonary finding can be protracted and may even require thoracotomy, thereby substantially delaying other treatment. In these circumstances, as in many medical scenarios, one must determine priority by asking (and answering) two questions. First, which is the more serious problem? Second, how does one problem modify the treatment recommendation for the other? A third question might be: Could the treatment of both be reasonably accommodated?

In the case of a pulmonary metastasis, the patient is not curable, and the treatment should maximize subjective well-being. Since the effects of uncontrolled head and neck cancer tend to be slow, but extremely debilitating from an appearance, airway, swallowing, or pain standpoint, such treatment may well be equivalent to the original recommendation. The prognosis of an advanced head and neck cancer may be worse than that of an early pulmonary lesion, in which case the former would be treated as planned and work-up of the latter deferred. In the case of an earlier, more curable head and neck lesion, possibly with several treatment options, there may be some flexibility and value in pursuing the lung lesion initially. Considerable judgment is required in this kind of decision, as well as an awareness of the relative natural histories, prognosis, and method of inflicting harm of the two problems at hand. In this regard the ability to correlate disease stage with relative treatment efficacy and morbidity is essential.

Although rare, a similar issue might arise in the case of a liver abnormality, common in the alcohol-imbibing population that gets head and neck cancer. Diagnostic scanning may not readily distinguish between cirrhosis, tumor, or other abnormalities.

No classification and staging system alone will provide clear-cut, invariably rigid instructions for patient management. As pointed out by Sisson, the ". . . shortcomings (of the TNM system) are as much a reflection of the complexity of the disease itself as a condemnation of the staging system."[7] It does, however, represent a common denominator through which information can be accrued, rarefied, and reapplied to a constantly changing discipline.

CLINICAL EVALUATION

General/Head and Neck—History and Physical Examination

A general knowledge of head and neck cancer is needed in order to put patient symptoms into perspective and provide an appropriate level of suspicion to focus further investigation or referral. While the anatomy involved by head and neck cancers is, for the most part, accessible to direct visual examination, formal endoscopy and examination under general anesthesia are often required to completely localize, measure, biopsy, or even detect most primary tumors.

The patient history reveals relative risk for head and neck cancer as well as medical facts pertinent to, and possibly limiting of, treatment. Exposure to carcinogens and information regarding prior or active medical problems are reviewed. Medical comorbidity is common in patients with head and neck cancer, often as a result of liver disease or chronic pulmonary disease, reflecting alcohol and tobacco use, respectively. An antecedent history of malignant or premalignant disease of the upper aerodigestive tract, lung, or esophagus, and the evaluations and treatment rendered, are crucial. A history of other malignancy is also germane, as this may modify life expectancy and thereby influence future treatment considerations. Cardiac, neurologic, renal, hematologic, and otologic diseases, and diabetes mellitus can limit surgical or chemotherapeutic treatment options, and may conceivably constitute a greater life threat than an early head and neck cancer. Family history is generally more indicative of a patient's social milieu rather than his or her cancer risk. Previous experience with a family member who had cancer, however, may substantially affect a given patient's perception and possible misconception of his or her own disease and its treatment. Available information pertaining to a patient's previous evaluation for the same or a related problem should be reviewed. It may be especially crucial to have biopsy material reassessed, in order to prevent any confusion about a prior diagnosis.

The symptoms of patients with head and neck cancer are neither esoteric nor exclusive, but they may be totally lacking. A patient may report his or her own observation of a "lump" in the neck, a "growth," or slowly healing "sore" in the mouth. When true symptoms are present, they may be nonspecific and poorly localized. Unilateral pain, dysarthria, hoarseness, and other forms of voice change, dysphagia, stridor, positional dyspnea, aspiration symptoms (choking), odynophagia, and any kind of bleeding are manifestations that alone or in combination may indicate a lesion in the upper aerodigestive tract, reflecting a loss of mucosal integrity, mass effect, or dysfunction of a portion of the dynamic anatomy involved. More localizing, but with many alternative possible explanations, would be unilateral nasal obstruction or bleeding, facial pain, serous otitis media (due to eustachian tube compromise), and orbital or ocular symptoms, indicating a possible lesion in the nose, paranasal sinuses, or nasopharynx. Otalgia (earache), a significant symptom in head and neck cancer patients, can be due to a referred stimulus from any of the nerves innervating the oral cavity, oropharynx, mandible, maxilla, hypopharynx, or larynx. Other nonotologic causes of ear pain include dental, cervical spine, and neurologic conditions. Unexplained, persistent otalgia in the presence of an unremarkable head and neck examination should be further evaluated. Lesions of the tongue base, pyriform sinus, and cervical esophagus can be particularly elusive to initial simple office physical examination techniques.

Cervical masses, single or multiple, may be associated with manifestations suggesting benign disease. However, these symptoms are never unique, and any neck mass in an adult should be viewed as malignant and probably metastatic until proved otherwise.[8] Concomitant sources of regional infection, fluctuation in size, tenderness and pain, a high jugular or midline location, oval shape, mobility, soft or cystic consistency, and bilaterality all suggest, but do not guarantee, benignancy in a cervical lymph node. A complete head and neck examination and symptom review are advisable. It is, furthermore, crucial to determine whether an isolated lump is a lymph node, another cervical structure, or a mass within a major salivary gland or the thyroid gland, all of which can be sources of neoplasia, but with very disparate natural histories and treatment implications.

Most primary malignancies will be discernible through complete office examination. A systematic approach, with good illumination, topical anesthesia if needed, and the practiced use of equipment, is desirable. Not to be omitted is a general evaluation of facial and neck symmetry, eyes, skin lesions, respiratory status, and various stigmata of systemic disease. Otoscopic ear examination and nasal cavity examination via nasal speculum are often performed next, followed by detailed visualization and palpation of all accessible mucosal surfaces of the nasopharynx, oral cavity, oropharynx, hypopharynx, and larynx. The assessment of symmetry is always helpful. A tongue retractor and various mirrors are generally used, coupled with coaxial illumination from either a direct or indirect source. Also available are an array of rigid and flexible fiberoptic telescopes, inserted through the nose or oral cavity, to facilitate examination of areas not well visualized through other means. The importance of digital, bimanual palpation of the oral cavity and oropharynx cannot be overemphasized. As the sage has often commented concerning the examiner's finger, "It's a cheap, informative tool, and hard to lose."

Palpation of the neck, noting both normal landmarks and abnormal contours or masses, requires practice, experience, and a good awareness of the underlying anatomy. Benign adenopathy is not infrequently encountered. "Worrisome" lymph nodes can be anywhere and will tend to be firm or hard, round, 2 cm or greater in size, possibly fixed (immobile) or partially fixed, and often single and unilateral. Palpable "normal" nodes are unusual in the supraclavicular or posterior triangle portions of the neck. The location and tissue of origin of any lump should be ascertained (i.e., distinguishing a high jugular lymph node from a mass in the tail of the parotid). Auscultation of the neck may suggest subglottic or tracheal airway compromise or a bruit associated with certain vascular tumors or occult carotid artery compromise.

Other Evaluations

Further investigation of a patient already ascertained to have head and neck cancer focuses on the lesion's histologic type, local extent, regional metastatic spread, and presence of distant dissemination. Medical parameters impacting on relevant available treatment options (and their comorbidity) are also determined.

Biopsy for histologic review of lesions in the oral cavity and in some parts of the nose, nasopharynx, and oropharynx can be performed in an office setting, as can the cytologic evaluation of a needle aspirate (fine-needle biopsy) from a neck mass. Generally, however, examination under anesthesia is both necessary and more informative. In addition to palpation of the oral cavity and neck, direct laryngoscopy (of the oropharynx, hypopharynx, and larynx), rigid esophagoscopy, nasopharyngoscopy, and bronchoscopy (including the trachea and subglottic airway) are carried out in some combination appropriate for the lesion at hand. Such "triple endoscopy" is important not only to assess a known lesion in greater detail but also to identify any other coincidental abnormalities, including second primary mucosal lesions of the upper aerodigestive tract or lung.[9-12] An accurate description of pretreatment tumor location and extent is essential to specify optimal treatment, assess response, and observe the post-treated patient in follow-up. Multiple biopsies by way of mapping the tumor may be contemplated, for instance, in the case of an early laryngeal cancer, for which a decision regarding partial versus total laryngectomy requires a precise determination of tumor extent. The presence or absence of tumor at a crucial possible resection margin (midline base of tongue, for example) might also be determined. "Tattooing" with India ink is useful in order to maintain an objective visual representation of the pretreatment tumor site and volume as it responds to radiation or chemotherapy. The tattoos, pinpoint dots around the tumor periphery, also assist a surgeon in recalling the area of concern during resection after pretreatment.

Blood work is performed as a baseline assessment of the relevant general medical parameters described previously and includes routine tests reflecting liver, renal, and hematologic function. Nutritional indicators, arterial blood gases, pulmonary function testing, and creatinine clearance are all considered. Various serologic "markers," including carcinoembryonic antigen

(CEA) and Epstein-Barr virus (EBV) antibody titers, can be useful in follow-up.

Imaging studies are an important, sometimes crucial, adjunct to clinical evaluation. A chest x-ray is routine in order to evaluate cardiopulmonary health and rule out parenchymal lesions. Barium swallow examination of the hypopharynx/esophagus is relevant and useful, but rarely takes the place of a good endoscopic examination. Anteroposterior (A-P) tomography of the larynx or sinuses may delineate tumor extension in these areas, perhaps below the vocal cords, or into the facial bones, respectively, and can be superior to computed tomography (CT) scanning for select purposes. Mandible x-rays will identify significant cortical bone invasion from an oral cavity or oropharyngeal tumor, but may not reveal tumor within the jaw due to extension through intrinsic foramina or tooth extraction sockets. A radionuclear bone scan of the jaw, when correlated with the patient's symptoms and physical findings, may suggest periosteal involvement or subclinical cortical bone erosion. Total body, brain, and liver scanning have a very low incidental yield in identifying distant metastases and are performed only if indicated by specific symptoms or other findings.

Axial and coronal CT scanning of the head and neck is essentially the imaging study of choice for most head and neck neoplasms. Cross-sectional images facilitate the anatomic evaluation of unexplained symptomatology associated with less advanced lesions and allow a noninvasive exploration of areas not otherwise examinable, such as the paranasal sinuses, parapharyngeal and pterygomaxillary spaces, orbits, and anterior skull base. The role of magnetic resonance imaging (MRI) will ultimately be similar to that of CT scanning. MRI non-radiation technology and high resolution are desirable, but its lack of universal availability and interpretive experience in the head and neck are, as yet, limiting. Soft tissue resolution, including that of the tumor-tissue interface, is occasionally superb, but bone delineation is poor. At present, MRI is most useful for representing the soft tissue extent of tumors that have transgressed the skull base or involve the parapharyngeal spaces. Its areas of superior applicability over CT scanning are in the process of becoming established.[13]

Arterial and vascular imaging, by either formal angiography or digital subtraction technique, is employed quite selectively in squamous cell carcinoma of the head and neck, primarily to discern carotid artery involvement and/or prepare for its reconstruction or resection in very selected cases. Ultrasound techniques, combined with CT scanning, can also suggest carotid artery invasion (as opposed to deviation) by tumor. None of these modalities is always accurate, however, and their use is judgmental. Arteriography is particularly useful with certain rare, nonepidermoid tumors of the head and neck, such as chemodectomas, angiofibromas, large or malignant hemangiomas, and some others. In these, angiography may be diagnostic and also provides a means of preoperative therapeutic embolization in order to lessen intraoperative bleeding.

TREATMENT FUNDAMENTALS

Surgery and radiation, alone or in combination, are the curative modalities in head and neck cancer. One may include with conventional resectional surgery various associated techniques for tissue removal or destruction, including endoscopic surgery, laser surgery, cryotherapy, electrocautery, and even phototherapy. Radiation may be delivered by external beam, interstitial implantation, or surface-contact exposure, each of which has technical variations. Chemotherapy by itself, in spite of its demonstrated ability to reduce or even eradicate clinically detectable squamous cell cancer, is not curative, and is currently undergoing vigorous assessment as adjunctive or synergistic treatment in association with surgery and radiation.

Research in the treatment of head and neck cancer centers, in large part, around ways of improving the efficacy or decreasing the morbidity of existing therapies. While the combination of radiation and surgery is well established as more effective against some advanced lesions, the optimum manner and sequence in which these are administered for a given cancer type, stage, and site is a continued area of controversy and review. "Conservation" surgery, the achieving of adequate tumor resection with less radical tissue removal or functional impairment, is a frequent topic of report, as are further-refined techniques in the reconstruction of tumor defects or the rehabilitation of functional deficits. Radiation sensitizers are pharmacologic agents capable of increasing the effect of ionizing radiation on hypoxic tumor cell masses, while maintaining or decreasing the normal tissue side effects. The use of hyperbaric oxygen has a similar rationale. Technologic improvements in the power and type of radiation have made possible the use of electron and neutron beam therapies, with selected applicability. An area of very active investigation concerns the twice-daily format for external beam therapy, in which either the conventional or higher dosages are delivered through an increased number of fractions administered more rapidly over compressed time periods ("hyperfractionation" and "accelerated fractionation"). The correlation of such clinical research inquiries with investigations into the basic science of tumor carcinogenesis, biology, evolution, and natural history is crucial to the perspective of an active practitioner in this field today, whether as a surgeon, radiation therapist, or medical oncologist.

The goals of cancer treatment are to eliminate the known tumor, deter its recurrence, and prevent the emergence of occult cancer cells. These objectives must be integrated with the goals of patient management, which are to do all of the previously mentioned with the maintenance of satisfactory physiologic function, reasonable appearance, social interaction, and rehabilitation for a lifestyle compatible with the patient's own priorities and standards. Nevertheless, one has no control over some of these goals and little influence over others. The art becomes one of exercising well-informed, accurately communicated judgment as to the best compromises to make.

As indicated by the natural history of these cancers, there is an expected pattern of spread for each type, site, and stage. Consequently, not only must definitive therapy be directed at the identifiable disease, but also "prophylactic," or "elective" therapy aimed at areas of possible cancer cell dispersal, based on the likelihood of this occurrence. The amount and combination of therapy are further tempered with a probability contrast between treatment morbidity, likelihood of efficacy, and the preservation of future options. The physiologic morbidity of either surgery or radiation in the head and neck area influences life-sustaining and socially necessary function and appearance, with secondary psychologic, domestic, and occupational consequences. Areas of potential physical impairment are listed in Table 2–2.

TABLE 2–2. AREAS OF POTENTIAL PHYSICAL IMPAIRMENT

Speech
    Phonation (larynx)
    Articulation (tongue, teeth, palate, lips)

Chewing (jaw, teeth, salivary lubrication, relevant musculature)

Swallowing
    Deglutition (tongue, palate, pharynx, esophagus, salivary lubrication)
    Airway protection (larynx, esophagus; coordinated reflexes and sensation)

Breathing (larynx, trachea)

Senses
    Taste
    Smell
    Vision
    Hearing

Secondary effects of above on **nutrition,** chronic **pulmonary health**

Appearance

It can be difficult to accurately convey to a patient the effects treatment will have on his or her future. Assessing a patient's motivation and powers of rehabilitation, both physical and emotional, compounds the task. And yet, the patient's informed desires regarding treatment must be elicited as another of the many factors influencing treatment planning. The advantages of a particular treatment concern its effect on the tumor, while the disadvantages relate to its effect on the patient.

Surgery

As contrasted with radiation, operative eradication of a tumor and its areas of potential spread offers a more expeditious treatment, avoiding both the immediate and long-term side effects of radiation. The tissue volume treated is less and is available for pathologic analysis, which allows a determination of treatment adequacy and a confirmation of pretreatment staging classification. Furthermore, radiation is preserved as a future treatment option, and the increased complication rate of surgery after radiation is avoided.

Technically, cancer operations on the head and neck anatomy seek to minimize direct handling of the tumor-bearing tissue itself by working through the adjacent normal tissue and commencing the procedure in the least involved area, progressing toward the region of the primary site. While a number of standard procedures are described for dealing with tumors of different locations and sizes, each patient is approached in an individualized manner. A wide margin around the primary tumor is desirable, but limited by the functional or cosmetic importance of the adjacent tissue, as well as the ability to surgically or prosthetically reconstruct the resulting defect. The extent of any surgical procedure must also relate to its relative importance and efficacy in cancer control. Hence, for example, it may be worthwhile to remove a small tumor of the lateral tongue, while the same lesion in the midline base of tongue would require a very extensive procedure with no better effectiveness than radiation. Reconstruction, both cosmetic and functional, is an integral component of surgical management and may involve more technically sophisticated procedures than the tumor site ablation.

Head and neck oncologic operations may be described in four identifiable but overlapping and integrated phases, namely exposure, exploration, resection, and reconstruction. The proportionate time and expertise required to accomplish each of these processes can vary widely, depending on the site in question. Likewise, there are often several alternative techniques available to complete the endeavor. While a detailed description of operative procedures is beyond the scope of the present discussion, some generalities will be developed.

For primary site resection, the oral cavity and oropharynx can be approached through the mouth. More often, however, exposure through a lip-splitting incision with facial flap retraction, or via midline or lateral mandibulotomy, is necessary. A degloving, or pull-through, procedure may alternatively be feasible. Integration of the exposure process with the need for mandibular resection is an overriding factor. In general, the choice of exposure technique depends on the size of the lesion, how far posterior the epicenter of resection is, and the need for partial or complete changes in jaw integrity. Previous surgery, radiation treatment, or surgery for recurrent disease, as well as plans for postoperative radiation or staged rehabilitative surgery, all affect technical decisions. Individual surgical expertise and the exigencies of unexpected intraoperative findings must also be factored in. As an example, a midline anterior mandibulotomy for approaching the tongue base would be preferable to an angle split if postoperative radiation is planned. Even though the former generally requires a lip incision and the manipulation of more uninvolved tissues, an angle mandibulotomy would be in the radiation portal, thereby increasing the risk of radiation healing difficulties. By and large, one-stage ablation/reconstructive operations are becoming the norm, involving longer operative times, potentially greater (but one-time) perioperative risk, and requiring increasingly sophisticated technical expertise or a team approach. Simple reconstructive techniques involving split-thickness or dermal skin, or local intraoral flaps, or even primary closure, are variously feasible. More sophisticated techniques, generally for larger defects and/or jaw reconstruction, involve pedicled myocutaneous flaps, with or without bony or prosthetic grafting or microvascular free-transfer of composite tissue aggregates from a distant part of the body. These can include skin, muscle, or bone in any combination, from sources such as the periscapular region or iliac crest/groin, and constitute the state-of-the-art in head and neck reconstruction.

Overall, the evolution of ablative surgery on the larynx, hypopharynx, and esophagus has seen a refinement in the amount of tissue removed with preservation of cancer treatment efficacy and organ function. The development of new techniques of local reconstruction has, of necessity, paralleled this trend. Many basic types and modifications of subtotal laryngectomy exist, with attempted optimization of postoperative airway, deglutition, pulmonary protection, and voice. Total laryngectomy remains a comparatively simple technical procedure, insofar as the airway is exteriorized rather than reconstructed, and only a conduit for swallowing need be created through simple primary repair of the pharyngotomy defect. Vocal rehabilitation is quite often nonsurgical and delayed, through the use of an electrolarynx vibration device externally, or the learning of esophageal speech by the patient. The surgical placement of a vocal prosthesis (which allows the shunting of air through the posterior tracheal wall into the neopharynx, thereby creating an audible vibration that can be formed into understandable speech) can be performed at the time of total laryngectomy (primary vocal reconstruction), but is more often done at least six months later (secondary vocal reconstruction), after a period of observation and attempt at learning esophageal speech. Reconstruction of the pharyngoesophagus after total laryngopharyngectomy or cervical esophagectomy remains a surgical challenge for which there are several techniques. Gastric transposition ("pullup") is a historically well-established procedure that requires combined abdominal, thoracic, and cervical manipulation and is believed by some to be excessively morbid in certain patients. Regional reconstruction using tubed or partially tubed myocutaneous flaps, with or without accessory skin grafting, can also be very successful. More recently the use of microvascular free skin-muscle tissues has found favor in some institutions, as has the transfer of a jejunal segment through vascular reanastomosis, this also involving entry into the abdominal cavity.

It must be pointed out that while developing and refining ways of resecting and reconstructing head and neck cancers is extremely important, it would be vastly preferable if cure rates could be advanced without the side effects of the more sophisticated, more radical operative procedures.

Cervical lymphadenectomy (neck dissection) is commonly combined with local surgical treatment, though not always for the same reasons in two different patients. Almost without exception, neck dissection is mandatory in cases of existing gross nodal disease, whether untreated, partially treated, or recurrent. Neck dissection might also be elected in cases in which the primary site has a high likelihood of occult lymphatic dissemination, particularly if surgery is the only treatment modality planned at the given therapeutic juncture in question. The need for cervical tissue modification in order to accommodate a planned reconstructive technique is germane, as also are the situations in which, because of physical stature or prior treatment, a neck at risk is not well evaluable. This is also true in the case of an unexpected intraoperative finding of metastatic disease. Contraindications might include uncontrollable local (primary site) or distant metastatic disease, short life expectancy, or massive or infiltrative nodal disease unaffected by radiation or chemotherapy.

The descriptive nomenclature of cervical lymph node ablations has been refined over the years, but remains inconsistently applied. The historically classic radical neck dissection, now referred to as *classical radical neck dissection*, was originally described by Crile in 1906.[14] The procedure involves the contiguous removal of the submandibular and submental compartment lymph nodes, the upper, middle, and lower deep jugular nodal chains, as well as the upper and lower posterior triangle nodes. Included in the process are the submandibular salivary gland, the tail of parotid, the sternocleidomastoid and omohyoid muscles, the internal jugular vein, the cervical plexus (mostly sensory) nerves, and the spinal accessory nerve. A modified radical neck dissection (RND) is identical, with the exception of the preservation of the spinal accessory nerve, thereby mitigating against one of the more significant consequences of a classical dissection, shoulder drop, weakness, and pain. Other side effects of RND surgery include facial swelling and neck deformity, regional numbness, occasionally painful neuroma formation, and a small, but significantly increased after radiation, risk of major complication, such as pharyngocutaneous fistulization, thoracic duct ("chyle") fistula, and carotid rupture. The term *modified neck dissection* is not a single procedure but rather an overall term referring to a number of variations of regional lymphadenectomy. A well-configured rational classification scheme has been proposed by Suen and Goepfert.[15] A functional neck dissection (referred to by some as a *conservation neck dissection*) seeks to remove essentially the same structures as a radical neck dissection, but with preservation of the spinal accessory nerve, internal jugular vein, and sternocleidomastoid muscle. This procedure was popularized by Bocca and has served to focus attention on the refinement of changing indications for the various regional lymph node procedures in an era when nonsurgical head and neck cancer treatment is also evolving rapidly.[16] The other forms of modified neck dissections are various selective neck dissections directed at specific regional nodal sites, such as the submandibular triangle dissection or the posterior neck dissection.[17]

Radiation

Radiation avoids the small but finite risk of perioperative mortality that remains in judiciously selected and carefully managed surgical patients. As no tissue is removed, the cosmetic effect can be minimal. Functional side effects do occur but are generally much less dramatic than with surgery. These side effects relate to the loss of mucosal lubrication (due to radiation effect on salivary gland function) and taste, chronic mucosal inflammation and fragility, and scarring, fibrosis, and edema around the area of treatment. These radiation reactions are not just confined to the mucosa but to all exposed tissues. Fibrosis of various muscles can cause dysfunction (trismus, vocal cord fixation). Chronic edema, adding to the deglutitory discomfort caused by salivary insufficiency, can also result in chronic dysphagia, dysphonia, and airway obstruction. The risk of soft tissue, cartilage or bone necrosis is small with present management and technical practice but must be weighed.

The logistics of radiation therapy, which involve daily treatments for five to eight weeks, are not one of its finer features. An advantage is the ability of radiation to treat multiple regions simultaneously in the case of coexistent multiple primary mucosal lesions. As elective treatment for occult lymphatic disease, either independently or in conjunction with surgery, radiotherapy carries relatively little morbidity and is effective. Its use in place of neck dissection surgery is a multifactorial decision, with site, stage, and individual considerations.

The dosage of radiation is determined by the site and volume of tumor, its proclivity for spread, and the intent of treatment (curative or palliative). Palliative dosages are likely to be lower, with smaller field sizes, in order to minimize side effects. Larger (T_3 or T_4) tumors tend to need higher dosages of 7000 rads (or cGy) or more, while smaller tumors (T_1 or T_2) may be cured with 6000 to 7000 rads. The treatment of the clinically negative neck (N_0) is traditionally with dosages of 5000 to 5500 rads. Some nodal areas will receive more if they overlay a primary tumor that is being treated concomitantly to a higher dosage. Dosages much higher than 7000 rads, if delivered externally, increase complications substantially. Although retreatment to a high cumulative dosage after delayed recurrence is generally not feasible, it can be attempted with very small field sizes. The nasopharynx, which generally lacks a surgical alternative for local recurrence, can be retreated with radiation.

Usually several different focus angles of the beam onto the tumor are used in order to lessen the deleterious effects of radiation on the interposed normal tissues. The fields (or portals) of delivery for external radiotherapy are simulated by computer to ensure an accurate dosage in the area of tumor and to allow the consistent daily administration of the beam. Regions needing additional treatment (radiation boost) are focused onto with smaller field sizes (shrinking field technique).

Higher dosages can also be delivered through the insertion or implantation of radioactive materials, such as gold or iridium, via seeds, needles, removable catheters, or surface contact. The interstitial technique (brachytherapy) is particularly useful in the tongue base, tonsil fossa, and oral cavity. Surface exposure is occasionally used to deliver additional radiation to the nasopharynx or to a maxillectomy cavity. Among others, an advantage of this highly localized boost technique is the relatively greater sparing of uninvolved tissues, which may have a favorable impact on postradiation surgery complication. With regard to lymphatic dissemination, Fletcher[18] has demonstrated that 5000 rads can control clinically undetectable (occult) microscopic nodal metastases if present. The availability and utilization of cervical irradiation may not, however, always preempt a decision for nodal exploration and dissection.

Combination Therapy

As a rule, surgical salvage (indicating the successful retreatment of a recurrent or persistent cancer after previous treatment) for radiation failure is more likely than radiation salvage after previous surgery. A recurrence after radiation is more likely to be at the epicenter of the original lesion, rather than at its periphery. Therefore a surgical procedure, albeit with functional and operative sequelae, is more likely to anatomically encompass the recurrence with a reasonable margin. Recurrence at the primary site after surgery, by contrast, will more likely develop submucosally at the periphery of the original tumor, in the margin of resection. The difficulty involved in discerning recurrent tumor from postoperative fibrosis is formidable and often results in diagnostic delay. Even if recurrence is suspected, the technical difficulties in obtaining tissue and histologic confirmation of metastasis from a previously operated site can be problematic. Furthermore, such a tumor in a scarred, distorted, and relatively avascular tissue field is likely to have multiple areas of sequestration and hypoxia. These features probably account for the resistance to radiation salvage noted in this setting.

While a segregated discussion of radiation and surgery lends a certain perspective, they are frequently employed together. As a very general guideline, in the absence of clinically identifiable lymphatic spread, small lesions (T_1 or T_2) are equally well served by either radiation or surgery, the choice based on relative morbidity for the site in question. Additional weight is given to radiation if there is a high risk of occult nodal disease. The alternative of surgery including neck dissection is possible. For large primary tumors (T_3 or T_4) or clinically evident nodal disease (N_1, N_2, N_3) combined treatment with radiation and surgery is indicated, with sequence and sites of emphasis determined by the staging and site particulars, perceived effectiveness, combined morbidity, and individual preference.

As previously suggested, the risk of surgical complications is increased by the previous administration of radiotherapy. Because of its deleterious effects on the microcirculation, healing may be significantly delayed, impaired, or even impossible after surgical manipulation of irradiated tissues. There is a consequent risk of wound infection, mucosal-cutaneous discontinuity, and even progressive tissue breakdown (necrosis), including major vessel rupture. These risks aside, previous radiation will also affect judgment as to the choice of or even the feasibility of any surgical procedure, placing limitations on technique, tissue preservation, reconstruction, and patient rehabilitation. For example, a previously irradiated mandible that must then undergo resection for a recurrence in the oral cavity has a generally poor chance of healing, thereby limiting the usefulness of immediate reconstructive procedures. Osteoradionecrosis of the mandible remains one of the more feared complications of head and neck cancer treatment and can occur spontaneously after radiation, due to pre-existent dental disease or following further manipulation by surgery. Laryngeal necrosis can also occur (at times forcing total laryngectomy, even in the absence of discernible malignancy) in order to salvage airway, deglutition, and pulmonary protection. As an aside, the use of adjunctive hyperbaric oxygen therapy in the treatment of tissue hypoxia due to radiation causing infectious or healing sequelae has shown some promise, but is not universally available.[19–21]

Chemotherapy[22–24]

A number of antineoplastic drugs are effective against epidermoid cancer of the head and neck. While chemotherapy does not have the capacity to cure this family of malignancies, it can bring about a considerable reduction in tumor cell population, volume, and density. As local control of more advanced cancers has improved with the use of combined radiation and surgery techniques, failure due to delayed or late-manifesting distant metastases has become a bigger problem. Systemic therapy would allow the possible eradication of tumor cells dispersed hematogenously or early tumor colonies in distant organs. By lessening the tumor volume at the primary and nodal sites, a subsequent curative therapy such as radiation may work better. Surgery, by encompassing a smaller tumor mass, could have greater latitude for larger margins of resection.[25] Alternatively, a lower tumor density at the margin may result in a decrease in tumor viability.

An actively investigated result of these mechanisms may be that pretreatment with chemotherapy ("induction" chemotherapy) would lessen the extent of subsequent treatment needed or even eliminate one of the combined modalities presently employed for advanced head and neck cancer. A more traditional but very important use for chemotherapy has been in the palliation of incurable individuals.

Methotrexate and bleomycin but particularly cisplatin and 5-fluorouracil are the most effective agents used in chemotherapy trials today. The principles of induction chemotherapy are to administer combinations of established drugs with differing mechanisms of antineoplastic action and nonoverlapping major toxicities in a dosage and timing sequence that takes advantage of each agent's action on the tumor cell cycle.

As an independent variable, adjuvant chemotherapy in head and neck cancer has not yet been conclusively shown to improve survival. While the degree of response to chemotherapy does correlate with survival, it is not clear that this trend is due to the chemotherapy itself or to the fortuitous biology of an individual tumor that renders it sensitive to both traditional treatment and chemotherapy. Well-designed, randomized, prospective clinical trials with long-term follow-up will help to determine the role for chemotherapy in the treatment of advanced head and neck cancer patients. It is speculated that when complete response (CR) rates can consistently exceed 50 per cent, because of refinements in drug selection and administration, a survival benefit will be apparent.[26] A practical role in early lesions is not envisioned.

REFERENCES

1. Cann, C.I., Fried, M.P., and Rothman, K.J.: Epidemiology of squamous cell cancer of the head and neck. Otolaryngol. Clin. North Am. *18:*367–388, 1985.
2. Silverberg, E., and Lubera, J.A.: Cancer Statistics, 1988. CA *38:*5–22, 1988.
3. Suen, J.Y., and Myers, E.N. (Eds.): Cancer of the Head and Neck, New York, Churchill Livingstone, 1981, p. 3.
4. Moolgavkar, S.H., and Knudson, A.G.: Mutation and cancer: A model for human carcinogenesis. JNCI *66:*1037–1052, 1981.
5. Beahrs, O.H., Henson, D.E., Hutter, R.V.P., and Myers, M.H.: Manual for Staging of Cancer. 3rd edition. American Joint Committee on Cancer. Philadelphia, J.B. Lippincott, 1988.
6. Sercarz, J., Ellison, D., Holmes, E.C., and Calcaterra, T.C.: Isolated pulmonary nodules in head and neck cancer patients. Ann. Otol. Rhinol. Laryngol. *98:*113–118, 1989.
7. Sisson, G.A., and Pelzer, H.J.: Staging system by sites: Problems and refinements. Otolaryngol. Clin. North Am. *18:*397–402, 1985.
8. Norris, C.M., Jr., and Miller, D.: The neck mass. *In* English, G.M. (Ed.): Otolaryngology. Philadelphia, Harper & Row, 1985.
9. Shikhani, A.H., Matanoski, G.M., Jones, M.M., et al.: Multiple primary malignancies in head and neck cancer. Arch. Otolaryngol. Head Neck Surg. *112:*1172–1179, 1986.
10. Shaha, A.R., Hoover, E.L., Mitrani, M., et al.: Synchronicity, multicentricity, and metachronicity of head and neck cancer. Head Neck Surg. *10:*225–228, 1988.
11. Atkins, J.P., Jr., Keane, W.M., Young, K.A., and Rowe, L.D.: Value of panendoscopy in determination of second primary cancer. Arch. Otlaryngol. *110:*533–534, 1984.
12. Atkinson, D., Fleming, S., and Weaver, A.: Triple endoscopy: A valuable procedure in head and neck surgery. Am. J. Surg. *144:*416–419, 1982.
13. Magnetic resonance imaging of the head and neck region. Present status and future potential. Council on Scientific Affairs. Report of the Panel on Magnetic Resonance Imaging. JAMA *260:*3313–3326, 1988.
14. Crile, G.: Excision of cancer of the head and neck. J. Am. Med. *47:*1780–1787, 1906.
15. Suen, J.Y., and Goepfert, H.: Editorial standardization of neck dissection nomenclature. Head Neck Surg. *10:*75, 1987.
16. Bocca, E., and Pignataro, O.: A conservation technique in radical neck dissection. Ann. Otol. Rhinol. Laryngol. *76:*975, 1967.
17. Suen, J.Y.: Cancer of the neck. *In* Myers, E.N., and Suen, J.Y. (Eds.): Cancer of the Head and Neck, 2nd edition. New York, Churchill Livingstone, 1989, pp. 221–254.
18. Fletcher, G.H.: Elective irradiation of subclinical disease in cancers of the head and neck. Cancer *29:*1450, 1972.
19. Davis, J.C., Dunn, J.M., Gates, G.A., and Heimbach, R.D.: Hyperbaric oxygen. A new adjunct in the management of radiation necrosis. Arch. Otolaryngol. *105:*58–61, 1979.
20. Patel, P., Raybould, T., and Maruyama, Y.: Osteoradionecrosis of the jaw bones at the University of Kentucky Medical Center. J. Ky. Med. Assoc. *87:*327–331, 1989.

21. Ferguson, B.J., Hudson, W.R., and Farmer, J.C., Jr.: Hyperbaric oxygen therapy for laryngeal radionecrosis. Ann. Otol. Rhinol. Laryngol. 96:1–6, 1987.
22. Ervin, T.J., Clark, J.R., Weichselbaum, R.R., et al.: An analysis of induction and adjuvant chemotherapy in the multidisciplinary treatment of squamous cell carcinoma of the head and neck. J. Clin. Oncol. 5:10–20, 1987.
23. Dreyfuss, A.I., Clark, J.R., Fallon, B.G., et al.: Cyclophosphamide, doxorubicin and cisplatin combination chemotherapy for advanced carcinomas of salivary gland origin. Cancer 60:2869–2872, 1987.
24. Dreyfuss, A.I., Clark, J.R., Wright, J.E., et al.: Continuous infusion high-dose leucovorin with 5-fluorouracil and cisplatin for untreated stage IV carcinoma of the head and neck. Ann. Intern. Med. 112:167–172, 1990.
25. Norris, C.M., Jr., Clark, J.R., Frei, E., III, et al.: Pathology of surgery after induction chemotherapy: An analysis of resectability and locoregional control. Laryngoscope 96:292–302, 1986.
26. Clark, J.R., Fallon, B.G., and Frei, E., III: Induction chemotherapy as initial treatment for advanced head and neck cancer: A model for the multidisciplinary treatment of solid tumors. In DeVita, V.T., Jr., Hellman, S., and Rosenberg, S.A. (Eds.): Important Advances in Oncology. Philadelphia, J.B. Lippincott, 1987, pp. 175–195.

FLOOR OF MOUTH AND TONGUE
by Charles M. Norris, Jr., M.D.

The oral cavity is subdivided into the mobile tongue (oral tongue, anterior two-thirds), floor of mouth, gingiva, hard palate, buccal mucosa, and retromolar trigone. Though the oral cavity is relatively accessible to self-examination, dental evaluation, and routine physical examination, even without subspecialty equipment or training, there are often delays in the diagnosis of oral cavity cancer, which arises out of confusion with traumatic, inflammatory, or infectious lesions.[1] Patients often do not seek medical help until more advanced symptoms are present.[2] The tongue base is anatomically part of the oropharynx, which also includes the tonsillar pillars, fossae and tonsils (if present), soft palate, and the pharyngeal walls below the nasopharynx (posterior edge of soft palate) and above the hypopharynx (pharyngoepiglottic fold).

Generally, the morbidity of treatment increases and the prognosis worsens as the disease progresses posteriorly from the oral cavity to the oropharynx and then to the hypopharynx. With the exception of the larynx, the oral cavity and oropharynx are the most common sites for squamous cell carcinoma of the head and neck. Excluding the lips, the mobile tongue and floor of mouth comprise over half of oral cavity sites in a head and neck cancer patient population[3] (Table 2–3). The patients tend to be males in the fifth and sixth decades, but the number of female and young adult cases has been increasingly established.[4–7]

Tobacco use of any kind, including snuff and chewing tobacco, and alcohol consumption are significant etiologic factors. Not infrequently oral cancers are associated with poor dentition, ongoing oral infection, or chronic trauma of any cause. The incidence of oral cavity cancer in nonsmoking

TABLE 2–3. STAGING OUTLINE—CANCER OF THE ORAL CAVITY AND OROPHARYNX (AJCC*)

Primary Tumor
General—for all sites
- T_X —No available information on primary tumor
- T_0 —No evidence of primary tumor
- T_{IS} —Carcinoma *in situ*

Fom/Ant. Tongue/Base of Tongue
- T_1 —Greatest diameter of primary tumor $\leq$ 2 cm
- T_2 —2 cm $\geq$ 4 cm
- T_3 —> 4 cm
- T_4 —Massive tumor, and/or extension/invasion into adjacent structures (cortex of mandible, pterygoid muscles, deep tongue muscle, skin, soft tissues of neck)

Nodal Metastasis (N)
- N_X —Nodes cannot be assessed
- N_0 —No clinically positive nodes
- N_1 —Single, clinically positive, ipsilateral node; $\leq$ 3 cm
- N_{2A}—Single, clinically positive, ipsilateral node; 3 cm $\geq$ 6 cm
- N_{2B}—Multiple, clinically positive, ipsilateral nodes; all $\leq$ 6 cm
- N_{2C}—Single or multiple, clinically positive, bilateral or contralateral, any/all $\leq$ 6 cm
- N_3 Any clinically positive node; > 6 cm

Distant Metastasis (M)
- M_X —Not assessed
- M_0 —No distant metastases identified
- M_1 —Distant metastasis present (specify site)

Stage Groupings
- Stage I —T_1 N_0 M_0
- Stage II —T_2 N_0 M_0
- State III—T_3 N_0 M_0
  - T_1, T_2 or T_3 N_1 M_0
- Stage IV—T_4 N_0 or N_1 M_0
  - Any T N_2 or N_3 M_0
  - Any T Any N M_1

*American Joint Committee on Cancer.[8]

younger individuals, particularly women, possibly relates to as yet uncharacterized deficiencies in epithelial cellular repair mechanisms, which are important in an area exposed to so many environmental factors.[5, 7]

The focus of this discussion is on epidermoid cancers of the floor of mouth and tongue, both oral and base, as common sites entailing a broad clinical spectrum of diagnostic, treatment, and management issues.

HISTOLOGY

Over 95 per cent of cancers of the floor of mouth and tongue (anterior and base) are epidermoid (squamous cell) carcinoma, with a trend toward less differentiation and higher grade as the lesion moves posteriorly. Various forms of leukoplakia may coexist or precede the evolution of a malignancy and can be histologically confusing.

Minor salivary gland malignancies, usually mucoepidermoid carcinoma (low- and high-grade), adenocarcinoma, or adenoid cystic carcinoma are rare, occurring more commonly in the palate. With the exception of low-grade mucoepidermoid carcinoma, these present a poor prognosis. Aggressive, complete primary surgery is necessary for cure in all but the smallest lesions, with radiation a meaningful adjuvant in the higher grade histologies or in cases of incomplete excision, perineural spread, or lymphatic metastasis. Nodal spread is generally rare, except in high-grade mucoepidermoid carcinomas, but the incidence of distant metastasis is high and remains a substantial cause of death in patients with locoregional control. Chemotherapy has no role in the initial curative treatment of resectable minor salivary gland malignancies but can provide a measure of palliation in appropriate cases.[9-11]

Verrucous carcinoma, an epithelial variant lesion, occurs rarely. In some cases these lesions have been believed to transform into a more anaplastic lesion, historically raising questions about the validity of radiation in their treatment. While true transformation remains controversial, verrucous carcinoma does appear to exist in a hybrid form with areas of invasive squamous cell carcinoma. Surgery is conceded to be the treatment of choice by most investigators, but radiation can be a reasonable alternative in selected patients.[12]

The lymphoid constituents of the tongue base, a part of Waldeyer's tonsillar ring, may give way to lymphoepithelioma, a highly radiosensitive variant of epidermoid carcinoma. Malignant lymphomas occur, which are usually extranodal non-Hodgkin's lesions of the diffuse histiocytic type.[13,14]

Malignant melanoma as well is a rare but recognized lesion in the oral cavity and oropharynx. Histologic review and confirmation is important, as benign melanotic lesions may precede or coexist with the malignant variety. Metastatic melanoma to the oral cavity (20 per cent of the malignancies in one review series)[15] must also be ruled out.[16]

CLINICAL FEATURES

Lesions in the oral cavity and oropharynx are often poorly delineated, with early, potentially extensive, submucosal spread. They are generally not limited by the anatomic midline, an observation with important surgical implications. There is no typical appearance of either early or late primary lesions. An exophytic (as opposed to ulcerated or infiltrative) growth pattern is generally more favorable, but not invariably so. The intimate anatomic relationship between the floor of mouth and tongue allows for the ready spread of disease from one to the other, hence a considerable coincidence of patterns of spread and other clinical features. Involvement of the intrinsic deep tongue musculature, or extension laterally into the pterygoid muscles, is prognostically ominous. Adherence, with fixation of an even small tumor to periosteum, may occur. The mandibular periosteum is a reasonably effective barrier to bony invasion, which directs tumor spread along its surface in an occult manner, possibly far away from the tumor's apparent epicenter. True cortical bony invasion is a late event, serious both prognostically and from the standpoint of treatment morbidity. Bony involvement may occur without erosion, by insinuation of tumor through dental sockets, around intact teeth, and along the mandibular branch of the lingual nerve.

Multiple subdivisions within the oral cavity and oropharynx become involved as tumor enlargement and spread continue. Lateral extension from lesions in the posterior oral cavity or oropharynx can invade the parapharyngeal space or neck directly, with involvement of the cranial nerves and carotid artery. Extension of primary tumor across the midline is particularly problematic, as this renders surgical treatment much more debilitating. Unilateral oral organ dysfunction or sensation loss is usually well tolerated, while bilateral impairment compounds the sequelae exponentially.

There is a notable propensity (> 30 per cent) for patients with oral cavity lesions to develop synchronous or asynchronous second primary cancers, both within the oral cavity and elsewhere in the upper aerodigestive tract.[4, 17–19]

Nodal metastases, occult or overt, are relatively less common with small (T_1, T_2) lesions in the floor of mouth[20] or mobile tongue but occur with increasing frequency as the site of the primary lesion moves posteriorly into the oropharynx or as its size increases.[21–23] This feature accounts for a correspondingly worse prognosis. Furthermore, patients with oropharyngeal lesions tend to present with a more advanced stage of disease.

Floor of mouth and anterior tongue lesions will tend to first metastasize to the submandibular and upper deep jugular nodes, while base of tongue metastases spread through the deep jugular chain, beginning with either the upper or middle nodal stations. A rich lymphatic network facilitates the contralateral spread of disease observed in all these sites, whether at presentation or in delayed recurrence of the untreated neck. This potential for bilateral lymphatic spread is considerable. In a landmark study on the usefulness of radiation in treating occult nodal metastasis, Fletcher demonstrated that almost half the patients presenting with ipsilateral nodal disease associated with floor of mouth cancer will develop contralateral metastasis if prophylactic treatment is not rendered.[24] Others have corroborated this observation.[25] While the anatomic pattern of early or presenting nodal metastasis is somewhat predictable, obstruction and diversion of lymphatic pathways by tumor or surgery can alter the distribution of nodes at risk.

Floor of mouth and mobile tongue lesions will involve detectable nodal disease in 30 to 38 per cent of cases.[21, 26] The tongue base, however, exhibits a much higher rate of associated metastasis, approaching 80 per cent, with almost one-third of patients having bilateral nodal disease.[21] Even in the N_0 neck, the incidence of occult metastasis is relatively high, ranging from 30 per cent up to probably 60 per cent as one moves from the anterior oral cavity (floor of mouth and mobile tongue) to the oropharynx.[25, 27, 28] Interestingly, Jesse and others noted that the delayed appearance of recurrent metastatic disease did not invariably affect the prognosis.[29] More and more recent studies, however, disagree with that conclusion.[30, 31]

DIAGNOSIS

Patients with early asymptomatic lesions of the floor of mouth or tongue may be identified on routine dental or incidental medical evaluation. Local pain, perhaps initially only when eating, may be present. Base of tongue lesions, relatively inaccessible to simple examination, are invariably asymptomatic in the early stages and often identified during the evaluation of a neck mass that proves to be metastatic.

Size progression and extension will lead to more persistent pain, including referred otalgia, as well as trismus and other dysfunctions of speech and swallowing due to infiltration of the deep tongue, pterygoid muscles, or palate. Loosening of teeth, bleeding, and halitosis, due to ulceration and tissue necrosis, are generally later symptoms.

Understandably, the more anterior the lesion, the easier and more reliable the assessment of tumor extent. Palpation, both internally and externally (bimanual), is of paramount importance and may be the only way to even detect a more posterior lesion. The distinction of direct tumor spread into the neck from ipsilateral metastasis can be difficult, as also can be the discernment of periosteal attachment from true bony invasion.[32] Computed tomography (CT) scanning and mandible x-rays, particularly the occlusal and submental views, are helpful. A negative bone scan is the most reassuring.[33]

Endoscopy and examination under anesthesia are advisable to fully evaluate primary site extent, especially of the tongue base, and the possibility of synchronous second primaries in other areas of the upper aerodigestive tract. As floor of mouth lesions often arise within or are associated with other areas of mucosal abnormality, including chronic leukoplakia, the diagnostic biopsy yield of earlier tumors may require multiple tissue samplings and/or pretreatment with toluidine blue. Identification of the patient with multifocal disease ("field cancerization") may significantly influence treatment decisions. Deep biopsies may be required to document a submucosal tongue base lesion, with an attendent risk of bleeding and absolute requirement for general anesthesia.

Evaluation of the teeth and jaw, whether directly involved by tumor or not, is advisable in order to plan for any jaw surgery or dental extractions prior to radiation therapy.

TREATMENT

General

When a satisfactory evaluation and staging of the disease and patient is completed, including any medical comorbidity influencing treatment decisions, a basic treatment plan is usually apparent, subject, of course, to individual application and acceptance.

Generally, since radiation techniques and surgery are both equally effective, the treatment of early stage primary lesions of the oral cavity or oropharynx is determined by perceptions of morbidity, including that related to speech, chewing/swallowing, and appearance. Because of the number of variables that influence these side effects, including, but not limited to, size, precise location, proximity to neighboring structures, midline orientation, and previous treatment effects, as well as those relating to an individual patient's desires and expectations, it is not possible to generalize treatment plans dogmatically. To a certain extent, as the tumor site moves posteriorly, the morbidity of surgery increases (e.g., lateral lesions of the mobile tongue versus tongue base). It is likely that patients will tend to underestimate the degree and duration of radiation side effects and overestimate the side effects of early stage surgery, many of which are transient or reasonably accommodated. A patient with multiple early oral primary cancers ("field cancerization") or multiple premalignant lesions may best be treated with surgical techniques, preserving radiation for significantly more advanced disease, unfavorable locations, or associated delayed metastases.

In the absence of nodal disease (N_0), T_1 lesions of the floor of mouth and tongue are usually best treated via wide excision. An exception might be in the case of a lesion incompletely removed previously for diagnosis (T_x), in which case the reliability of assessing subsequent excisional adequacy by frozen section will be poor. Some groups[34] have drawn particular attention to anterior tongue lesions as being more serious than historically considered, citing undertreatment due to understaging as a cause of treatment failure. Unfortunately, it is difficult to generalize from published data because of the diversity of reporting styles and treatment approaches and the lack of uniform staging, even within established guidelines. Other staging measures, such as vascular and perineural invasion, the nature of the stromal inflammatory infiltrate surrounding the tumor, and various measures of circulatory and systemic immune function have been investigated in order to further refine indices for local and regional treatment.[1, 35–38]

T_2 lesions of the floor of mouth and oral tongue are a therapeutic challenge and remain controversial. Because the morbidity of surgery is not always severe it becomes more noteworthy, and the higher likelihood of nodal disease requires assessment for treatment of the neck. More posterior lesions should be handled with primary site excision and planned prophylactic radiation to the neck, or radiation alone to nodes and primary, with a dosage boost (possibly through interstitial implantation) to the primary site. More anterior lesions could be handled similarly, although radiation might be avoided if bilateral supraomohyoid neck dissections are performed and no microscopic evidence of occult metastasis is identified. Particularly favorable (exophytic) T_2 lesions can be approached with primary site surgery alone, with various parameters of tumor aggressiveness (mitoses; vascular, lymphatic, and neural invasion) that determine the need for postoperative local and nodal irradiation. On the other hand, midline floor of mouth lesions risk a disproportionate amount of tongue restriction and bilateral occult nodal disease if treated surgically. Radiation, therefore, might be given preference. Crissman[1] has identified two populations within the T_2N_0 (stage II) group with divergent natural histories based on the level of histologic invasion. His conclusion is that superficial lesions will behave like T_1s, with good results from local excision only, while the deeper lesions require disproportionately more extensive treatment, including nodal areas at risk.

Treatment of the clinically negative neck in early stage lesions of the floor of mouth and oral tongue entails various options. The yield (i.e., presence of histologic nodal metastasis) of elective neck dissection for T_1 and T_2 floor of mouth carcinomas is low,[20] although supraomohyoid dissection is believed to represent a good staging maneuver and, taken together with a histologic evaluation of the primary disease, can affect a decision on postoperative radiation therapy.[39] Reliance on salvage treatment for delayed recurrence in a previously untreated neck is not universally endorsed. N_0 disease is less reassuring in oral tongue, and certainly in base of tongue, lesions of any stage. The incidence of occult metastasis in both is high.[30, 31,]

[40, 41] Some authors think that anterior oral tongue lesions should be treated as aggressively as posterior oral or tongue base lesions, with elective treatment, including the contralateral neck, at least with radiation.[30, 42] Surgery on the ipsilateral neck (supraomohyoid or radical neck dissection) might be elected for technical reasons of primary site exposure, resection margin, or reconstruction (e.g., to accommodate a distant flap).

T_1 and T_2, N_0 lesions of the tongue base will most often be treated with radiation, including external treatment of both neck and primary site, and usually an interstitial implant to the tongue base. Because of the significant morbidity of surgery, T_3 tongue base lesions, especially if they cross the midline, can be treated similarly, with radical or modified neck dissections reserved for treating pre-existent palpable nodal metastasis, i.e., N_1 through N_3. The presence of adenopathy with small primary tongue base lesions is believed to obligate surgery on the neck, particularly if greater than N_1 size. Neck dissection can be concomitantly performed with an interstitial implant radiation boost. There is a surprisingly high percentage of false-positive adenopathy turned up at surgery for floor of mouth lesions,[1, 2] possibly out of confusion with other submandibular triangle structures.

Advanced primary lesions (T_3, T_4) and/or associated nodal disease (N_1, N_2, N_3), i.e., stages III and IV cancers at any of these sites, have most often required combined treatment, traditionally by both radiation and surgery, in various patterns and sequences. The role for adjunctive chemotherapy, either as initial treatment and/or as final treatment, remains controversial, and with regard to the oral cavity and oropharynx has not yet been shown to permit a curtailing of traditional treatment type or extent. Surgical exposure can be difficult, especially posteriorly, compounding morbidity and reconstructive aspects. In floor of mouth lesions attached to periosteum, the concern for radiation effects on bone may prompt surgical treatment, whereas the same size lesion away from the jaw would preferentially be treated with radiation.

As noted, posterior lesions, even early ones, have an increased likelihood of occult nodal metastasis. Not infrequently, surgical findings result in the need for postoperative radiation. Among the lymphatic drainage pathways are nodes inaccessible to standard surgical techniques (i.e., retropharyngeal and parapharyngeal), or for which contralateral surgical treatment would be considered excessive. Even aggressive radical surgery for early stage lesions of the oropharynx may not remove all gross and subclinical disease, and consequently radiation would be appropriate.

The need for and type of treatment of one site (primary or neck) may direct treatment of the other area. It is useful, therefore, to identify which aspect of the patient's disease poses the greatest threat in terms of the risks of treatment failure and options for treatment of a recurrence. Clinically overt nodal metastasis, with either oral cavity or oropharyngeal primaries, confers an advanced staging and generally requires combined treatment. Some will advocate radiation alone for unilateral N_1 neck disease in conjunction with primary site treatment, but the number of such proponents is few. Combined treatment does not necessarily entail combined T_x of both primary and nodal disease. For example, a small oropharyngeal primary with ipsilateral nodal disease may be treated with radiation and implant to cure the primary lesion and sterilize the contralateral neck, with surgery (neck dissection) to control the known nodal disease. More advanced primaries will require surgery as well to optimize cure potential.

Extremely advanced disease may be determined to be an incurable situation, for which aggressive, potentially debilitating treatment may not be in the best interest of preserving the quality of the patient's existence for the limited time he or she may have. As such, nonsurgical techniques for palliation may be recommended, in an effort to minimize morbidity and preserve some control of tumor for a period of time.

Surgery—Primary Site

Surgery on anteriorly located structures may be attempted transorally. Dentition can get in the way, however, and be severely limiting. Primary closure, especially of the mobile tongue following partial glossectomy, but also of the buccal mucosa or floor of mouth, is often possible. If not, split thickness or dermal skin grafting is feasible. A variety of local, intraoral flaps have been defined, allowing the transfer of tissue from one area of the oral cavity to another (buccal mucosal flaps, tongue advancement). The floor of mouth presents the added considerations of the nearby lingual and hypoglossal nerves to be preserved if feasible. The Wharton's salivary ducts, sublingual, and submandibular glands may be included in the resection or preserved with reimplantation, as appropriate. Periosteal involvement may dictate a sagittal or marginal (or "rim") mandibulectomy, which can be performed intraorally, although with some difficulty. Many surgeons think that any lesion within a centimeter of the mandible should include the adjacent periosteum and bone in any resection planned.

For larger or less accessible anterior (oral cavity) lesions, and for most posterior (oropharyngeal) lesions, intraoral surgery is limiting, and a transcervical approach for exposure, with or without mandible or lip splitting procedures, will be required. Segmental mandibulectomy will always require an approach from outside the oral cavity. Reconstruction can require elaborate means, including the transfer of distant tissue such as a pectoralis major myocutaneous (muscle-skin pedicle) flap, bone graft, or artificial prosthesis (jaw plate). The reconstructive endeavors may constitute as formidable a group of procedures as the tumor extirpation itself.

The preoperative assessment of resectability can be difficult and in some cases impossible. Margins are limited by the confined anatomy of the oral cavity and oropharynx. When the boundaries of resection are increased, even if anatomically feasible, significant increases in patient morbidity usually result. Frozen section analysis of the margins taken during surgery, appropriately oriented and related to the tumor-patient defect, is essential but still not an absolute guarantee of the adequacy of resection.

Postoperative radiation, advocated by some as reasonable back-up for an area of incompletely excised tumor, should not be relied on. Often, postoperative radiation is already part of the treatment plan. The tongue base and lower pharynx are particularly treacherous areas and may require adjunctive total laryngectomy in order to avoid postoperative aspiration problems. Some surgeons consider this inappropriately excessive initial treatment for a lesion that is likely incurable. However, for the palliation of recurrent disease, total laryngectomy may actually provide relief from pain and aspiration, as well as allow the resumption of oral intake.

Surgery—Nodal Metastasis

The surgical treatment of known nodal disease is generally via radical neck dissection, possibly with preservation of the spinal accessory nerve (modified radical neck dissection). Such surgery entails the removal of all major nodal groups in the cervical region, obligating coincident removal of the internal jugular vein, sternocleidomastoid muscle, and cervical sensory nerves. Other forms of less radical neck dissection are occasionally appropriate, including the supraomohyoid dissection (generally only for contralateral prophylaxis or ipsilateral staging) or functional neck dissection (for treatment of a clinically positive contralateral neck with preservation of that internal jugular vein). The so-called "anterior" neck dissection would have little applicability in oral cavity cancer treatment due to the high risk of submandibular triangle metastasis. Treatment of clinically uninvolved nodal areas is usually by radiation. However, the requisites of primary site resection and/or reconstruction may greatly facilitate or even require the coincident carrying out of neck dissection surgery. For example, if a pectoralis flap will be needed to reconstruct a major soft tissue or jaw defect, ipsilateral modified radical neck dissection (MRND) will be carried out, even in the pretreatment absence of overt nodal disease.

Radiation

Radiation, if elected for primary site treatment, can be delivered by external beam technique, interstitial implantation (brachytherapy), or by combined external/implant methods. Treatment of nodal disease, either occult or evident, is incorporated into the plan. Generally a minimum of 6000 to 7000 rads must be delivered to ensure the 80 to 85 per cent cure rate of T_1 to T_2 oral cavity/oropharyngeal lesions. Adjuvant treatment of a previously excised primary site or nodal disease prophylaxis requires 4500 to 5500 rads. Areas within the field of a primary lesion being treated for cure by radiation alone will get more. Areas of known nodal disease will often be treated with postradiation neck dissection. If this is not planned, neck dosages will have to be higher, at least 6000 rads, with a resultant increase in side effects. The spinal cord must be blocked out of the treatment field after 4500 to 5000 rads. In general, nodal prophylaxis by radiation should at least be considered for all but the smallest oral cavity lesions and for most oropharyngeal lesions. A substantial boost of radiation dosage to the primary site can be delivered without additional exposure of uninvolved external structures via the interstitial implant of radioactive material directly into the tumor. This procedure can be performed at the same sitting as neck dissection. Some radiation centers, such as the University of Florida, are well-known and adept proponents of interstitial technique and recognize its superiority over exclusively external radiation administration.[43-45] Others (Massachusetts General Hospital) favor the use of an external or internal "cone-down" boosting to augment the dosage to a disease site at unusual risk or in need of a higher dosage of treatment (usually the primary site).[46] Twice-daily treatment schemata are also becoming popular for certain areas (such as the tongue base), where improved control of advanced tumors without the morbidity of surgery is particularly desirable.[47, 48]

Combined Therapy

Combined therapy is generally the rule for oral cavity/oropharyngeal lesions in the following circumstances:

Large Primary of OC/OP:
- surgery first on primary ± neck
- with clinically negative neck, radiation second, to neck + primary

Small Primary of OC/OP:
- radiation first to primary + neck
- with clinically positive neck, surgery second on neck ± radiation implant of primary

Major Primary + Metastatic Neck Disease:
- surgery + radiation, w/radiation first if resectability in question;

OR
- chemotherapy + surgery + radiation

Recurrent Disease, Primary +/or Neck Disease:
- \> surgery *or* radiation, for "salvage" of either location after previous failure with other modality, unless palliative only, +/or chemotherapy.

OUTCOME

As with most sites in the head and neck, early, i.e., T_1 and T_2 disease of the oral cavity and T_1 disease of the oropharynx, without nodal involvement, have a reasonably good chance for cure. Second primary cancers are a problem in oral cavity malignancy. The addition of either nodal disease (especially N_2 or N_3), an advanced primary, or a recurrence after previous treatment represents a significant determinant in decreasing survival and incorporates a substantial (roughly 20 per cent) risk of distant (usually pulmonary) metastasis. Fewer than one-third of patients who fail single modality treatment are salvaged. Overall survival (5 years) for oral cavity tumors is in the 40 to 50 per cent range, while oropharyngeal lesions fare more poorly, at about 20 to 35 per cent. The base of tongue, pharyngeal walls, and any tumor involving bone are particularly deadly. The treatment of advanced tumors in either site leaves survivors with major, possibly in and of itself, life-threatening morbidity.

Floor of Mouth

In series for which surgery was the primary approach, with radiation for salvage or adjuvant treatment, Crissman[1] and Shaha[2] have demonstrated quite similar results, citing 5-year cure and 2-year survival, respectively: stage I—91 per cent, 88 per cent; stage II—73 per cent, 80 per cent; stage III—

60 per cent, 66 per cent; stage IV—33 per cent, 32 per cent. Within the stage III groups there is generally a prognostic distinction between the T_1, N_1 patients (more favorable) and those with more advanced primary disease. A substantial detriment is conferred by adenopathy greater than N_1, having an already poor outcome. In a primarily radiation-treated series, Million's group[45] reports local control of the floor of mouth site, at 2-years minimum, as follows: T_1—88 per cent; T_2—94 per cent; T_3—68 per cent. T_4s were not considered candidates for primary radiation treatment. Eight of 15 patients with recurrence after XRT were salvaged by surgery. These reports are a good example of the difficulty inherent in comparing various treatment data, exhibiting a range of statistical and therapy techniques. There is a seeming trend for some series to report on the disease-free interval or survival, determinate or otherwise, while other reports examine local control, independent of distant and sometimes regional metastasis or intercurrent morbidity.

Mobile Tongue

For anterior tongue cancer, as reported by Leipzig[34] and Marks,[49] respectively, the following cure rate by stage is noted: stage I—67 per cent, 88 per cent; stage II—48 per cent, 59 per cent; stages II, IV—33 per cent, 56 per cent. The better figures of Marks are compiled after a two-year follow-up, while those of Leipzig entail a minimum of three years and include a number of salvage attempts. The disparity is in keeping with observations that recurrence plateaus are not achieved for three years in many head and neck sites.

Base of Tongue

In a series treated with preoperative radiation and aggressive surgery, Thawley[19] reported survival at 5 years: stages I, II—75 per cent; stage III—54 per cent; stage IV—35 per cent. Twenty per cent of the stages III and IV patients got distant metastatic disease, with which they were presumably alive at the time of analysis. Parsons'[47] report described 5-year determinate survival for base of tongue carcinoma treated by primary radiation techniques, external and interstitial, with surgery reserved for radiation failure. For stages I, II, III, and IV, respectively, survivals were 100 per cent, 100 per cent, 86 per cent, and 24 per cent. Patients with T_1 to T_3, N_{2A} to N_{3A} disease were striated as more favorable, whereas those with T_4 and/or N_{3B} disease were unfavorable, with a 40 per cent and 10 per cent actuarial survival, respectively. Combined therapy is most often endorsed for advanced stage tongue carcinoma, whether anterior or base. While local control is improved, a survival superiority is not clearly demonstrated. At least for the base of tongue, wherein the surgical morbidity of treatment can be extreme, the argument for primary radiation, with surgical salvage for recurrence, can be advanced from a quality-of-life perspective.[44]

Callery,[4] in a multifactorial evaluation of treatment trends for tongue cancer at the Memorial Sloan-Kettering Hospital, made some telling, though not surprising, observations. Site of lesion was a statistically significant determinate of 5-year cure for stages I and II disease (anterior—71 per cent; base—30 per cent), but not for stages III and IV disease. While advanced stage anterior tongue lesions did fare better (31 per cent versus 16 per cent) than those of the tongue base, the difference was not statistically significant. The presence of nodal disease, regardless of primary site or overall patient stage, was also a cure determinant (30 per cent if N[+]; 56 per cent if N[−]). While combined treatment with surgery and radiation did bring about an improved cure rate for both sites, this difference was not statistically significant when compared with surgical treatment alone. A trend toward decreasing radicality of surgery was noted.

FOLLOW-UP

Close post-treatment follow-up of the head and neck cancer patient is important for many more reasons than the risk of recurrence. Aside from the risk of second primary neoplasms previously alluded to, there are multiple potential treatment sequelae that can have ongoing deleterious effects. Cure of the cancer by no means guarantees the future health and stability, physical or emotional, of the patient.

From a practical standpoint, it is unusual for an aggressively treated patient rendered disease-free (no evidence of disease [NED]) to develop a detectable recurrence during the first six months of follow-up surveillance. These months are generally devoted to the rehabilitation and recovery of the patient and determining a new "status quo," from which future departures must be investigated and explained. Follow-up with complete head and neck examination is usually monthly for the first year, bimonthly for the second year, subsequently lengthened by one-month increments each year until five years, at which point biannual examination is appropriate. Periodic chest x-rays are obtained twice yearly for the first three years and as otherwise indicated, then yearly. Periodic blood work, including thyroid function testing, liver functions, hematologic profile, and nutritional parameters where indicated, is also indicated. Education and self-confidence are vital goals during the early post-treatment years in order for the patient to become comfortable assessing and dealing with future symptoms, identifying those that are significant, and not getting overly distraught at those that are not.

Radiation xerostomia, skin change, and taste aberration are permanent and render the patient extra-sensitive to physical irritation in the respective regions so affected. Sensitivity to dry air, spicy foodstuffs, and further sun damage is noted. More insidious may be the development of dental infectious complications, with the attendent risk of jaw necrosis. Poor healing of seemingly innocuous injury to mucosa or skin is seen, for instance, due to an ill-fitting denture or insect bite. The effects of surgery are often mechanical, but can have more removed implications. While there may be ostensibly stable elements of dysarthria and dysphagia in a patient who has undergone oropharyngeal resection, subtle aspiration and/or increasing patient frustration with the demands of providing adequate nutrition may eventuate in chronic pulmonary debility or systemic inanition, with multiple health implications. The problem will be compounded in the infrequent presence of even minor post-tracheotomy sequelae, such as the loss of laryngeal elevation or laryngotracheal stenosis. Postsurgical scar contracture can evolve over a protracted period, which leads to progressive mechanical stresses or limitations that progress after an initial period of improvement. Shoulder dysfunction after radical neck dissection can be progressive, causing a deterioration in a patient's employability, recreational activities, appearance, or pain that results in both physical and psychologic consequences. Often this is seen after an apparent initial period of adjustment, through physical rehabilitation or postural adaptation. Likewise the effects of voice loss, even if rehabilitated, can progressively wear away at a patient's self-confidence. The threat of suicide after laryngectomy is very real. Post-treatment depression after any sequence of therapy is nearly universal and can become manifested in a variety of ways. Delayed airway obstruction can occur not only overtly, or precipitated by upper respiratory infection or manipulation (e.g., by endotracheal intubation), but also more subtly. An occasional patient, probably more than is realized, will develop manifestations of obstructive sleep apnea following the surgical and/or radiotherapeutic modification of the upper aerodigestive tract.[50, 51] Whether through conflict with a spouse because of loud snoring, degraded employment performance or physical inactivity due to excessive daytime somnolence, or major hypoxic insult, a definite link to previous head and neck cancer treatment may exist.

Another area of ongoing concern in the follow-up period is the continued comorbidity of many of the patients who are susceptible to head and neck cancer in the first place. Many patients do *not* stop smoking or using alcohol after treatment, compounding treatment sequelae as well as perpetuating liver, vascular, and pulmonary disease. Dependency on narcotics, sleeping medication, tranquilizers, alcohol, or recreational drugs is a risk often difficult to detect. Good communication among a patient's family and treating physicians is crucial.

Recurrences, particularly local or regional recurrences in areas of prior treatment, can be difficult to identify. A high index of suspicion is necessary, tempered by the feasibility of diagnostic biopsy and options for further treatment. When necessary, confirmatory biopsy by needle or tissue sampling is performed, often under general anesthesia. In the event of a recurrence of second primary lesion, complete restaging is essential before formulating a treatment plan or a determination of incurability. The second time around, patients are usually sicker, the options fewer, and morbidity considerably higher. Distant metastasis is most often incidentally identified on routine chest x-ray. Occasionally a new pain will prompt the bone scan/x-ray determination of bony metastasis. Neurologic symptoms or hepatic deterioration are rare but possible indications of metastatic involvement.

Finally, the occurrence of head and neck cancer does not confer immunity on an individual to other medical diseases, including malignancy. Other sources of metastatic disease should be considered, for example, bowel symptoms attended to, breast self-examinations continued, and so forth. Many successfully treated head and neck cancer patients come to view the head and neck team, and often the surgeon alone, as their primary medical manager. If this is so, a low threshold for obtaining consultative help is mandatory. Better still is the maintenance of the patient's own medical physician in an active role.

In few other fields of oncology must so many variables be considered in formulating a treatment recommendation than in head and neck cancer, particularly for advanced disease. At all sites of the disease, functional, cosmetic, and social issues are to be respected. The medical status of the patient, and location, stage, and natural history of the disease are integral. A multidisciplinary approach is the norm. Patient education is measured not as a function of the time spent talking with him or her or the number of consultants to whom he or she is exposed, but rather in achieving a true perspective in terms with which the patient can identify. Patient participation in healthcare decisions is expected. Decisions concerning the quantity and quality of future life must be accorded the patient, particularly when the most effective treatment may also be the most threatening to one's physical and psychologic integrity.

A very important early determination, following complete and accurate staging, is whether or not the patient's disease is curable to a meaningful extent, or worthy only of a palliative approach. The way in which this information is presented to the patient can be crucial and is always difficult. Preserving hope while at the same time giving a realistic appraisal requires a delicate, personal balance as well as some familiarity with the patient through prior contact or communication with other clinicians involved.

REFERENCES

1. Crissman, J.D., Gluckman, J., Whiteley, J., and Quenelle, D.: Squamous-cell carcinoma of the floor of the mouth. Head Neck Surg. *3:*2–7, 1980.
2. Shaha, A.R., Spiro, R.H., Shah, J.P., and Strong, E.W.: Squamous carcinoma of the floor of mouth. Am. J. Surg. *148:*455–459, 1984.
3. MacComb, W.S., Fletcher, G.H., and Healey, J.E. Jr.: Intra-oral cavity. *In* MacComb, W.S., and Fletcher, G.H. (Eds.): Cancer of the Head and Neck. Baltimore, Williams & Wilkins, 1967, pp. 89–151.
4. Callery, C.D., Spiro, R.H., and Strong, E.W.: Changing trends in the management of squamous carcinoma of the tongue. Am. J. Surg. *148:*449–454, 1984.
5. Wey, P.D., Lotz, M.J., and Triedman, L.J.: Oral cancer in women nonusers of tobacco and alcohol. Cancer *60:*1644–1650, 1987.
6. Son, Y.H., and Kapp, D.S.: Oral cavity and oropharyngeal cancer in a younger population. *55:*441–444, 1985.
7. Cusumano, R.J., and Persky, M.S.: Squamous cell carcinoma of the oral cavity and oropharynx in young adults. Head Neck Surg. *10:*229–234, 1988.
8. Beahrs, O.H., Henson, D.E., Hutter, R.V.P., and Myers, M.H. (Eds.): Manual for Staging of Cancer, 3rd edition. Philadelphia, J.B. Lippincott, 1988.
9. Goldblatt, L.L., and Ellis, G.L.: Salivary gland tumors of the tongue. Cancer *60:*74–81, 1987.
10. DeVries, E.J., Johnson, J.T., Myers, E.N., et al.: Base of tongue salivary gland tumors. Head Neck Surg. *9:*329–331, 1987.
11. Kessler, D.J., Mickel, R.A., and Calcaterra, T.C.: Malignant salivary gland tumors of the base of the tongue. Arch. Otolaryngol. *111:*664–666, 1985.
12. Medina, J.E., Dichtel, W., and Luna, M.A.: Verrucous-squamous carcinomas of the oral cavity. Arch. Otolaryngol. *110:*437–440, 1984.
13. Fierstein, J.T., and Thawley, S.E.: Lymphoma of the head and neck. Laryngoscope *88:*582–593, 1978.
14. Banfi, A., Bonnadonna, G., Basso Ricci, S., et al.: Malignant lymphomas of Waldeyer's ring: Natural history and survival after radiotherapy. Br. Med. J. *600:*140–152, 1972.
15. Trodahl, J.N., and Sprague, W.G.: Benign and malignant melanocytic lesions of the oral mucosa. An analysis of 135 cases. Cancer *25:*812–823, 1970.
16. Rapini, R.P., Golitz, L.E., Greer, R.O. Jr., et al.: Primary malignant melanoma of the oral cavity. Cancer *55:*1543–1551, 1985.
17. Gilbert, E.H., Goffinet, D.R., and Bagshaw, M.A.: Carcinoma of the oral tongue and floor of mouth: Fifteen years experience with linear accelerator therapy. Cancer *35:*1517–1524, 1975.
18. Shibuya, H., Hisamitsu, S., Shioiri, S., et al.: Multiple primary cancer risk in patients with squamous cell carcinoma of the oral cavity. Cancer *60:*3083–3086, 1987.
19. Thawley, S.E., Simpson, J.R., Marks, J.E., et al.: Preoperative irradiation and surgery for carcinoma of the base of the tongue. Ann. Otol. Rhinol. Laryngol. *92:*485–490, 1983.

20. Patterson, H.C., Dobie, R.A., and Cummings, C.W.: Treatment of the clinically negative neck in floor of mouth carcinoma. Laryngoscope 94:820–824, 1984.
21. Lindberg, R.D.: Distribution of cervical lymph node metastasis from squamous cell carcinoma of the upper respiratory and digestive tracts. Cancer 29:1446–1450, 1972.
22. Mendelson, B.C., Woods, J.E., and Beahrs, O.H.: Neck dissection in the treatment of carcinoma of the anterior two-thirds of the tongue. Surg. Gynecol. Obstet. 143:75–80, 1976.
23. Spiro, R.H., and Strong, E.W.: Epidermoid cancer of the mobile tongue. Treatment by partial glossectomy alone. Am. J. Surg. 122:707–710, 1971.
24. Fletcher, G.H.: Elective irradiation of subclinical disease in cancers of the head and neck. Cancer 29:1450–1454, 1972.
25. Million, R.R.: Elective neck irradiation for $T_x N_0$ squamous carcinoma of the oral tongue and floor of mouth. Cancer 34:149–155, 1974.
26. DiTroia, J.F.: Nodal metastasis and prognosis in carcinoma of the oral cavity. Otolaryngol. Clin. North Am. 5:333–342, 1972.
27. Southwick, H.W., Slaughter, D.P., and Trevino, E.T.: Elective neck dissection for intra-oral cancer. Arch. Surg. 80:905–910, 1960.
28. Simons, J.N., Masson, J.K., and Beahrs, O.H.: Results of radical treatment for intra-oral cancer. Am. J. Surg. 106:819–825, 1963.
29. Jesse, R.H., Barkley, H.T. Jr., Lindberg, R.D., et al.: Cancer of the oral cavity: Is elective neck dissection beneficial? Am. J. Surg. 120:505–508, 1970.
30. Teichgraeber, J.F., and Clairmont, A.A.: The incidence of occult metastases for cancer of the oral tongue and floor of the mouth: Treatment rationale. Head Neck Surg. 7:15–21, 1984.
31. Cunningham, M.J., Johnson, J.T., Myers, E.N., et al.: Cervical lymph node metastasis after local excision of early squamous cell carcinoma of the oral cavity. Am. J. Surg. 152:361–366, 1986.
32. Marchetta, F.C., Sako, K., and Murphy, J.B.: The periosteum of the mandible and intraoral carcinoma. Am. J. Surg. 122:711–713, 1971.
33. Weisman, R.A., and Kimmelman, C.P.: Bone scanning in the assessment of mandibular invasion by oral cavity carcinomas. Laryngoscope 92:1–4, 1982.
34. Leipzig, B., Cummings, C.W., Chung, C.T., et al.: Carcinoma of the anterior tongue. Ann. Otol. Rhinol. Laryngol. 91:94–97, 1982.
35. Close, L.G., Burns, D.K., Reisch, J., and Schaefer, S.D.: Microvascular invasion in cancer of the oral cavity and oropharynx. Arch. Otolaryngol. Head Neck Surg. 113:1191–1195, 1987.
36. Eskinazi, D.P., Perna, J.J., and Mihail, R.: Mononuclear cell subsets in patients with oral cancer. Cancer 60:376–381, 1987.
37. Moore, C., Flynn, M.B., and Greenberg, R.A.: Evaluation of size in prognosis of oral cancer. Cancer 58:158–162, 1986.
38. Yamamoto, E., Kohama, G-I, Sunakawa, H., et al.: Mode of invasion, bleomycin sensitivity, and clinical course in squamous cell carcinoma of the oral cavity. Cancer 51:2175–2180, 1983.
39. Donegan, J.O., Gluckman, J.L., and Crissman, J.D.: The role of suprahyoid neck dissection in the management of cancer of the tongue and floor of mouth. Head Neck Surg. 4:209–212, 1982.
40. Bradfield, J.S., and Scruggs, R.P.: Carcinoma of the mobile tongue: Incidence of cervical metastases in early lesions related to method of primary treatment. Laryngoscope 93:1332–1336, 1983.
41. Ballantyne, A.J.: Current controversies in the management of cancer of the tongue and floor of mouth. In Kogan, A.R., and Miles, J.W. (Eds.): Head and Neck Oncology: Controversies in Cancer Management. Boston, G.K. Hall & Co., 1981, pp. 87–97.
42. Leipzig, B., and Hokanson, J.A.: Treatment of cervical lymph nodes in carcinoma of the tongue. Head Neck Surg. 5:3–9, 1982.
43. Mendenhall, W.M., VanCise, W.S., Bova, F.J., and Million, R.R.: Analysis of time-dose factors in squamous cell carcinoma of the tongue and floor of mouth treated with radiation therapy alone. Int. J. Radiat. Oncol. Biol. Phys. 7:1005–1011, 1981.
44. Riley, R.W., Fee, W.E. Jr., Goffinet, D., et al.: Squamous cell carcinoma of the base of the tongue. Otolaryngol. Head Neck Surg. 91:143–150, 1983.
45. Million, R.R., Cassisi, N.J., and Wittes, R.E.: Cancer in the head and neck. In DeVita, V.T., Hellman, S., and Rosenberg, S.A. (Eds.): Cancer: Principles and Practice of Oncology. Philadelphia, J.B. Lippincott, 1982, pp. 301–395.
46. Wang, C.C.: Radiotherapeutic management and results of T_1N_0, T_2N_0 carcinoma of the oral tongue: Evaluation of boost techniques. Int. J. Radiat. Oncol. Biol. Phys. 17:287–291, 1989.
47. Parsons, J.T., Cassisi, N.J., and Million, R.R.: Results of twice-a-day irradiation of squamous cell carcinomas of the head and neck. Int. J. Radiat. Oncol. Biol. Phys. 10:2041–2051, 1984.

48. Wang, C.C., Blitzer, P.H., and Suit, H.D.: Twice-a-day radiation therapy for cancer of the head and neck. Cancer 55:2100–2104, 1985.
49. Marks, J.E., Lee, F., Freeman, R.B., et al.: Carcinoma of the oral tongue: A study of patient selection and treatment results. Laryngoscope 91:1548–1559, 1981.
50. Panje, W.R., and Homes, D.K.: Mandibulectomy without reconstruction can cause sleep apnea. Laryngoscope 94:1591–1594, 1984.
51. Herlihy, J.P., Whitlock, W.L., Dietrich, R.A., and Shaw, T.: Sleep apnea syndrome after irradiation of the neck. Arch. Otolaryngol. Head Neck Surg. 115:1467–1469, 1989.

LARYNX
by Charles M. Norris, Jr., M.D.

HISTOLOGY

Excluding the skin, laryngeal cancer is the most common malignancy in the adult upper aerodigestive tract. With rare exception, squamous cell (epidermoid) carcinoma, arising from a mucosal surface, is the predominant histology. As in the oral cavity, carcinoma *in situ* may precede, coexist with, or be confused with invasive lesions. Multiple other histologies have been encountered,[1] some occasionally, some rarely, and at times with profound treatment implications.

Variant epidermoid cancers in the larynx include verrucous carcinoma, pseudosarcoma, carcinosarcoma, and others. Verrucous carcinoma[2,3] is a lesion for which the histologic appearance alone does not establish the diagnosis. The gross appearance of a discrete, exophytic lesion, with multiple horn-like projections, coupled with a very well-differentiated microscopic appearance, is typical. A T_1 or T_2 presentation is the rule, and nodal spread is rare. However, the distinction of verrucous carcinoma is significant, as radiation treatment may not be as efficacious as with conventional squamous cell carcinoma, thereby increasing the importance of surgery. Pseudosarcoma (carcinosarcoma, sarcomatoid carcinoma, spindle cell carcinoma, and others)[4,5] represents a stromal spindle cell reaction to a squamous cell carcinoma that mimics a true sarcoma.

Laryngeal melanoma is extremely rare (fewer than 3 cases in 35 years at Memorial Hospital). The lesions tend to be supraglottic, with poor survival, but with fairly good local control.[6]

Neuroendocrine (carcinoid) lesions of the larynx are equally rare and likewise aggressive, with a tendency toward failure by distant metastasis and a requirement for surgical treatment of the primary site.[7-10]

True sarcomas are exceedingly rare.[11-17] Small cell (oat cell) carcinomas have been recognized with increasing frequency[18-20] but remain unusual, as are malignancies arising from the minor salivary glands of the supraglottic region.[21-25] Lymphomas,[26-29] benign cartilage tumors, and other neoplastic conditions[30] have been reported as well.

Metastatic malignancy to the larynx has been reported from, in order of frequency, disseminated cutaneous melanoma, renal cell carcinoma, breast carcinomas, lung malignancies, prostate adenocarcinoma, gastrointestinal adenocarcinomas, and others. Submucosal involvement of the supraglottic larynx is typical.[31-33] Leukemic infiltration, likewise, has been noted. These entities are infrequently discovered prior to autopsy.

Anatomically, physiologically, and with regard to clinical pathogenesis, the larynx may be apportioned into three subdivisions: glottic, supraglottic, and subglottic, which are delineated within an outer framework of cartilaginous structures (thyroid, cricoid, epiglottis), muscles (intrinsic and extrinsic groups), and ligaments (cricothyroid and thyrohyoid). This laryngeal framework is intimately associated with the base of tongue, hypopharyngeal walls, cervical esophagus, and upper trachea, all of which may serve as areas of extension for infiltrative lesions. The study of horizontal and coronal laryngeal sections has greatly expanded the practical awareness of tumor spread mechanisms.[34-37]

Glottic

The glottic portion of the larynx includes the true vocal cords and anterior commissura (excluding the arytenoid region). The superior surface of the true vocal cords extends laterally to form the floor of the laryngeal ventricle, the lateral aspect of which divides the glottis from the supraglottic larynx. The undersurface of the true cords extends obliquely inferiorly (the conus elasticus) for 4 to 6 mm, demarcating the subglottis at its junction with the trachea. The glottic larynx primarily subserves the functions of phonation, airway protection during deglutition and coughing, and as an important pulmonary cleaning mechanism. The vocal cords close during deglutition to protect the airway from aspiration and open variably during respiration to transmit and regulate airflow. Symptoms of cancers in the glottic portion of the larynx occur early in their natural history, and hence the opportunity exists for earlier diagnosis. The true vocal cords are dynamic mucosa-lined muscles, but lymphatics are sparse, thereby accounting for the clinical rarity of associated nodal spread. In contradistinction to supraglottic or hypopharyngeal carcinoma, nodal metastasis in glottic cancer is clinically rare, occurs late, and usually occurs only with longstanding advanced local disease. The relative prognosis of glottic carcinoma is correspondingly better, both overall and stage for stage.

Locally, glottic cancers tend most often to extend either anteriorly or superiorly. The anatomic barrier against spread of anterior lesions into the thyroid cartilage is poor at the anterior commissura, and cartilage invasion can be very difficult to determine, whether endoscopically or via imaging techniques. Limitation of vocal cord mobility, due to deep muscle invasion and thyroid cartilage invasion, represents poor prognostic features with direct treatment implications. Glottic cancers tend to be moderately or well differentiated, enlarging slowly at first. There is virtually no barrier to the spread of lesions locally into the supraglottic portion, however, whereupon more rapid extension may occur. Submucosal spread in the paraglottic or pre-epiglottic fat planes can be difficult to detect. Other mechanisms of vocal cord fixation include cricoarytenoid joint invasion and recurrent laryngeal nerve involvement. Nodal metastasis is rare in lesions confined to glottic structures, even with vocalis muscle fixation. Larger lesions, usually with extension into the supraglottis, will spread to the ipsilateral jugular chain lymphatics. Likewise, true subglottic extension, or penetration through the anterior commissura, will increase the likelihood of metastasis to pretracheal and paratracheal nodes.

Supraglottic

The false vocal cords, arytenoid region and posterior commissura, epiglottis, and aryepiglottic folds make up the supraglottic portion of the larynx. The supraglottis borders superiorly with the oropharynx and posterolaterally with the hypopharynx (pyriform sinuses), into and from both of which malignancies can extend. Functioning as an air passage, as well as a divertor and sphincter to protect the airway, this part of the larynx is physiologically important. However, supraglottic malignancy is often silent, thereby generally presenting at a more advanced stage. There is a much higher likelihood of occult and palpable nodal metastasis in supraglottic lesions, as well as few barriers to extension of the primary tumor site. These features account for the worse prognosis observed as tumor location moves away from the true vocal cords. Glottic lesions that have spread to supraglottic structures begin to assume this worse biologic behavior. Supraglottic tumors may infiltrate in any direction, including into the glottis, pyriform sinus, tongue base, and pre-epiglottic space. Lymphatic spread is generally to the upper and mid-jugular chain nodes, with submandibular and posterior triangle involvement rare. Larger and midline invasive lesions risk a significant chance of contralateral nodal involvement, a consideration for treatment planning.

Subglottic

The subglottis is the mucosal lining of the airway below the true vocal cords and above the first tracheal ring, basically within the cricoid cartilage. Primary carcinomas are rare. Subglottic involvement is usually through submucosal extension of a glottic or supraglottic tumor. As an air conduit, symptoms from tumor involvement of this area include stridor and possibly hemoptysis. Because of its anatomic proximity to the tracheal walls and the cricopharyngeal region of the esophagus, subglottic malignancies entail a risk of esophageal involvement. Furthermore, a rich lymphatic network in this region drains into the paratracheal and superior mediastinal nodes, which place difficult demands on surgical treatment. True primary subglottic lesions are rarely very large, as they will attract attention from airway obstruction.

As with all cancers, pretreatment staging, correlated with subsequent findings, tumor behavior, and eventual outcome, is important.[38] In addition to the formulation of treatment guidelines, a staging system provides a means for comparison of clinically identifiable variables and subsequent histological confirmation.[39] A staging outline for laryngeal carcinoma is depicted in Table 2–4.

TABLE 2–4. STAGING OUTLINE—CANCER OF THE LARYNX (AJCC*)

Larynx
Glottic
- T_1 —Confined to true vocal cords; normal mobility; includes anterior or posterior commissura
- T_2 —Supraglottic or subglottic extension; normal or impaired mobility
- T_3 —Confined to larynx proper; cord fixation
- T_4 —Cartilage destruction and/or extension out of larynx

Supraglottic
- T_1 —Confined to site of origin; normal mobility
- T_2 —Extension to glottis or adjacent supraglottic site; normal or impaired mobility
- T_3 —Confined to larynx proper; cord fixation and/or extension into hypopharynx or pre-epiglottic space
- T_4 —Massive tumor; cartilage destruction and/or extension out of larynx

Subglottic
- T_1 —Confined to subglottic region
- T_2 —Glottic extension; normal or impaired mobility
- T_3 —Confined to larynx proper; cord fixation
- T_4 —Massive tumor; cartilage destruction and/or extension out of larynx

Nodal Metastasis
- N_X —Nodes cannot be assessed
- N_0 —No clinically positive nodes
- N_1 —Single, clinically positive, ipsilateral node; ≤ 3 cm
- N_{2A} —Single, clinically positive, ipsilateral node; 3 cm $\geq$ 6 cm
- N_{2B} —Multiple, clinically positive, ipsilateral nodes; ≤ 6 cm
- N_{2C} —Single or multiple, clinically positive, bilateral or contralateral nodes; any/all ≤ 6 cm
- N_3 —Any clinically positive node; > 6 cm

Distant Metastasis
- M_X —Not assessed
- M_0 —No distant metastases present
  - Specify site: PUL—pulmonary
  - OSS—osseous
  - BRA—brain
  - LYM—lymph nodes (noncervical)
  - MAR—bone marrow
  - PLE—pleura
  - SKI—skin
  - OTH—other

Stage Groupings
- Stage I —T_1 N_0 M_0
- Stage II —T_2 N_0 M_0
- Stage III —T_3 N_0 M_0
  - T_1, T_2, or T_3 N_1 M_0
- Stage IV —T_4 N_0 or N_1 M_0
  - Any T N_2 or N_3 M_0
  - Any T Any N M_1

*American Joint Committee on Cancer.[40]

EPIDEMIOLOGY[41]

Squamous cell carcinoma of the larynx is the classic smoker's cancer of the head and neck that generally occurs after years of cigarette use. Its occurrence in nonsmokers is extremely unusual. Alcohol does not appear to be a significant independent or synergistic etiologic cofactor, in marked contrast to the situation in the oral cavity, hypopharynx, or esophagus. Males continue to predominate. While the incidence of lung cancer in women has increased substantially over the last several decades, only a small increase in the female population with laryngeal cancer has been observed.[42] Individuals who stop smoking would appear to have the same risk of tobacco-related cancer of the upper aerodigestive tract as ongoing smokers for approximately the first five years of abstention. At 10 years of abstention the risk in exsmokers will apparently approach that in individuals who had never smoked.[43] The possible risk associated with chronic gastroesophageal reflux has recently received a lot of attention.[44,45]

CLINICAL FEATURES

True vocal cord (glottic) carcinomas tend to cause hoarseness early in their course. Nevertheless, a voice change may still be obscured in a patient with longstanding hoarseness, productive cough, vocal abuse, and the like. Focal or referred pain (usually to the ear) and airway compromise reflect disease that has significantly progressed.

In supraglottic cancer, pain, either ill-defined or associated with swallowing (odynophagia), is more common, possibly associated with dysphagia, aspiration, halitosis (due to tumor surface infection or necrosis) or globus ("lump-in-throat") symptoms. The voice change in supraglottic lesions is not hoarseness (dysphonia), but rather a form of dysarthria, as though one were speaking with marbles caught in the throat. The term "hot potato voice" is sometimes used. Not uncommonly, the patient's perception of a (metastatic) mass in the neck will be the first inkling of a problem.

Subglottic symptoms are usually overshadowed by those of a primary site in the glottis or supraglottis from which tumor extension has occurred. Stridor may be present, possibly in the absence of easily identifiable subglottic pathology. An occasional patient will have been treated for wheezing, asthma, or a chronic obstructive pulmonary disease (COPD) exacerbation before the site of the lesion becomes apparent. The stridor of a subglottic mass will tend to be biphasic (inspiratory and expiratory), especially if the glottis is involved, not exclusively expiratory, as in the case of reactive airway disease. Airway obstruction due to supraglottic lesions, on the other hand, will be inspiratory and represent a generally far-advanced stage of disease.

DIAGNOSIS

Office inspection of the larynx had traditionally required a coaxial lighting source and visualization via angled mirrors. Flexible fiberoptic instrumentation now greatly facilitates examination by those not expert in indirect mirror technique. The overall perspective of view and limitations of either method suggest that they best be viewed as complementary rather than exclusive.

Aside from identification of the laryngeal lesion, an assessment of factors referable to its staging is advisable. Vocal cord motion, for example, is much better assessed in an awake, cooperative patient, prior to any formal biopsy, which may impair mobility due to edema. Changes in mobility may be subtle and vary in character, depending on whether they are caused by muscle invasion, bulk effect, or cricoarytenoid joint involvement. The precise location, extent, and areas of infiltration of the primary tumor are estimated, in part as may be suggested by exophytic or submucosal distortions of the known normal anatomy. Pre-epiglottic space or thyroid cartilage invasion is difficult to ascertain on physical examination, but may be suspected by epiglottic or vallecular distortion, by direct palpation of tumor extension into the neck, or by widening of the thyroid laminae (Schall sign).

Imaging studies, particularly in advanced laryngeal cancer, are important. With some important limitations, transverse CT scanning, when combined with other clinical parameters, has had considerable impact on staging accuracy.[46-49] Anteroposterior laryngeal tomography will occasionally give a better composite perspective of the vertical extent of disease than coronal CT reconstructions, but is used relatively rarely. The role and strengths of magnetic resonance image (MRI) scanning are still undergoing evolution and evaluation. Even on well-composed CT scans, early cartilage or pre-epiglottic space invasion can be difficult to identify. More advanced disease, however, is well depicted. Subglottic extension, or direct involvement of the cervical soft tissue, is generally quite clear-cut. In supraglottic primary tumors, tongue base, pre-epiglottic, or direct neck extension are sought out. Information about nodal metastatic disease may also be gleaned from a CT scan. Palpably occult disease, particularly in an obese patient, or involvement of vital structures by recognizable, semifixed adenopathy, may be suspected.

Lindberg's representation of nodal disease on presentation for supraglottic carcinoma[50] documents the 55 percentage rate of clinically apparent metastasis. Upper and middle deep jugular nodes predominate, and there is a fair incidence (16 per cent) of contralateral disease. An untreated N_0 neck will have a one in three[51] likelihood of developing subsequent nodal disease. Note that the staging system in use at the time of Lindberg's review is different from the most recent modification. Lesions confined to the true glottic structures have a very low incidence of associated adenopathy, either evident or occult. Even large, advanced T_3 and T_4 glottic lesions will only present with nodal mets in 20 to 30 per cent.[50] In spite of a tendency to drain into paratracheal and mediastinal lymphatics, toward which treatment must be directed, subglottic lesions do not usually present with clinically apparent metastasis (10 per cent).[52]

Endoscopy in laryngeal malignancy is mandatory. Imaging studies should be done prior to biopsy procedures, and may facilitate airway management in the presence of luminal tumor, lest over-instrumentation or intubation precipitate obstruction. Pulmonary function testing is needed if conservation surgery is contemplated. Chest x-ray is necessary to review any associated pulmonary functional disease, or identify a possible coexistent lung cancer. Direct laryngoscopic examination is often performed as well as bronchoscopy and esophagoscopy (so-called "triple endoscopy") in order to completely map the primary tumor as well as seek out possible second primary lesions.[53] Adequate tissue sampling should be confirmed by frozen section, which also may suggest an unusual histology, for which additional tissue or special histochemical handling may be indicated. Not all suspect lesions, of course, will prove to be malignant. Various degrees of hyperplasia, dysplasia, keratoses, papillomata, and even some infectious diseases (fungal, acid-fast) may mimic cancer on gross examination.

As in the oral cavity, the larynx is exposed to considerable functional trauma and environmental insult. Leukoplakia, keratoses, and various forms of dysplasia[54] are common, and may antedate the development of frank malignancy. Carcinoma *in situ* may exist either independently or in association with invasive carcinoma. The diagnosis of either can be deceptive. Careful follow-up of patients with suspicious findings or preliminary biopsy results is critical.[55] Any focal or generalized areas of mucosal change within the larynx of a smoker should prompt consideration for endoscopic investigation.

TREATMENT

To a certain extent, the treatment approach to laryngeal cancer can be segregated into that for "early" stage disease, with single modality therapy and generally good result, and that for "advanced" stage disease, more commonly by multimodality treatment with a poorer prognosis. Progress, as in any cancer field, entails the curing of more individuals by existing modality manipulation, or by decreasing the morbidity of equally effective treatment. Organ-sparing, usually of the primary disease site (the larynx), or major function maintenance (the voice), comprises a goal of induction chemotherapy in head and neck cancer.

As with other sites in the head and neck, and especially for advanced laryngeal cancer, therapeutic decisions must account for the patient's interests regarding effects on laryngeal function. While phonation is the most apparent concern, it is less important physiologically than airflow or pulmonary protection during deglutition. Furthermore, while alaryngeal speech can be learned or assisted through a variety of means, other functions are less able to be re-established following anatomic alteration by surgery. Chronic aspiration can be lethal in both short-term and long-term. These perspectives can be difficult to render to a patient faced with losing his or her voice. Preliminary consultation with a laryngectomee patient may be helpful, and should be considered prior to the rendering of a final treatment plan. Research and treatment techniques in laryngeal malignancy seek to achieve more result with less therapy or at least the same result with fewer side effects. Consequently, surgery that spares portions of the functional laryngeal anatomy ("conservation" laryngeal surgery) is a constantly refined, and requested, treatment modality.[56] Hyperfraction radiation and induction chemotherapy may also allow effective nonsurgical cure for advanced lesions. Patient selection is crucial but cannot be accomplished without accurate tumor staging or an awareness of tumor biology.

The rare primary subglottic carcinoma[57,58] is treated similarly to glottic lesions, though conservation surgery is not often feasible, and radiation is less effective. Generally total laryngectomy and an extended mediastinal radiation portal are required, with a poorer prognosis, stage for stage. Worse still is the outlook for a patient with a rare minor salivary gland malignancy of the subglottic larynx, the treatment of which is often aggressive and unsuccessful, though with a protracted course.[59]

The treatment of "early" laryngeal lesions,[60–62] generally T_1 and some T_2, in the absence of overt nodal disease (N_0), is generally successful and equally affected by either surgery or radiation alone. As a result, the choice is determined largely by the morbidity anticipated. In the glottic area, given the minimal likelihood of occult nodal disease, limited surgery on the primary lesion may be possible, provided that the multifunctional integrity of the larynx can be maintained. Radiation would then be reserved for recurrent disease or second primaries. Generally, however, vocal quality after limited-field radiation to the larynx, particularly for glottic lesions, is far superior to that which follows conservation surgery. Small glottic lesions confined to the tendinous part of the vocal cord can be excised with excellent functional preservation using endoscopic carbon dioxide laser technique.[63–65] This approach might also be taken with small supraglottic cancers clearly confined to the upper half of the epiglottis (epiglottidectomy). Larger (still T_1 or T_2) glottic lesions, those involving the anterior commissure, or lesions with any trace of limited cord mobility would be better treated with either an external surgical approach, i.e., partial laryngectomy, or radiation. At least 6000 rads is considered necessary, this dosage generally well tolerated since the treatment field is so small, being confined to the glottic larynx itself.

The treatment of glottic laryngeal cancer is only rarely determined by cervical nodal considerations. Clinically evident nodal metastases in association with early laryngeal lesions would be handled with neck dissection after radiation for primary site cure. In this instance, the radiation portal would include all the lymphatics bilaterally at risk.[66]

More advanced glottic lesions could require the addition of a conservation surgical procedure, if anatomically feasible and provided the patient is otherwise an acceptable candidate for the postoperative recovery of airway preservation and swallowing functions, as well as voice production.

Partial laryngectomy procedures[56, 67–76] have been developed in virtually all permutations:

Supraglottic laryngectomy (horizontal partial)[72, 73]

Vocal cordectomy[69, 70]

Anterior commissure resection[69]

Vertical partial laryngectomy, frontolateral and extended frontolateral partial laryngectomy[70, 71, 74]

Near-total laryngectomy[75, 76]

The importance of accurate, pretreatment clinical staging is emphasized here particularly, as an underestimate of local disease extension risks inappropriate treatment. If a patient has been prepared for partial laryngectomy and intra-operative findings mandate more extensive surgery, the patient should have given consent for a contingency total laryngectomy, or else the surgeon will end up doing less than optimal surgery where other modalities may have sufficed. Patient selection not only requires physiologic evaluation, but also a frank and informative discussion between physician and patient. By contrast, clinical overstaging is relatively unlikely to occur.

What one must retain sight of is that the surgical care of a patient and cancer involves much more than the sophisticated, technically challenging removal and reconstruction of an important piece of the human anatomy. Rehabilitation, with a return to normalcy or near-normalcy, is equally, if not more, important. To a large extent, even sophisticated surgery is a mere technical exercise, wherein the art resides in determining when and on whom it should be performed, and in handling the unexpected.

Early supraglottic lesions[66, 77–81] are anatomically amenable to conservative surgical techniques, but the likelihood of occult local extension and/or nodal metastasis requires treatment encompassing both the primary site and neck. This will often be by external radiation to both, including at least 6600 rads to the primary. Supraglottic laryngectomy alone is less commonly performed at this time. More often, this procedure would be envisioned for a more extensive T_2 lesion, in which case planned postoperative radiotherapy would be appropriate. Neck dissection would be incorporated in the presence of nodal disease. Patients who are candidates for such surgery also require unusually good pulmonary function, as they must learn to swallow in the absence of most of their protective airway reflexes. Given advances in the efficacy of radiation therapy and the enlightenment of patient expectations, the role for partial laryngectomy in a potentially radiocurable lesion is currently defined ever more narrowly.

Advanced (T_3 or T_4)[82, 83] lesions, of either the glottic or supraglottic larynx generally, require total laryngectomy and postoperative x-ray therapy to both the neck and larynx fields. The higher likelihood of nodal disease would require associated neck dissection in conjunction with laryngectomy, whether metastases were recognized clinically or not. An exception might be the case of a T_3 glottic lesion, especially with bilateral endolaryngeal involvement, with negative findings at exploration for the laryngectomy. Very occasional, highly selected patients have been successfully treated with conservation surgery and postoperative radiation for T_3 glottic tumors.[84–86] Positive nodal metastases, whether identified preoperatively or intraoperatively, require neck dissection. The addition of cervical nodal radiation is advised for suspect, but unconfirmed, nodal mets (based on primary site location and extent), whether surgery is otherwise planned or not.

Present clinical research in laryngeal cancer centers on nonsurgical therapy for T_3 lesions. Hyperfractionation radiotherapy, in some hands,[87, 88] would appear to offer a reasonable cure potential, but remains controversial, as the associated morbidity does not always differ substantially from surgery, and may even be worse. Induction chemotherapy resulting in a confirmed histologic complete response and followed by definitive radiation to the larynx and neck also offers reasonable larynx-sparing therapy.[89–92] This combination treatment formula is presently undergoing intensive prospective clinical evaluation.[90] T_4 lesions at either glottic or supraglottic sites have a limited chance for cure. The optimum opportunity requires at least radical surgery (total laryngectomy and neck dissection) and postoperative radiation. As in other sites, the contributory role of cytoreductive chemotherapy, as either induction or adjuvant treatment, remains to be legitimized.

Traditionally, the treatment of recurrent laryngeal disease after radiation failure has required total laryngectomy, usually with ipsilateral neck dissection. In the supraglottic larynx, there is little argument. However, the role of partial laryngectomy after radiation failure in glottic carcinoma has become controversial.[93–95] In selected patients with unilateral endolaryngeal involvement, conservation surgery may be possible. The drawbacks include a considerable difficulty with determination of the extent of disease preoperatively. Even intraoperative evaluation by gross inspection and frozen section can be misleading. Other pitfalls include complications with post-radiation healing and persistent edema or fibrosis, which can compromise what laryngeal function has been preserved.

OUTCOME

To simplify somewhat, the fate of a patient with glottic carcinoma is most significantly affected by the presence of vocal cord fixation, which almost halves the cure rate of 95 per cent achievable in T_1, and 80 to 85 per cent achievable in T_2 glottic lesions. The addition of clinically perceptible nodal metastases has the same effect. Advanced (T_3 or T_4) lesions with nodal mets entail a less than 30 per cent five-year survival rate. Supraglottic laryngeal cancer is generally more lethal, stage for stage, for both early and more advanced lesions, with or without positive adenopathy. Survival rates are generally 10 to 25 per cent worse than the corresponding glottic lesion. The prognosis in primary subglottic cancer is generally poor.

REFERENCES

1. Ferlito, A.: Histologic classification of larynx and hypopharyngeal cancers and their clinical implications. Pathologic aspects of 2,052 malignant neoplasms diagnosed at the ORL Department of Padua University from 1966 to 1976. Acta Otolaryngol. [suppl.] (Stockh) *342*:1–88, 1976.
2. Lundgren, J.A.V., Van Nostrand, P., Harwood, A.R., et al.: Verrucous carcinoma (Ackerman's tumor) of the larynx: Diagnostic and therapeutic considerations. Head Neck Surg. *9*:19–26, 1986.
3. Ferlito, A.: Diagnosis and treatment of verrucous squamous cell carcinoma: A critical review. Ann. Otol. Rhinol. Laryngol. *94*:575–579, 1985.
4. Giordano, A.M., Ewing, S., Adams, G., and Maisel, R.: Laryngeal pseudosarcoma. Laryngoscope *93*:735–740, 1983.
5. Lambert, P.R., Ward, P.H., and Berci, G.: Pseudosarcoma of the larynx. Arch. Otolaryngol. *106*:700–708, 1980.
6. Reuter, V.E., and Woodruff, J.M.: Melanoma of the larynx. Laryngoscope *94*:389–393, 1986.
7. Woodruff, J.M., Shah, J.P., Huvos, A.G., et al.: Neuroendocrine carcinomas of the larynx. Am. J. Surg. Pathol. *9*:771–790, 1985.
8. Stanley, R.J., Scheithauer, B.W., Weiland, L.H., and Neel, H.B., III.: Neural and neuroendocrine tumors of the larynx. Ann. Otol. Rhinol. Laryngol. *96*:630–638, 1987.
9. Wenig, B.M., Hyams, V.J., and Heffner, D.K.: Moderately differentiated neuroendocrine carcinoma of the larynx. A clinicopathologic study of 54 cases. Cancer *62*:2658–2676, 1988.
10. Baugh, R.F., Wolf, G.T., Lloyd, R.V., et al.: Carcinoid (neuroendocrine carcinoma) of the larynx. Ann. Otol. Rhinol. Laryngol. *96*:315–321, 1987.
11. Gorenstein, A., Neel, H.B., III, Weiland, L.H., and Devine, K.D.: Sarcomas of the larynx. Arch. Otolaryngol. *106*:8–12, 1980.
12. Dahm, L.J., Schaeffer, S.D., Carder, H.M., and Vellios, F.: Osteosarcoma of the soft tissue of the larynx. Cancer *42*:2343–2351, 1978.
13. Ferlito, A., Nicolai, P., and Caruso, G.: Angiosarcoma of the larynx. Ann. Otol. Rhinol. Laryngol. *94*:93–95, 1985.
14. Meis, J.M., Mackay, B., and Goepfert, H.: Liposarcoma of the larynx. Arch. Otolaryngol. Head Neck Surg. *112*:1289–1292, 1986.
15. Lavertu, P., and Tucker, H.M.: Chondrosarcoma of the larynx. Ann. Otol. Rhinol. Laryngol. *93*:452–456, 1984.
16. Leonetti, J.P., Collins, S.L., Jablokow, V., and Lewy, R.: Laryngeal chondrosarcoma as a late-appearing cause of "idiopathic" vocal cord paralysis. Otolaryngol. Head Neck Surg. *97*:391–395, 1987.
17. Dodd-o, J.M., Wieneke, K.F., and Rosman, P.M.: Laryngeal rhabdomyosarcoma. Cancer *59*:1012–1018, 1987.
18. Posner, M.R., Weichselbaum, R.R., Carrol, E., et al.: Small cell carcinomas of the larynx: Results of combined modality treatments. Laryngoscope *93*:946–948, 1983.
19. Ferlito, A.: Diagnosis and treatment of small cell carcinoma of the larynx: A critical review. Ann. Otol. Rhinol. Laryngol. *95*:590–600, 1986.
20. Baugh, R.F., Wolf, G.T., Beals, T.F., et al.: Small cell carcinoma of the larynx: Results of therapy. Laryngoscope *96*:1283–1290, 1986.
21. Batsakis, J.G., Rice, D.H., and Solomon, A.R.: The pathology of head and neck tumors:

Squamous and mucous-gland carcinomas of the nasal cavity, paranasal sinuses, and larynx. Head Neck Surg. 2:497–508, 1980.
22. Spiro, R.H., Lewis, J.S., Hajdu, S.I., et al.: Mucous gland tumors of the larynx and laryngopharynx. Ann. Otol. Rhinol. Laryngol. 85:498–503, 1976.
23. Gatti, W.M., and Erkman-Balis, B.: Mucoepidermoid carcinoma of the larynx. Arch. Otolaryngol. 106:52–53, 1980.
24. Houle, J., Joseph, P., and Batsakis, J.G.: Primary adenocarcinoma of the larynx. J. Laryngol. 90:1159–1163, 1976.
25. Bloom, J., Behar, A.J., Zikk, D., and Shanon, E.: Adenocarcinoma of the epiglottis. Arch. Otolaryngol. Head Neck Surg. 113:1330–1333, 1987.
26. Anderson, H.A., Maisel, R.H., and Cantrell, R.W.: Isolated laryngeal lymphoma. Laryngoscope 86:1251–1257, 1976.
27. McClatchey, K.D., and Schnitzer, B.: Pathology of lymphoreticular disorders. In Thawley, S.E., and Panje, W.R. (Eds.): Comprehensive Management of Head and Neck Tumors. Philadelphia, W.B. Saunders, 1987.
28. Morgan, K., MacLennan, K.A., Narula, A., et al.: Non-Hodgkin's lymphoma of the larynx. Cancer 64:1123–1127, 1989.
29. Ferlito, A., Nicolai, P., Recher, G., and Narne, S.: Primary laryngeal malignant fibrous histiocytoma: Review of the literature and report of seven cases. Laryngoscope 93:1351–1358, 1983.
30. Maniglia, A.J., and Xue, J.W.: Plasmacytoma of the larynx. Laryngoscope 93:741–744, 1983.
31. Freeland, A.P., Van Nostrand, A.W.P., and Jahn, A.F.: Metastases to the larynx. J. Otolaryngol. 8:448–456, 1979.
32. Ferlito, A., Caruso, G., and Recher, G.: Secondary laryngeal tumors. Report of seven cases with review of the literature. Arch. Otolaryngol. Head Neck Surg. 114:635–639, 1988.
33. Ferlito, A., Pesavento, G., Meli, S., et al.: Metastasis to the larynx revealing a renal cell carcinoma. J. Laryngol. Otol. 101:843–850, 1987.
34. Lam, K.H.: Extralaryngeal spread of cancer of the larynx: A study with whole-organ sections. Head Neck Surg. 5:410–424, 1983.
35. Tucker, G.F., Jr.: The anatomy of laryngeal cancer. Can. J. Otolaryngol. 3:417–431, 1974.
36. Brandenburg, J.H., Condon, K.G., and Frank, T.W.: Coronal sections of larynges from radiation therapy failures: A clinical-pathologic study. Otolaryngol. Head Neck Surg. 95:213–218, 1986.
37. Kirchner, J.A.: Two hundred laryngeal cancers: Patterns of growth and spread as seen in serial section. Laryngoscope 87:474–482, 1977.
38. Bocca, E., Calearo, C., De Vincentiis, I., et al.: Occult metastases in cancer of the larynx and their relationship to clinical and histological aspects of the primary tumor: A four-year multicentric research. Laryngoscope 94:1086–1090, 1984.
39. Pillsbury, H.R.C., and Kirchner, J.A.: Clinical vs. histopathologic staging in laryngeal cancer. Arch. Otolaryngol. 105:157–159, 1979.
40. Beahrs, O.H., Henson, D.E., Hutter, R.V.P., and Myers, M.H. (Eds.): Manual for Staging of Cancer, 3rd edition. Philadelphia, J.B. Lippincott, 1988.
41. Rothman, K.J., Cann, C.I., Flanders, D., and Fried, M.P.: Epidemiology of laryngeal cancer. Epidemiol. Rev. 2:195–209, 1980.
42. Devesa, S.S., and Silverman, D.T.: Cancer incidence and mortality trends in the United States: 1935–1974. J. Natl. Cancer Inst. 60:545–571, 1978.
43. Wynder, E.L.: The epidemiology of cancers of the upper alimentary and upper respiratory tracts. Laryngoscope 88 (suppl. 8):50–51, 1978.
44. Morrison, M.D.: Is chronic gastroesophageal reflux a causative factor in glottic carcinoma? Otolaryngol. Head Neck Surg. 99:370–373, 1988.
45. Ward, P.H., and Hanson, D.G.: Reflux as an etiological factor of carcinoma of the laryngopharynx. Laryngoscope 98:1195–1199, 1988.
46. Katsantonis, G.P., Archer, C.R., Rosenblum, B.N., et al.: The degree to which accuracy of preoperative staging of laryngeal carcinoma has been enhanced by computed tomography. Otolaryngol. Head Neck Surg. 95:52–62, 1986.
47. Hoover, L.A., Calcaterra, T.C., Walter, G.A., and Larrson, S.G.: Preoperative CT scan evaluation for laryngeal carcinoma: Correlation with pathological findings. Laryngoscope 94:310–315, 1984.
48. Isaacs, J.H., Jr., Mancuso, A.A., Mendenhall, W.M., and Parsons, J.T.: Deep spread patterns in CT staging of T_{2-4} squamous cell laryngeal carcinoma. Otolaryngol. Head Neck Surg. 99:455–464, 1988.
49. Werber, J.L., and Lucente, F.E.: Computed tomography in patients with laryngeal carcinoma: A clinical perspective. Ann. Otol. Rhinol. Laryngol. 98:55–58, 1989.
50. Lindberg, R.D.: Distribution of cervical lymph node metastases from squamous cell carcinoma of the upper respiratory and digestive tracts. Cancer 29:1446–1450, 1972.
51. Ogura, J.H., Biller, H.F., and Wette, R.: Elective neck dissection for pharyngeal and laryngeal cancers: An evaluation. Ann. Otol. Rhinol. Laryngol. 80:646–651, 1971.

52. Lederman, M.: Place de la radiothérapie dans le traitement du cancer du larynx. Ann. Radiol. 4:433–454, 1961.
53. Wagenfeld, D.J.H., Harwood, A.R., Bryce, D.P., et al.: Second primary respiratory tract neoplasms in supraglottic carcinoma. Arch. Otolaryngol. 107:135–137, 1981.
54. Goodman, M.L.: Keratosis (leukoplakia) of the larynx. Otolaryngol. Clin. North Am. 17:179–183, 1984.
55. Crissman, J.D., Zarbo, R.J., Drozdowicz, S., et al.: Carcinoma in situ and microinvasive squamous carcinoma of the laryngeal glottis. Arch. Otolaryngol. Head Neck Surg. 114:299–307.
56. Maceri, D.R., Lampe, H.B., Makielski, K.H., et al.: Conservation laryngeal surgery: A critical analysis. Arch. Otolaryngol. 111:361–365, 1985.
57. Shaha, A.R., and Shah, J.P.: Carcinoma of the subglottic larynx. Am. J. Surg. 144:456–458, 1982.
58. Berger, G., Harwood, A.R., Bryce, D.P., and van Nostrand, A.W.: Primary subglottic carcinoma masquerading clinically as T_1 glottic carcinoma—a report of nine cases. J. Otolaryngol. 14:1–6, 1985.
59. Donovan, D.T., and Conley, J.: Adenoid cystic carcinoma of the subglottic region. Ann. Otol. Rhinol. Laryngol. 92:491–495, 1983.
60. Kaplan, M.J., Johns, M.E., McLean, W.C., et al.: Stage II glottic carcinoma: Prognostic factors and management. Laryngoscope 93:725–728, 1983.
61. Gilbert, R.W., Birt, D., Shulman, H., et al.: Correlation of tumor volume with local control in laryngeal carcinoma treated by radiotherapy. Ann. Otol. Rhinol. Laryngol. 96:514–518, 1987.
62. Kaiser, T.N., Sessions, D.G., and Harvey, J.E.: Natural history of treated T_1N_0 squamous cell carcinoma of the glottis. Ann. Otol. Rhinol. Laryngol. 98:217–219, 1989.
63. Ossoff, R.H., Sisson, G.A., and Shapshay, S.M.: Endoscopic management of selected early vocal cord carcinoma. Ann. Otol. Rhinol. Laryngol. 94:560–564, 1985.
64. Koufman, J.A.: The endoscopic management of early squamous carcinoma of the vocal cord with the carbon dioxide surgical laser: Clinical experience and a proposed subclassification. Otolaryngol. Head Neck Surg. 95:531–537, 1986.
65. Davis, R.K., Shapshay, S.M., Strong, M.S., and Hyams, V.J.: Transoral partial supraglottic resection using the CO_2 laser. Laryngoscope 93:429–432, 1983.
66. Marks, J.E., Breaux, S., Smith, P.G., et al.: The need for elective irradiation of occult lymphatic metastases from cancers of the larynx and pyriform sinus. Head Neck Surg. 8:3–8, 1985.
67. Pearson, B.W.: Subtotal laryngectomy. Laryngoscope 91:1904–1912, 1981.
68. Kirchner, J.A.: Pathways and pitfalls in partial laryngectomy. Ann. Otol. Rhinol. Laryngol. 93:301–305, 1984.
69. Bailey, B.J., and Biller, H.F. (Eds.): Surgery of the Larynx. Philadelphia, W.B. Saunders, 1985.
70. Lore, J.M., Jr.: An Atlas of Head and Neck Surgery, volume 2, 2nd edition. Philadelphia, W.B. Saunders, 1973.
71. Norris, C.M.: Technique of extended fronto-lateral partial laryngectomy. Laryngoscope 68:1240–1250, 1958.
72. Bocca, E., Pignataro, O., and Oldini, C.: Supraglottic laryngectomy: 30 years of experience. Ann. Otol. Rhinol. Laryngol. 92:14–18, 1983.
73. Burstein, F.D., and Calcaterra, T.C.: Supraglottic laryngectomy: Series report and analysis of results. Laryngoscope 95:833–836, 1985.
74. Mohr, R.M., Quenelle, D.J., and Shumrick, D.A.: Vertico-frontolateral laryngectomy (hemilaryngectomy). Arch. Otolaryngol. 109:384–395, 1983.
75. DeSanto, L.W., Pearson, B.W., and Olsen, K.D.: Utility of near-total laryngectomy for supraglottic, pharyngeal, base-of-tongue, and other cancers. Ann. Otol. Rhinol. Laryngol. 98:2–7, 1989.
76. Biller, H.F., and Lawson, W.: Partial laryngectomy for transglottic cancers. Ann. Otol. Rhinol. Laryngol. 93:297–300, 1984.
77. DeSanto, L.W.: Cancer of the supraglottic larynx: A review of 260 patients. Otolaryngol. Head Neck Surg. 93:705–711, 1985.
78. Levendag, P., Sessions, R., Vikram, B., et al.: The problem of neck relapse in early stage supraglottic larynx cancer. Cancer 63:345–348, 1989.
79. Spaulding, C.A., Krochak, R.J., Hahn, S.S., and Constable, W.C.: Radiotherapeutic management of cancer of the supraglottis. Cancer 57:1292–1298, 1986.
80. Robbins, K.T., Davidson, W., Peters, L.J., and Goepfert, H.: Conservation surgery for T_2 and T_3 carcinomas of the supraglottic larynx. Arch. Otolaryngol. Head Neck Surg. 114:421–426, 1988.
81. Spaulding, C.A., Constable, W.C., Levine, P.A., and Cantrell, R.W.: Partial laryngectomy and radiotherapy for supraglottic cancer: A conservative approach. Ann. Otol. Rhinol. Laryngol. 98:125–129, 1989.

82. Yuen, A., Medina, J.E., Goepfert, H., and Fletcher, G.: Management of stage T_3 and T_4 glottic carcinomas. Am. J. Surg. *148:*467–472, 1984.
83. Seiden, A.M., Mantravadi, R.P., Haas, R.B., and Applebaum, E.L.: Advanced supraglottic carcinoma: A comparative study of sequential treatment policies. Head Neck Surg. *7:*22–27, 1984.
84. Pearson, B.W., Woods, R.D., and Hartman, D.E.: Extended hemilaryngectomy for T_3 glottic carcinoma with preservation of speech and swallowing. Laryngoscope *90:*1950–1961, 1980.
85. Kessler, D.J., Trapp, T.K., and Calcaterra, T.C.: The treatment of T_3 glottic carcinoma with vertical partial laryngectomy. Arch. Otolaryngol. Head Neck Surg. *113:*1196–1199, 1987.
86. Biller, H.F., and Lawson, W.: Partial laryngectomy for vocal cord cancer with marked limitation or fixation of the vocal cord. Laryngoscope *96:*61–64, 1986.
87. Parsons, J.T., Cassisi, N.J., and Million, R.R.: Results of twice-a-day irradiation of squamous cell carcinomas of the head and neck. Int. J. Radiat. Oncol. Biol. Phys. *10:*2041–2051, 1984.
88. Wang, C.C., Blitzer, P.H., and Suit, H.D.: Twice-a-day radiation therapy for cancer of the head and neck. Cancer *55:*2100–2104, 1985.
89. Dreyfuss, A.I., Clark, J.R., Wright, J.E., et al.: Continuous infusion high-dose leucovorin with 5-fluorouracil and cisplatin for untreated stage IV carcinoma of the head and neck. Ann. Intern. Med. *112:*167–172, 1990.
90. Dimery, I.W., Kramer, A.M., Choksi, A.J., and Hong, W.K.: Neoadjuvant chemotherapy and radiotherapy in larynx preservation. Am. J. Clin. Oncol. *12:*173–177, 1989.
91. Jacobs, C., Goffinet, D.R., Goffinet, L., et al.: Chemotherapy as a substitute for surgery in the treatment of advanced resectable head and neck cancer. A report from the Northern California Oncology Group. Cancer *60:*1178–1183, 1987.
92. Clark, J.R., Dreyfuss, A.I., Busse, P.M., et al.: Continuous infusion cisplatin, 5-FU and high-dose leucovorin: An induction therapy for SCCHN with high rates of complete response and radiotherapy alone as primary site management. *In* Salmon, S.E. (Ed.): Adjuvant Therapy of Cancer VI. New York, Grune & Stratton, 1990, pp. 71–81.
93. Burns, H., Bryce, D.P., and Van Nostrand, A.W.P.: Conservation surgery in laryngeal cancer and its role following failed radiotherapy. Arch. Otolaryngol. *105:*234–239, 1979.
94. Croll, G.A., Van Den Broek, P., Tiwari, R.M., et al.: Vertical partial laryngectomy for recurrent glottic carcinoma after irradiation. Head Neck Surg *7:*390–393, 1985.
95. Strauss, M.: Hemilaryngectomy rescue for radiation failure in early glottic carcinoma. Laryngoscope *98:*317–320, 1988.

HYPOPHARYNX AND CERVICAL ESOPHAGUS
by Charles M. Norris, Jr., M.D.

An independent discussion of malignancies of the hypopharynx and cervical esophagus is somewhat redundant, as there is considerable similarity in the anatomic, physiologic, and treatment considerations for tumors in these areas to those of the larynx and oropharynx. Tumor extension from one anatomic region into another is a common determinant for the extent of surgical treatment. Cancers of the hypopharynx and esophagus are distinctive for an often surreptitious evolution to advanced stages with relatively modest symptomatology.

The hypopharynx extends from the inferior border of the oropharynx to just above the cricopharyngeal muscle portion of the upper alimentary tract. Included are the pyriform sinuses, the posterior pharyngeal wall, and the postcricoid portion of the larynx. The hypopharynx surrounds the larynx and its aryepiglottic folds and epiglottis anatomically separate it from the pyriform sinuses (hypopharynx) and tongue base (oropharynx). Because tumors will frequently straddle boundaries, to name and classify a lesion can be difficult. The medial wall of the pyriform sinus represents, in effect, the lateral wall of the larynx. The anterior and anterolateral portion of the pyriform sinuses are contained within the thyroid cartilage ala, which allows for its direct invasion. Generally, a visual estimation of the epicenter of the tumor is taken as the site of origin, though such basis for designation may be tempered by observations on the clinical behavior of the tumor.

The cervical esophagus has its uppermost border at, and includes, the cricopharyngeal muscle region, which comprises the functional upper esophageal sphincter. This area represents a substantial narrowing of the hypopharyngeal lumen, so that tumors that impinge on the cricopharyngeal vicinity will require pharyngoesophageal reconstruction during surgery, in order to reinstate alimentary integrity and/or prevent stricture formation. The same applies even if only the desirable margin of resection involves the cricopharyngeal muscle or if the circumferential extent of resection is substantial. Radiation to this area, furthermore, can cause strictures that mandate surgical or dilation therapy. The lower border of the cervical esophagus is generally taken as the thoracic inlet.

CLINICAL FEATURES

Epithelial malignancies of the hypopharynx and cervical esophagus are generally similar clinically and, with the possible exception of some salivary gland histologies and melanoma, represent the deadliest group of tumors in the head and neck. They tend to occur with advanced disease and nodal involvement. Nonepidermoid malignancies are rare. The cervical esophagus is known particularly for the submucosal extension of tumors for great distances from the visually apparent margin. Direct invasion of the trachea, which shares a common wall with the esophagus, is not uncommon. The potential for mediastinal nodal metastasis is an additional poor prognostic feature.

As with other head and neck mucosal sites, epidermoid carcinoma of the hypopharynx and cervical esophagus is often the result of the prolonged and excessive use of alcohol and inhaled tobacco products. While postcricoid cancer is relatively rare, it has been associated in women with the Plummer-Vinson syndrome.

In the preliminary evaluation of these patients, a barium swallow is often performed. This study, however, can vastly underestimate the extent of disease, and by no means replaces the need for direct evaluation. Endoscopy must determine at least the mucosal margins of the lesion, direct involvement of the larynx or trachea, as well as indicating a need for esophageal reconstruction. Flexible endoscopy of the hypopharynx has significant limitations and should not be substituted for rigid examination under anesthesia. Computed tomography (CT) scanning[1] is also useful for suggestion of laryngeal, tracheal, or prevertebral fascia involvement and mediastinal or nodal disease, particularly in someone with a large neck. In the event that distal endoscopy is not possible due to obstructing or friable disease (risking perforation), a CT scan can help delineate the inferior margin of the tumor. Clinical staging must be correlated with the known biologic behavior of tumors in this area in order to formulate a treatment plan.[2]

TREATMENT AND OUTCOME[3, 4]

Early tumors (T_1 and some T_2 primaries), although rare, are generally treated with external x-ray therapy to the primary, areas of anticipated spread, and both the cervical and upper mediastinal node regions.[5] The occasional small lesion confined to the lateral wall of the pyriform sinus or pharynx may lend itself to complete excision by lateral pharyngectomy with primary or flap reconstruction. Similarly, the rare localized lesion of the cervical esophagus that is substantially below the cricopharyngeal muscle will permit a larynx-sparing surgical approach. Notwithstanding, the likelihood of metastatic nodal disease dictates some form of nodal treatment, usually at least elective dosages of radiation.

More advanced stages of primary site disease generally require combined treatment, which involves radical pharyngolaryngectomy or laryngoesophagectomy with appropriate reconstruction.[6-14] Advanced disease of the hypopharynx and cervical esophagus carries such a high probability of at least occult nodal disease,[15] that radical or modified radical neck dissections would also be performed at the time of surgery. Postoperative external radiation of an approximate dosage of 6000 rads would be the general rule, which generally begins 3 to 6 weeks following surgery. The ability of a patient to heal, recuperate, start his or her rehabilitation, and get on with radiation is crucial to the success of combined treatment rendered in this sequence. Important factors include the patient's nutrition and medical status, the choice and technical achievement of a single-stage ablative and reconstructive surgical procedure, and the avoidance of postoperative complications in order to avoid additional delay in further treatment. If the patient's surgical tolerance status or the resectability of the tumor is questionable, preoperative radiation with associated hyperalimentation measures can be considered, allowing for staged surgical procedures subsequently. By virtue of cytoreduction and gross tumor shrinkage, unresectable tumors may become resectable during chemotherapy, which thereby permits surgery on an as-yet unirradiated patient. This is an attractive alternative to the surgeon but, as noted, may not result in any improvement in long-term survival.[16] Induction chemotherapy with a goal of increasing survival and/or decreasing treatment morbidity by preserving function has yet to find a clearly defined role. The presumption that following chemotherapy with combined, aggressive surgery and radiation will improve curability has not been proven (see further discussion in following section). Furthermore, in some studies, cancers of the hypopharynx did not tend to respond as well to chemotherapeutic cytoreduction.[17] Generally, for earlier lesions, an approach utilizing concomitant, overlapping, or repeated sequential combination therapy with chemotherapy and radiation is undergoing trial study, with a primary goal to avoid laryngoesophagectomy surgery.[18, 19]

Overall survival in this group of tumor patients is generally less than 30 per cent. The rare early stage lesion without involved adenopathy may be cured 60 to 70 per cent of the time. Even the apparently successful control of local (primary site with or without extension) and regional (nodal) disease for a period of time may eventuate in survival failure due to blood-borne metastases. Delayed distant metastasis along with second sites of primary cancer[20] is a possibility in any patient with head and neck malignancy. The former represents an invariably incurable situation and is particularly common in advanced hypopharyngeal lesions and in tumors of any head and neck origin with associated advanced nodal involvement. The evolution of distant metastasis, of course, requires that the patient be successfully treated initially for the local and regional disease with which he or she presented. As local and regional control and treatment results have improved as a result of combined therapies, the proportion of patients who succumb to delayed distant disease has increased. This fact, in part, accounts for the desirability for some form of systemic (whole body) therapy, like chemotherapy.

A patient's motivation to avoid the loss of laryngeal function is understandably great. The rationale to avoid surgery, while a proportionate level of cure is maintained, is presently being explored through the use of hyperfractionated radiation schedules and/or induction chemotherapy. It is somewhat paradoxically true that a patient may be better off, both objectively and subjectively, following radical surgery, even if only for palliation. The elimination of pain or obstruction to breathing and swallowing may well not be achieved by radiation alone. Surgical salvage after full-dosage radiation carries with it a substantially increased complication rate. However, based on his or her own personal standards and philosophy, a patient may well elect a traditionally less effective or experimental treatment plan in order to modify what is viewed as unacceptable morbidity.

REFERENCES

1. Hirano, M., Kurita, S., Cho, J.S., and Tanaka, H.: Computed tomography in determining laryngeal involvement of hypopharyngeal carcinoma. Ann. Otol. Rhinol. Laryngol. 97:476–482, 1988.
2. Sulfaro, S., Barzan, L., Querin, F., et al.: T staging of laryngohypopharyngeal carcinoma. Arch. Otolaryngol. Head Neck Surg. 115:613–620, 1989.
3. Mendenhall, W.M., Parsons, J.T., Devine, J.W., et al.: Squamous cell carcinoma of the pyriform sinus treated with surgery and/or radiotherapy. Head Neck Surg. 10:88–92, 1987.
4. Collin, C.F., and Spiro, R.H.: Carcinoma of the cervical esophagus: Changing therapeutic trends. Am. J. Surg. 148:460–466, 1984.
5. Mendenhall, W.M., Parsons, J.T., Vogel, S.B., et al.: Carcinoma of the cervical esophagus treated with radiation therapy. Laryngoscope 98:769–771, 1988.
6. Teichgraeber, J.F., and McConnel, F.M.S.: Treatment of posterior pharyngeal wall carcinoma. Otolaryngol. Head Neck Surg. 94:287–290, 1986.
7. Marks, J.E., Smith, P.G., and Sessions, D.G.: Pharyngeal wall cancer. Arch. Otolaryngol. 11:79–85, 1985.
8. Vandenbrouck, C., Eschwege, F., De La Rochfordiere, A., et al.: Squamous cell carcinoma of the pyriform sinus: Retrospective study of 351 cases treated at the Institut Gustave-Roussy. Head Neck Surg. 10:4–13, 1987.
9. Dumich, P.S., Pearson, B.W., and Weiland, L.H.: Suitability of near-total laryngopharyngectomy in piriform carcinoma. Arch. Otolaryngol. 110:664–669, 1984.
10. Langer, M., Choi, N.C., Orlow, E., et al.: Radiation therapy alone or in combination with surgery in the treatment of carcinoma of the esophagus. Cancer 58:1208–1213, 1986.
11. Pingree, T.F., Davis, R.K., Reichman, O., and Derrick, L.: Treatment of hypopharyngeal carcinoma: A 10-year review of 1,362 cases. Laryngoscope 97:901–904, 1987.

12. Yates, A., and Crumley, R.L.: Surgical treatment of pyriform sinus cancer: A retrospective study. Laryngoscope *94:*1586–1590, 1984.
13. Driscoll, W.G., Nagorsky, M.J., Cantrell, R.W., and Johns, M.E.: Carcinoma of the pyriform sinus: Analysis of 102 cases. Laryngoscope *93:*556–560, 1983.
14. Harrison, D.F.N.: Surgical management of hypopharyngeal cancer. Arch. Otolaryngol. *105:*149–152, 1979.
15. Lefebvre, J.L., Castelain, B., De La Torre, J.C., et al.: Lymph node invasion in hypopharynx and lateral epilarynx carcinoma: A prognostic factor. Head Neck Surg. *10:*14–18, 1987.
16. Advani, S.H., Saikia, T.K., Swaroop, S., et al.: Anterior chemotherapy in esophageal cancer. Cancer *56:*1502–1506, 1985.
17. Strong, E.W., Wolf, G., and Vickram, B.: Adjuvant chemotherapy for advanced head and neck squamous carcinoma. Final report of the head and neck contracts program. Cancer *60:*301–311, 1987.
18. Coia, L.R., Engstrom, P.F., and Paul, A.: Nonsurgical management of esophageal cancer. Report of a study of combined radiotherapy and chemotherapy. J. Clin. Oncol. *5:*1783–1790, 1987.
19. Keane, T.J., Harwood, A.R., Elhakim, T., et al.: Radical radiation therapy with 5-fluorouracil infusion and mitomycin C for oesophageal squamous carcinoma. Radiother. Oncol. *4:*205–210, 1985.
20. Fogel, T.D., Harrison, L.B., and Son, Y.H.: Subsequent upper aerodigestive malignancies following treatment of esophageal cancer. Cancer *55:*1882–1885, 1985.

ROLE OF NEOADJUVANT CHEMOTHERAPY IN HEAD AND NECK CANCER

by Charles M. Norris, Jr., M.D.

Although there is much enthusiasm and an enormous amount of experience being accumulated and results reported on the use of chemotherapy as an adjunct to the curative-intent therapy of previously untreated, primarily advanced stage head and neck cancer patients, its role remains to be legitimized by consensus. The activity of various antineoplastic agents, alone or in combination, against squamous cell cancers is well established as is chemotherapy's heretofore more conventional role in disease palliation. Phase I and II studies have progressed, correlate with basic science investigations. The overriding question remains of whether there can be possible improved survival with the addition of chemotherapy to conventional treatment, whether classic or modified.

The rationale initially espoused for the justification of induction chemotherapy was the observed activity of certain agents in recurrent, previously treated patients; the combination of drugs that involve nonoverlapping toxicities and that are administered in a manner that takes advantage of established cellular mechanisms; the putative improvement in local and regional treatment by surgery and/or radiation after initial regression (and corresponding stage reduction) of the tumor by chemotherapy; the conversion of unresectable disease to resectable disease after initial chemotherapy;

and the earliest treatment, hopefully with eradication, of any already-established distant micrometastases. More recently, the opportunity to reduce local morbidity while preserving the efficacy of treatment has been advanced. The administration of induction chemotherapy according to strict protocol in a multidisciplinary cancer treatment setting is crucial in order to fully assess outcome and to attribute cause and effect.

Beginning 15 years ago, initial studies with methotrexate and leucovorin were initiated at the Dana-Farber Cancer Institute/New England Deaconess Head and Neck Clinic with interesting and promising results.[1,2] Subsequent protocols have involved cisplatin/5-fluorouracil/bleomycin, cisplatin/5-fluorouracil, and, most recently, cisplatin/5-fluorouracil/leucovorin. Eligible patients have evaluable stage IV or advanced stage III disease, with T_3N_0 tonsil lesions and T_1N_1 lesions anywhere excluded. Appropriate medical criteria as well as standard informed consent rituals must be satisfied. Following a complete multidisciplinary assessment and staging with biopsy and complete endoscopy, as well as primary site tattooing when feasible, chemotherapy is initiated according to protocol formula. Response is assessed after each cycle and graded as CR (complete response), which indicates the complete disappearance of all clinically detectable tumor; PR (partial response), which indicates a 50 per cent clinical reduction of tumor volume; or NR (non-response), which indicates anything less than a PR. The term "histologic CR" designates those tumor sites that, upon post-chemotherapy rebiopsy, show no light microscopic evidence of malignancy.

With experience that accrues in the administration and evaluation of chemotherapy impact, a number of refinements have been realized. Generally, three cycles of chemotherapy are optimum, acute and delayed toxicities are increasingly better recognized and controlled, and the clinical limitations in determining a CR have been acknowledged so that repeat biopsy histology from areas of accessible disease are now becoming a standard. (Even a small but notable incidence of clinical PRs without histologic tumor residual has been determined.) Additionally, the synergistic cytotoxicity of certain combinations has been realized, the superiority of continuous infusion cisplatin (versus bolus) administration has been noted, and the enhancement of 5-fluorouracil cytotoxicity by leucovorin has been established.

The decade has seen a progressive refinement of combination chemotherapy protocols for the initial (induction) treatment of advanced head and neck cancer, with increased rates observed of clinically complete response as well as a substantial and increasing rate of histologic tumor clearing by light microscopy (histologic CR). It has become a well-established fact that a response to cytoreductive chemotherapy as initial treatment, particularly a complete response, is associated with a substantially and significantly improved statistical chance of tumor-free survival. However, while response predicts for cure, it is far from clear that cause and effect are at work as opposed to a selection, by chemotherapy, of those patients who would otherwise have done as well with conventional surgery and radiation combinations. A correlation between radiation response and chemotherapy response is well-documented clinically,[3,4] as are some of the potential mechanisms of chemotherapy resistance *in vitro*.[5-7] The extreme heterogeneity of head and neck cancer continues to complicate prognostic comparisons.

While improved survivorship would be an acknowledged endpoint of any cancer treatment regimen, therapies that maintain cure rates with lesser morbidity are also worthwhile, particularly in the head and neck, wherein local treatment can result in substantial functional and cosmetic debility. Both of these aspects of progress, survival with cure and lower long-term morbidity, are currently relevant, actively investigated goals in this arena.

Prospective studies of induction chemotherapy have yet to document an overall survival advantage attributable to induction chemotherapy.[8-15] By and large, however, these studies have been flawed in one or another major way, including small patient numbers, brief follow-up periods, poor response rates to suboptimal chemotherapy regimens, or compromised locoregional treatment by radiation and/or surgery. There remains a conviction among many in the field that with a well-controlled study of an active combination regimen a survival benefit could be realized resulting from chemotherapy. A single study[16] in which patients who responded to induction chemotherapy regimen of platinum-bleomycin-methotrexate were randomized to receive, or not, additional (adjuvant) chemotherapy after completing courses of chemotherapy and radiation with or without surgery, showed a significant failure-free survival advantage for initial partial responders who received additional chemotherapy. However, this remains the only prospective demonstration that chemotherapy can alter the natural history of this disease. It is speculated that a consistent CR rate of 50 per cent will need to be realized before a survival advantage as a result of induction chemotherapy can be demonstrated.[17]

As the survival impact of chemotherapy in squamous cell carcinoma of the head and neck (SCCHN) plays out in prospective trials, the goal of morbidity limitation, specifically via functional organ preservation, is to receive increased attention. Quality of life is becoming an increasingly determinate goal of cancer therapy. Issues involved include the identification during induction chemotherapy of those patients whose chance of cure may reasonably be maintained through lesser local therapies, usually radiation instead of surgery, thereby preserving vital primary site organ function (e.g., larynx; tongue base).[18, 19]

There is legitimate concern that pursuing investigation of these two goals may be to a certain extent contradictory in that a potential for induction chemotherapy to actually improve survival in this disease may not be realizable if local and regional therapy is not maintained at a maximum level. Traditionally, in earlier studies, local treatment was not modified, either in extent or distribution, after induction chemotherapy. More recently, a modification of local treatment in the most favorable chemotherapy responders is becoming the norm, without a substantive worsening but also without a substantive improvement in survival. At the time of writing, a very interesting and ongoing prospective study through the VA Hospitals system addresses the question of laryngeal preservation.[15] This larynx-sparing approach using induction chemotherapy has predictably resulted in an observed increased incidence of local failure, which requires salvage total laryngectomy. However, while a survival improvement overall has not been demonstrated, a number of patients have been treated without laryngectomy and without an overall worsening of prognosis. A decreased incidence of distant metastatic failure has also been noted.

Local and regional treatment side effects, whether by surgery, radiation, or both, are not substantially affected by antecedent chemotherapy, though some technical problems are noted with the accuracy of intraoperative frozen-section analysis.[20]

The latest combined Dana-Farber Cancer Institute/New England Deaconess Head and Neck Clinic protocol[21, 22] for induction chemotherapy in advanced squamous cell cancer of the head and neck (PFL) involves the administration of three 28-day cycles of cisplatin—25 mg/m^2/day on days 1–5, leucovorin—500 mg/m^2/day on days 1–6, and 5-fluorouracil—800 mg/m^2/day on days 2–6. Interim analysis of 46 patients (May, 1990) has determined a complete response rate of 65 per cent, the highest yet reported in such studies and double that of a recent previous study utilizing cisplatin/5-fluorouracil only. Most of the clinical CRs have also been determined through rebiopsy to be histologic CRs as well. These figures represent a significant improvement over the 28 percentage CR rate achieved in a previous protocol utilizing cisplatin/5-fluorouracil/bleomycin. A projected 2-year overall failure-free survival rate of 61 per cent in the latest data compares favorably with that of 50 per cent in earlier protocols and 30 per cent in historical controls. Again, however, in the absence of controlled prospective studies with consistently high CR rates, a survival advantage attributable to chemotherapy alone is impossible to confirm. Future chemotherapy refinements will continue to focus on further enhancement of the CR rate, with the combined goals of increased survivorship and decreased morbidity.

As alluded to previously, decreasing the morbidity of locoregional treatment is emerging as a mandated priority of cancer therapy in this decade. More and more often, patients who achieve a primary-site CR are being managed without primary-site surgical ablation but rather by radiation techniques, external beam and interstitial. Studies have demonstrated no change in prognosis in this subset, an observation not established in prior studies that achieve lower CR rates. Interestingly, in our own most recent series (PFL), while a substantial amount of therapeutic surgery continues to be performed (64 per cent of patients now versus 58 per cent in prior studies—not a significant difference), significantly fewer primary site resections (22 per cent) are being performed, with the majority of patients (78 per cent) receiving radiation as initial, definitive, local therapy. This contrasts with the 46 percentage rate of primary site resections implemented in prior Dana-Farber/New England Deaconess studies ($p = 0.004$). The majority of the procedures are nodal dissections that only occur in 64 per cent of patients after PFL, as contrasted with 49 per cent in prior studies ($p = 0.08$). Our present approach to nodal disease is to perform neck dissections on all patients who show greater than N_1 adenopathy, regardless of response to chemotherapy or radiation (if administered preoperatively). Patients with metastatic adenopathy that occurs with N_1 disease who achieve a complete response to induction chemotherapy are usually treated by radiation alone. Neck dissection is performed for less than a CR, or if primary site surgery is necessary anyway. A shifting pattern of failure somewhat away from the local (primary) site has been correspondingly observed.[18]

Future directions in the use of chemotherapy as induction or adjuvant treatment in head and neck cancer are aimed at the goals of increased survivorship coupled with decreased morbidity through the sparing of vital organ function. Generally, these directives will be approached through efforts at improving the rate of clinical and histologic CRs to chemotherapy. At the Dana-Farber Cancer Institute, as well as other centers, basic studies in biochemistry and cell biology are ongoing in an effort to define new drugs (dye complexes, antifolate analogs, antimitochondrial agents, and immunotoxins) and/or sensitizing factors for existing drug protocols (fluosol/oxygen, pentoxifylline, micronutrients). The molecular bases for various mechanisms of drug resistance and oncogene expression will, in head and neck cancer as in all fields of oncology, add to our insight into clinical efficacy of the pharmacologic manipulation of patients and their disease. Simple improvements in the administration of drugs with fewer side effects will also represent progress, for example, in the limitation of mucositis and its sequelae, as well as in other patient support parameters, including nutrition. Clinically, a further refined approach to the determination of need for, and carrying out of, necessary surgery will be developed, correlate with the development of better, clinically useful parameters of chemotherapy response. The paramount role of surgery continues in the salvage of the hopefully fewer failures of chemotherapy/radiation. Finally, the extension of chemotherapeutic awareness into other head and neck histologies, particularly salivary gland malignancies,[23] is undergoing evaluation, as also is the rapidly evolving field of chemoprevention,[24] involving the use of beta carotene and other vitamin constituents.

REFERENCES

1. Pitman, S.W., Miller, D., and Weichselbaum, R.: Initial adjuvant therapy in advanced squamous cell carcinoma of the head and neck employing weekly high dose methotrexate with leucovorin rescue. Laryngoscope *88*:632–638, 1978.
2. Ervin, T.J., Kirkwood, J., Weichselbaum, R.R., et al.: Improved survival for patients with advanced carcinoma of the head and neck treated with methotrexate-leucovorin prior to definitive radiotherapy or surgery. Laryngoscope *91*:1181–1190, 1981.
3. Weichselbaum, R.R., Beckett, M.A., Vijayakumar, S., et al.: Radioresistent tumor cell lines derived from head and neck radiation failures. Head Neck *11*:343–348, 1989.
4. Ensley, J.F., Jacobs, J.R., Weaver, A., et al.: Correlation between response to cisplatinum-combination chemotherapy and subsequent radiotherapy in previously untreated patients with advanced squamous cell cancers of the head and neck. Cancer *54*:811–814, 1984.
5. Rosowsky, A., Wright, J.E., Cucchi, C.A., et al.: Phenotypic heterogeneity in cultured human head and neck squamous cell carcinoma lines with low-level methotrexate resistance. Cancer Res. *45*:6205–6212, 1985.
6. Komiyama, S., Matsui, K., Kudoh, S., et al.: Establishment of tumor cell lines from a patient with head and neck cancer and their different sensitivities to anti-cancer agents. Cancer *63*:675–681, 1989.
7. Teicher, B.A., Holden, S.A., Kelley, M.J., et al.: Characterization of a human squamous cell line resistant to cis-diamminedichloroplatinum (II). Cancer Res. *47*:388–393, 1987.
8. Stell, P.M., Dalby, J.E., Strickland, P., et al.: Sequential chemotherapy and radiotherapy in advanced head and neck cancer. Clin. Radiol. *34*:463–467, 1983.
9. Kun, L.E., Toohill, R.J., Holoye, P.Y., et al.: A randomized study of adjuvant chemotherapy for cancer of the upper aerodigestive tract. Int. J. Radiat. Oncol. Biol. Phys. *12*:173–178, 1986.
10. Toohill, R.J., Anderson, T., Byhardt, R.W., et al.: Cisplatin and fluorouracil as neoadjuvant therapy in head and neck cancer: A preliminary report. Arch. Otolaryngol. Head Neck Surg. *113*:758–761, 1987.
11. Head and Neck Contracts Program. Adjuvant chemotherapy for advanced head and neck squamous carcinoma. Final report of the Head and Neck Contracts Program. Cancer *60*:301–311, 1987.
12. Martin, M., Mazeron, J.J., Brun, B., et al.: Neo-adjuvant polychemotherapy of head and neck cancer: Results of a randomized study (abstr.) Proc. Am. Soc. Clin. Oncol. *7*:590, 1988.
13. Carugati, A., Pradier, R., and de la Torre, A.: Combination chemotherapy pre radical treatment for head and neck squamous cell carcinoma (Abstr.) Proc. Am. Soc. Clin. Oncol. *7*:589, 1988.
14. Schuller, D.E., Metch, B., Stein, D.W., et al.: Preoperative chemotherapy in advanced

resectable head and neck cancer: Final report of Southwest Oncology Group. Laryngoscope 98:1205–1211, 1988.
15. Dimery, I.W., Kramer, A.M., Choksi, A.J., and Hong, W.K.: Neoadjuvant chemotherapy and radiotherapy in larynx preservation. Am. J. Clin. Oncol. 12:173–177, 1989.
16. Ervin, T.J., Clark, J.R., Weichselbaum, R.R., et al.: An analysis of induction and adjuvant chemotherapy in the multidisciplinary treatment of squamous-cell carcinoma of the head and neck. J. Clin. Oncol. 5:10–20, 1987.
17. Clark, J.C., Fallon, B.G., and Frei, E., III: Induction chemotherapy as initial treatment for advanced head and neck cancer: A model for the multidisciplinary treatment of solid tumors. In DeVita, V.T., Jr., Hellman, S., and Rosenberg, S.A. (Eds.): Important Advances in Oncology. Philadelphia, J.B. Lippincott, 1987, pp. 175–195.
18. Clark, J.R., Dreyfuss, A.I., Busse, P.M., et al.: Continuous infusion cisplatin, %-FU and high-dose leucovorin: An induction therapy for SCCHN with high rates of complete response and radiotherapy alone as primary site management. In Salmon, S.E. (Ed.): Adjuvant Therapy of Cancer, VI. New York, Grune & Stratton, 1990, pp. 71–81.
19. Jacobs, C., Goffinet, D.R., Goffinet, L., et al.: Chemotherapy as a substitute for surgery in the treatment of advanced resectable head and neck cancer. A report from the Northern California Oncology Group. Cancer 60:1178–1183, 1987.
20. Norris, C.M., Jr., Clark, J.R., Frei, E., III, et al.: Pathology of surgery after induction chemotherapy: An analysis of resectability and locoregional control. Laryngoscope 96:292–302, 1986.
21. Dreyfuss, A.I., Clark, J.R., Wright, J.E., et al.: continuous infusion high-dose leucovorin with 5-fluorouracil and cisplatin for untreated stage IV carcinoma of the head and neck. Ann. Intern. Med. 112:167–172, 1990.
22. Clark, J.R., Dreyfuss, A.I., Norris, C.M., Jr., et al.: Continuous infusion cisplatin, 5-FU and high-dose leucovorin (PFL): Favorable early results as induction therapy for squamous cell carcinoma of the head and neck (SCCHN). ASCO Proceedings 9:666, 1990.
23. Dreyfuss, A.I., Clark, J.R., Fallon, B.G., et al.: Cyclophosphamide, doxorubicin and cisplatin combination chemotherapy for advanced carcinomas of salivary gland origin. Cancer 60:2869–2872, 1987.
24. Lippman, S.M., Lee, J.S., Lotan, R., and Hong, W.K.: Chemoprevention of upper aerodigestive tract cancers. Head Neck 12:5–20, 1990.

NASOPHARYNGEAL CARCINOMA
by James W. Lucarini, M.D., and
Daniel Miller, M.D.

INTRODUCTION

Nasopharyngeal carcinoma is unique among head and neck malignancies because of its singular epidemiologic, genetic, etiologic, and demographic properties. The nasopharynx is a difficult area to examine and careful inspection must be motivated by a high index of suspicion. It is unusual for the tumor to be detected on routine evaluation of this area. More often patients have unilateral secretory otitis or a cervical mass of uncertain etiology. Except for very advanced local tumors, the T-stage has little correlation with the nodal staging and is not by itself of prognostic significance. Furthermore, this epithelial tumor offers a range of histologic features that distinguish it from the differentiated squamous cell carcinomas typical of head and neck cancer. Its proven association with Epstein-Barr virus

(EBV), its proclivity for people of southern Chinese ancestry, and its association with specific histocompatibility antigens distinguish it from other tumors and offer a unique insight into the cellular and molecular biology of cancer.

CLINICAL ANATOMY

The nasopharynx is a roughly quadrilateral space posterior to the nasal cavities and is bounded by the soft palate inferiorly, the basiocciput and sphenoid superiorly, the first two cervical vertebrae posteriorly, and the choanae anteriorly. Given these boundaries, it lies in close proximity to the nasal cavities and the oropharynx. The eustachian tube orifices lie laterally, each surrounded by the cartilaginous torus tubarius and the fossa of Rosenmüller. Laterally lies the posterior parapharyngeal space with its carotid sheath, cranial nerves IX through XII, and the cervical sympathetic ganglia. The foramen lacerum and foramen ovale of the skull base offer avenues of neoplastic extension to cranial nerves III through VI. Lymphatic drainage is to the jugulodigastric and spinal accessory nodes via the retropharyngeal nodes. The lack of lymphatic compartmentalization in this area accounts for the relative frequency of bilateral cervical metastases.

RISK FACTORS

Nasopharyngeal carcinoma is most prevalent in southern Chinese individuals, especially those from the province of Kwantung.[1,2] The incidence is somewhat reduced by emigration, but Americans of southern Chinese heritage still share a significantly higher risk than Caucasians.[3] While the incidence is low among the Japanese and Northern Chinese, it is higher in Indians. Risk of nasopharyngeal carcinoma has been linked to Epstein-Barr virus (EBV). Antibodies to the virus are elevated in individuals with the disease and the malignant cells contain the viral DNA patterns.[4-7] Certain histocompatibility antigens have been linked to the cancer and point to genetic factors. Two such antigens are $HLA-A_2$ and $HLA-BSIN_2$.[8,9] Environmental factors have been implicated, such as the nitrosamines from salted fish in the southern Chinese diet.[10] The relevance of these exposures has been controversial.[11]

SIGNS AND SYMPTOMS

The most common occurring complaint is the presence of a mass in the neck, which represents cervical metastasis.[12,13] Also very common is unilateral hearing loss.[14] In advanced cases local tumor invasion may lead to pain, headache, nasal obstruction, epistaxis, abnormal speech, trismus, proptosis, and various cranial neuropathies.

The findings parallel the symptoms. Cervical adenopathy is noted most commonly in the superior jugular chain, although the tumor has a relatively high rate of metastasis to the posterior triangle and supraclavicular areas compared with other head and neck malignancies. Bilateral metastasis is common, as mentioned. Serous effusion is often unilateral and resistant to medical treatment. This finding in an adult should always alert the clinician to the possibility of a nasopharyngeal malignancy. The tumor itself is usually an ulceration or mass noted in the fossa of Rosenmüller or the posterosuperior wall of the nasopharynx. The encroachment on the eustachian tube orifice leads to middle ear effusion. The size of the primary mass correlates poorly with the extent of adenopathy, as some very small tumors present with massive bilateral cervical nodes. In advanced local disease, invasion of the skull base may lead to a variety of cranial neuropathies.[15, 16] Tumor invasion of the foramen lacerum leads to involvement of cranial nerves III, IV, and VI. The jugular foramen is a second avenue for invasion, which affects cranial nerves IX, X, and XI.

DIAGNOSTIC WORK-UP

History and physical examination are most important both for suspicion and detection of the disease. Careful examination of the nasopharynx with a mirror or with fiberoptics is necessary in order to determine the extent of primary site disease. Otologic and cervical examinations should focus on detection of serous effusion and cervical adenopathy. In addition, nasopharyngoscopy and biopsy under general anesthesia are needed to determine the extent of local disease as well as the histologic type.

Radiologic evaluation should include computed tomography (CT) in order to assess local extent of disease (Fig. 2–1), as well as potential skull base bony invasion, which is an indicator of poor prognosis. CT scanning is

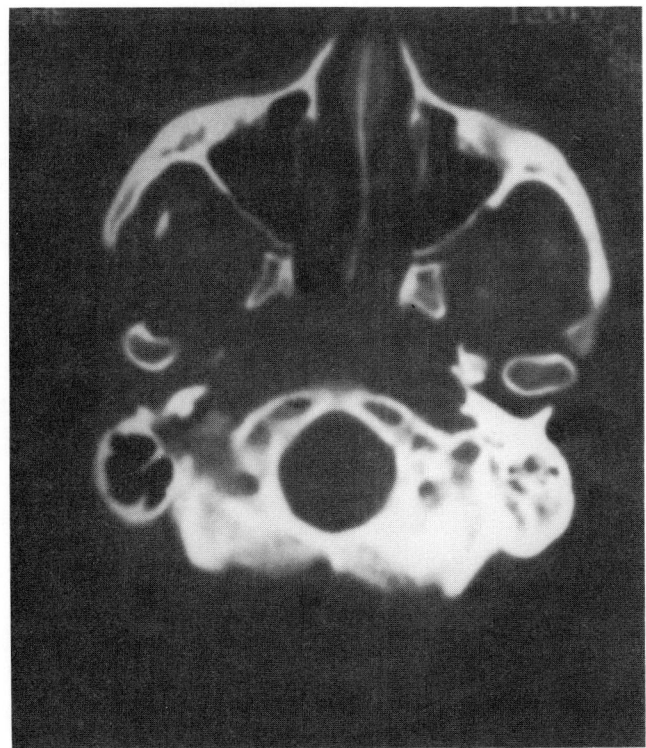

Figure 2–1. CT scan of patient with nasopharyngeal carcinoma exhibiting an extensive soft tissue mass in the nasopharynx.

useful in planning radiotherapy as well.[17] While magnetic resonance imaging (MRI) with gadolinium appears to offer superior soft tissue detail, it is not as useful in assessment of bony involvement. Gallium and bone scanning have not been found to be of additional benefit in delineating the tumor.

Antibody titers to Epstein-Barr virus (EBV) capsid antigen and diffused early antigen have been used in screening high-risk individuals.[18, 19] These titers are elevated in patients with nasopharyngeal carcinoma compared with controls.[20] In addition, recurrent disease can be heralded by a rise in titers prior to detection of clinical disease.[21] Testing is useful for tumors of undifferentiated and nonkeratizing types because antibody titers are relatively low in keratinizing squamous cell carcinoma of the nasopharynx.[22] Antibody titers to EBV-induced membrane antigen appear to predict prognosis when measured at presentation.[20] Low titers are initially seen in patients who develop clinical progression of disease at three years.

Routine evaluation should also include CBC, liver profile, and chest films, since early metastases to bone, lung, and liver have been noted in over half of patients with advanced cervical disease.[23]

HISTOLOGY

The World Health Organization (WHO) divides nasopharyngeal carcinomas into three histologies.[24] This works well for purposes of categorization, although there is probably a continuum between the three pure types. Differentiated squamous cell carcinoma occurs in about a quarter of cases. This is WHO type 1 histology and is typical of other squamous cell carcinomas of the head and neck.[20] Transitional cell or nonkeratinizing carcinomas are labeled WHO type 2. Anaplastic or so-called lymphoepitheliomas are labeled WHO type 3. The latter two types appear to have more common features and behave differently than type 1 tumors. The more undifferentiated carcinomas are more highly associated with elevated EBV titers and early and larger cervical metastases.[13, 14, 16, 25-27] However, they are more sensitive to radiotherapy and tend toward longer disease-free intervals following treatment. In addition, we have noted a tendency for these tumors to respond more readily to induction chemotherapy.[28]

Lymphomas are found much less frequently in the nasopharynx, while other rare malignancies include adenocarcinoma, plasmacytoma, sarcoma, and melanoma. Lymphomas can be difficult to distinguish from undifferentiated carcinomas and require electron microscopy and staining for lymphocytic cell markers.[29] These cancers are usually of B cell, large cell type with a diffuse growth pattern.

STAGING

The TNM staging of nasopharyngeal carcinoma, according to the American Joint Committee on Cancer Staging,[30] is outlined in Table 2-5. It is useful for prognostication and planning of therapy. Cervical adenopathy is staged as for other squamous cell carcinomas of the head and neck. Most staging systems omit important prognostic factors and are therefore limited. For example, the American Joint Committee on Cancer Staging (AJCC) does

TABLE 2–5. TNM STAGING FOR NASOPHARYNGEAL CARCINOMA ACCORDING TO THE AMERICAN JOINT COMMITTEE ON CANCER STAGING[3]

Primary Tumor (T)
- T_X—Primary tumor cannot be assessed
- T_0—No evidence of primary tumor
- Tis—Carcinoma *in situ*
- T_1—Tumor limited to one subsite of nasopharynx
- T_2—Tumor invades more than one subsite of nasopharynx
- T_3—Tumor invades the nasal cavity and/or oropharynx
- T_4—Tumor invades skull base and/or cranial nerves

Nodal Involvement (N)
- N_x—Minimum requirements to assess regional nodes not met
- N_0—No clinically positive nodes
- N_1—Single clinically positive homolateral node 3 cm or less in diameter
- N_2—Metastasis in a single ipsilateral lymph node, more than 3 cm but not more than 6 cm in greatest dimension; or multiple ipsilateral lymph nodes, none more than 6 cm in greatest dimension; or bilateral or contralateral lymph nodes, none more than 6 cm in greatest dimension
- N_{2a}—Metastasis in a single ipsilateral lymph node more than 3 cm but not more than 6 cm in greatest dimension
- N_{2b}—Metastasis in multiple ipsilateral lymph nodes, none more than 6 cm in greatest dimension
- N_{2c}—Metastasis in bilateral or contralateral lymph nodes, none more than 6 cm in greatest dimension
- N_3—Metastasis in a lymph node more than 6 cm in greatest dimension

Metastasis (M)
- M_0—No metastases present
- M_1—Metastases clinically demonstrable

Stage Grouping

Stage I	T_1,	N_0,	M_0
Stage II	T_2,	N_0,	M_0
Stage III	T_3,	N_0,	M_0
	T_1 or T_2 or T_3,	N_1,	M_0
Stage IV	T_4,	N_0 or N_1,	M_0
	Any T,	N_2 or N_3,	M_0
	Any T,	any N,	M_1

not take into account fixation of nodes or the level of nodes in the neck. Fixed nodes and inferiorly located nodes appear to adversely affect survival.[16] These factors are included in other classifications.[31, 22] On the other hand, bilateral or contralateral cervical disease does not by itself appear to affect survival compared with unilateral involvement.[16] Recently, the AJCC revised its nodal staging to reflect this idea. Ho's staging system[32] appears to be most useful prognostically, although it is not used widely in the United States. T-staging does not appear to predict survival unless advanced disease (T_4) is noted.[33, 34]

STANDARD THERAPY

External beam radiation is the mainstay of treatment. These tumors are highly radiosensitive in both the primary site and neck. Treatment planning must include protection of vital structures such as the cervical spinal cord and brain. Spinal cord and retinal exposure should not exceed 4500 rads.

Early lesions should be treated so as to include adjacent regions and the cervical nodes at risk. Advanced T_3 and T_4 lesions require irradiation of the nasal cavities, oropharynx, and any involved intracranial structures. Megavoltage or cobalt-60 gamma rays have been utilized with lateral opposed fields along with an anterior field for treatment of the lower cervical area. Fractional dosages of 170 to 180 rads five times weekly usually minimize mucositis. A minimum total dosage of 6500 rads to the primary site and cervical areas is utilized. Higher dosages are necessary for advanced lesions and keratinizing squamous cell carcinomas. Patients with residual disease can receive boosting with a cone-down technique that delivers over 90 Gy.[35] In addition, intracavitary radium or cesium can be used to increase local tumor dosage with little effect on the surrounding normal structures.[36] Side effects and complications of therapy include xerostomia, dental caries, serous otitis, trismus, neuropathy of cranial nerves IX through XII, transverse radiation myelitis, hypothalamic and pituitary dysfunction, hypothyroidism, retinopathy, and optic nerve injury.[27, 37, 38] These effects can often be mitigated by appropriate shielding and careful treatment planning.

Overall five-year survival ranges from 25 to 57 per cent.[27, 35, 39, 40] Primary site control ranges from 66 to 80 per cent, while nodal metastatic control ranges from 82 to 91 per cent.[23, 27, 41] In Wang's series of 185 patients, five-year survival rates for T_1, T_2, T_3, and T_4 lesions were 60 per cent, 48 per cent, 27 per cent, and 29 per cent, respectively.[42] Transitional and undifferentiated tumors appear more favorable than squamous cell carcinomas in some series[27, 42] while not in others.[39, 43] After therapy, elevated antibody titers to EBV antigens herald recurrent disease, offering a sensitive method of detection.[21] Earlier recurrences are usually associated with poorer prognosis.[44]

Management of cervical metastasis is determined somewhat by histology and outcome after radiation therapy. For transitional and undifferentiated carcinomas, even N_3 adenopathy appears to respond adequately to radiation therapy alone. Residual cervical disease following irradiation should be treated with neck dissection. Squamous cell carcinoma of the nasopharynx behaves much like its counterpart originating in other head and neck sites. N_2 and N_3 adenopathy is best managed by combination irradiation and neck dissection.

PALLIATIVE THERAPY

En bloc resection of the nasopharynx is not feasible and rarely useful in treating these cancers primarily. Radiation failures are occasionally amenable to surgical extirpation. Angiography is first performed in order to assess vascular supply to the tumor as well as potential involvement of the internal carotid artery. The tumor should involve only one wall of the nasopharynx and not invade the cavernous sinus. The techniques include the infratemporal fossa[45] and the transparotid temporal bone[46] approaches to the base of skull. The procedures are divided into stages. First, subtemporal craniectomy is done to evaluate pericarotid extension and resectability. At the same time a retrogasserian rhizotomy can be performed as needed for pain control. Carotid ligation is then performed with electroencephalographic monitoring to assess potential tolerance of carotid resection. At a second stage the tumor is extirpated; this procedure includes removal of the temporal bone, upper mandible, glenoid fossa, and the pterygoid plates. Recurrences in the neck alone can be treated with neck dissection.

Chemotherapy may be useful in some patients with metastatic disease as a palliative measure.

THERAPEUTIC FRONTIERS

We have reached a plateau in treating nasopharyngeal carcinoma with radiotherapy. In order to achieve higher control and cure rates systemic therapy will be necessary, especially in advanced locoregional disease, in which distant metastasis is common.

Patients with nasopharyngeal carcinoma have been noted to have depressed T cell immunity,[45] which suggests that immunotherapy may play a role in future adjunctive treatment. The possibility of a vaccine has been suggested by noting the induction of cytotoxic antibodies to EBV with use of a membrane glycoprotein from infected cells.[47] Specific induction of the immune system as well as monoclonal antibody production remain areas of investigation in treating this tumor.

Induction and adjuvant chemotherapy using cisplatin, 5-fluorouracil, leucovorin, cyclophosphamide, bleomycin, methotrexate, and vincristine have been investigated, with improved local control in some series[48] but not in others.[36]

Recent use of induction chemotherapy for untreated advanced nasopharyngeal carcinoma offers significant promise.[28] Twenty-four patients with previously untreated stage IV nasopharyngeal carcinoma were treated with combinations of cisplatin, bleomycin, 5-fluorouracil, methotrexate, and leucovorin over two to four months followed by standard radiation therapy and neck dissection when appropriate. With a total response rate of 75 per cent, a complete remission was noted in 29 per cent and partial remissions were noted in 46 per cent. The failure-free two-year survival rate for this series of advanced cases was 57 per cent, which represents a very favorable figure compared with other series in which radiation therapy alone was utilized. Furthermore, responsiveness to chemotherapy was associated with favorable treatment outcome after radiotherapy.

It is apparent that response to chemotherapy correlates with survival after locoregional therapy.[28, 49] An increase in the proportion of complete responses relative to partial responses very likely will improve survival, since

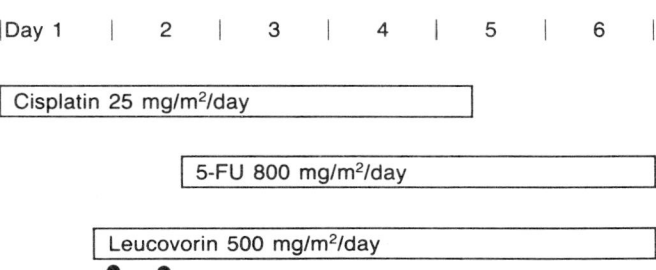

Figure 2–2. Induction chemotherapy utilizing cisplatin, 5-FU, and leucovorin. ● = blood samples obtained at 0 and 18 hours. Cycle length: 28 days; administration: intravenous, 24-hour continuous infusion of all drugs. (From Miller, D.: Nasopharyngeal cancer. *In* Gates, G. A. [Ed.]: Current Therapy in Otolaryngology—Head and Neck Surgery, 4th edition. Toronto, B. C. Decker, 1990.).

partial and lesser responses predict a poorer prognosis. More active chemotherapeutic regimens might accomplish a higher percentage rate of complete remission.

More recently, an induction protocol utilizing cisplatin, 5-fluorouracil, and leucovorin for stage III and IV squamous cell carcinoma of the head and neck has resulted in clinical responses in 78 per cent of 46 patients (Fig. 2–2).[50] Here complete remissions occurred in 65 per cent and the partial remissions in 13 per cent. After surgery or radiotherapy 80 per cent of patients were disease-free. Although follow-up evaluation is still limited, the increased activity of this regimen warrants further investigation into possible improved local control and failure-free survival in nasopharyngeal as well as other head and neck carcinomas.

CONCLUSION

Nasopharyngeal carcinoma presents challenges to the head and neck surgical oncologist. Diagnosis rests on clinical suspicion of a variety of often subtle symptoms. At the same time, early diagnosis allows detection of disease during its most curable stages. Therefore, aggressive office evaluation of the nasopharynx and early nasopharyngoscopy and biopsy are warranted in adults with unilateral serous otitis or cervical masses of unknown etiology. Radiotherapeutic management of these early lesions results in a high rate of cure.

The other challenge is to improve cure in patients with advanced disease. With current irradiation techniques having reached a plateau in controlling local disease and with the relatively high rate of distant metastasis, adjuvant therapy will be needed in the future in order to improve locoregional control and reduce systemic failures. Recent studies in which induction chemotherapy was used prior to standard treatment indicate that these goals may be approached by investigation of active drug regimens that offer high rates of complete remissions.

REFERENCES

1. Ho, J.H.: An epidemiologic and clinical study of nasopharyngeal carcinoma. Int. J. Radiat. Oncol. Bio. Phys. *4:*183, 1978.
2. Shanmugaratnam, K.: Nasopharynx. *In* Schottenfeld, D., and Fraumeni, J.F., Jr. (Eds.): Cancer Epidemiology and Prevention. Philadelphia, W.B. Saunders, 1982, pp. 536–553.
3. Buell, P.: Nasopharynx cancer in Chinese in California. Br. J. Cancer *19:*459, 1965.
4. de-Thé, G., Ho, J.H.C., Ablashi, D.V., et al.: Nasopharyngeal carcinoma IX-Antibodies to EBNA and correlation with response to other EBV antigens in Chinese patients. Int. J. Cancer *16:*713–721, 1975.
5. Henle, W., Ho, H.C., and Kwan, H.C.: Antibodies to Epstein-Barr virus related antigens in nasopharyngeal carcinoma: Comparison of active cases with long term survivors. J. Natl. Cancer Instit. *51:*361–369, 1973.
6. Ho, H.C., Ng, M.H., Kwan, H.C., and Chan, J.C.W.: Epstein-Barr virus-specific IgA and IgG serum antibodies in nasopharyngeal carcinoma. Br. J. Cancer *34:*655, 1976.
7. Klein, G., Giovanella, B.C., Lindahl, T., et al.: Direct evidence for the presence of Epstein-Barr virus DNA and nuclear antigen in malignant epithelial cells from patients with poorly differentiated carcinoma of the nasopharynx. Proc. Natl. Acad. Sci. *71:*4737, 1974.
8. Simons, M.H., Wee, G.B., Day, N.E., et al.: Immunogenetic aspects of nasopharyngeal carcinoma: I. Differences in HL-A antigen profiles between patients and control groups. Int. J. Cancer *13:*122, 1974.

9. Simons, M.H., Wee, G.B., Goh, E.H., et al.: Immunogenetic aspects of nasopharyngeal carcinoma: IV. Increased risk in Chinese of nasopharyngeal carcinoma associated with a Chinese-related HLA profile (A_2, Singapore 2). J. Natl. Cancer Inst. 57:977, 1976.
10. Armstrong, R.W., Armstrong, M.J., Yu, M.C., and Henderson, B.E.: Salted fish and inhalants as risk factors for nasopharyngeal carcinoma in Malaysian Chinese. Cancer Res. 43:2967, 1983.
11. Henderson, B.E., Louie, E., SooHoo Jing, J.S., et al.: Risk factors associated with nasopharyngeal carcinoma. N. Engl. J. Med. 295:1101, 1976.
12. Lindberg, R.D.: Distribution of cervical lymph node metastases from squamous cell carcinoma of the upper respiratory and digestive tracts. Cancer 29:1446, 1972.
13. Neel, H.B., III, Taylor, W.F., Prasad, U., et al.: Clinical presentation and diagnosis of nasopharyngeal carcinoma: Current status. *In* Neel, H.B. III, Taylor, W.F., Prasad, U., et al. (Eds.): Nasopharyngeal Carcinoma: Current Concepts. Kuala Lumpur, University of Malaya, 1983.
14. Dickson, R.I.: Nasopharyngeal carcinoma: An evaluation of 209 patients. Laryngoscope 91:333, 1981.
15. Hara, H.J.: Cancer of the nasopharynx: Review of the literature (Report of 72 Cases). Laryngoscope 79:1315, 1969.
16. Scanlon, P.W., Rhodes, R.E., Jr., Woolner, L.B., et al.: Cancer of the nasopharynx: 142 patients treated in the 11-year period 1950–1960. Am. J. Roentgenol. 99:313, 1967.
17. Hopping, S.B., Keller, J.D., Goodman, M.L., and Montgomery, W.W.: Nasopharyngeal masses in adults. Ann. Otol. Rhinol. Laryngol. 92:137–140, 1983.
18. Ablashi, D.V., Levine, P.H., Prasad, U., et al.: Application of field and laboratory studies to the control of NPC: Report from the Fourth International Symposium on Nasopharyngeal Carcinoma. Cancer Res. 43:2375, 1983.
19. Pearson, G.R., Weiland, L.H., Neel, H.B., et al.: Application of Epstein-Barr virus (EBV) serology to the diagnosis of North American nasopharyngeal carcinoma. Cancer 51:260, 1983.
20. Neel, H.B., III, Pearson, G.R., Weiland, L.H., et al.: Application of Epstein-Barr virus serology to the diagnosis and staging of North American patients with nasopharyngeal carcinoma. Otolaryngol. Head Neck Surg. 91:255, 1983.
21. Henle, W., Ho, J.H., Henle, G., et al.: Nasopharyngeal carcinoma: Significance of changes in Epstein-Barr virus-related antibody patterns following therapy. Int. J. Cancer 20:663, 1977.
22. Neel, H.B., III, Pearson, G.R., and Taylor, W.: Antibodies to Epstein-Barr virus in patients with nasopharyngeal carcinoma and in comparison groups. Ann. Otol. Rhinol. Laryngol. 93:477–482, 1984.
23. Bedwinek, J.M., Perez, C.A., and Keys, D.J.: Analysis of failures after definitive irradiation for epidermoid carcinoma of the nasopharynx. Cancer 45:2725, 1980.
24. Shanmugaratnam, K., and Sobin, L.H.: Histological typing of upper respiratory tract tumors. International Histologic Typing of Tumors. Geneva, World Health Organization, 1978.
25. Applebaum, E.L., Mantravadi, P., and Haas, R.: Lymphoepithelioma of the nasopharynx. Laryngoscope 92:510, 1982.
26. Bloom, M.S.: Cancer of the nasopharynx with special reference to the significance of histopathology. Laryngoscope 71:1207, 1961.
27. Hoppe, R.T., Goffinet, D.R., and Bagshaw, M.A.: Carcinoma of the nasopharynx: Eighteen years' experience with megavoltage radiation therapy. Cancer 37:2605, 1976.
28. Clark, J.R., Norris, C.M., Jr., Dreyfuss, A.I., et al.: Nasopharyngeal carcinoma: The Dana-Farber Cancer Institute experience with 24 patients treated with induction chemotherapy and radiotherapy. Ann. Otol. Rhinol. Laryngol. 96:608–614, 1987.
29. Banks, P.M.: Diagnostic applications of an immunoperoxidase method in hematopathology. J. Histochem. Cytochem. 27:1192, 1979.
30. Beahrs, O.H., Henson, D.E., Hutter, R.V.P., Myers, M.H. (Eds.): American Joint Committee for Cancer Staging and End Result Reporting: Manual for Staging of Cancer. 3rd ed. Philadelphia, J.B. Lippincott, 1988.
31. Harmer, M.H.: TNM Classification of Malignant Tumours, ed. 3. Geneva, Union Internationale Contre le Cancer, 1978.
32. Ho, J.H.: Stage classification of nasopharyngeal carcinoma: A review. IARC Sci. Publ. 20:99, 1978.
33. Baker, S.R.: Nasopharyngeal carcinoma: Clinical course and results of therapy. Head Neck Surg. 3:8–14, 1980.
34. Neel, H.B., III, Taylor, W.F., and Pearson, G.R.: Prognostic determinants and a new view of staging for patients with nasopharyngeal carcinoma. Ann. Otol. Rhinol. Laryngol. 94:529–537, 1985.
35. Qin, D., Hu, Y., Jiehua, Y., et al.: Analysis of 1379 patients with nasopharyngeal carcinoma treated by radiation. Cancer 61:1117–1124, 1988.

36. Wang, C.C., Busse, J., and Gitterman, M.: A simple afterloading applicator for intracavitary irradiation for carcinoma of the nasopharynx. Radiology *115:*737, 1975.
37. Parsons, J.T., Fitzgerald, C.R., Hood, C.I., et al.: The effects of irradiation on the eye and optic nerve. Int. J. Radiat. Oncol. Biol. Phys. *9:*609, 1983.
38. Samaan, N.A., Vieto, R., Schultz, P.N., et al.: Hypothalamic, pituitary and thyroid dysfunction after radiotherapy to the head and neck. Int. J. Radiat. Oncol. Biol. Phys. *8:*1857, 1982.
39. Moench, H.C., and Phillips, T.L.: Carcinoma of the nasopharynx: Review of 146 patients with emphasis on radiation dose and time factors. Am. J. Surg. *124:*515, 1972.
40. Shanmugaratnam, K., Chan, S.H., de-The, G., et al.: Histopathology of nasopharyngeal carcinoma. Cancer *44:*1029–1044, 1979.
41. Mesic, J.B., Fletcher, G.H., and Goepfert, H.: Megavoltage irradiation of epithelial tumors of the nasopharynx. Int. J. Radiat. Oncol. Biol. Phys. *7:*447, 1981.
42. Wang, C.C.: Radiation therapy for head and neck neoplasms: Indications, techniques and results. Boston, John Wright-PSG Inc, 1983.
43. Perez, C.A., Ackerman, L.V., Mill, W.B., et al.: Cancer of the nasopharynx: Factors influencing prognosis. Cancer *24:*1, 1969.
44. Meyer, J.E., and Wang, C.C.: Carcinoma of the nasopharynx: Factors influencing results of therapy. Radiology *100:*385, 1971.
45. Fisch, U.: The infratemporal fossa approach for nasopharyngeal tumors. Laryngoscope *93:*36, 1983.
46. Panje, W.R., and McCabe, B.F.: Transparotid approach to the skull base. *In* Sasaki, C., McCabe, B., and Kirchner, J. (Eds.): Surgery of the Skull Base. Philadelphia, J.B. Lippincott, 1984, pp. 125–140.
47. Hsu, M., and Lin, B.: Characterization of T cell subsets using monoclonal antibodies in nasopharyngeal carcinoma patients. Ann. Otol. Rhinol. Laryngol. *95:*298–301, 1986.
48. Rahima, M., Rakowsky, E., Barzilay, J., and Sidi, J.: Carcinoma of the nasopharynx: An analysis of 91 cases and a comparison of differing treatment approaches. Cancer *58:*843–849, 1986.
49. Ervin, T.J., Clark, J.C., Weichselbaum, R.R., et al.: An analysis of induction and adjuvant chemotherapy in the multidisciplinary treatment of squamous-cell carcinoma of the head and neck. J. Clin. Oncol. *5:*10–20, 1987.
50. Dreyfuss, A.I., Clark, J.R., Wright, J.E., et al.: Continuous infusion high-dose leucovorin with 5-fluorouracil and cisplatin for untreated stage IV carcinoma of the head and neck. Ann. Intern. Med. *112:*167–172, 1990.
51. Miller, D.D.: Nasopharyngeal cancer. *In* Gates, G.A. (Ed.): Current Therapy in Otolaryngology—Head and Neck Surgery, 4th ed. Toronto, B.C. Decker, 1990.

3

ESOPHAGEAL CARCINOMA

by F. Henry Ellis, Jr., M.D., Ph.D.

Carcinoma of the esophagus is not a common disease in the United States in comparison with its high incidence in some nearly endemic areas of the world. Only an estimated 10,900 carcinomas of the esophagus, 4 per cent of all digestive tract cancers, occurred during 1991.[1] However, if malignant tumors that involve the esophagogastric junction are included, the total number of cases will be nearly doubled because carcinoma of the gastric cardia, which will be discussed in a later chapter, has not shared in the overall decline of gastric malignancies. The incidence of carcinoma of the esophagus is increasing among black men in the United States, and there is suggestive evidence that the incidence of adenocarcinoma in patients with Barrett's esophagus is also on the increase.

Although the overall prognosis for patients with carcinoma of the esophagus remains poor, it is considerably better than it was in the past, and, in my opinion, current pessimism regarding therapy has been overstated. Untreated patients survive a relatively short time, usually four months or less, after the diagnosis of cancer. Long-term survival is rare, even with current forms of therapy, because it is estimated that more than half of the lesions have metastasized before a diagnosis has been made. On the other hand, patients with this disease are currently seeking medical care sooner than in past years. This fact, coupled with a more aggressive surgical approach that has increased operability and resectability rates and has produced lower mortality and morbidity rates, has led to an improvement in overall postoperative survival statistics. Today, operation provides the most effective palliation of dysphagia, the main symptom of the disease. Patients live longer, and there are more long-term survivors after resection than after other forms of treatment. The emphasis in this chapter is on the surgical management of carcinoma of the esophagus.

DEMOGRAPHY

Carcinoma of the esophagus occurs predominantly in men by a ratio of 3 or 4 to 1 and affects individuals in older age groups, primarily in the seventh and eighth decades of life, although young adults are not exempt. In the United States the death rate for carcinoma of the esophagus among white men is 3.5 per 100,000 and among black men is 13.3 per 100,000.[2] The highest incidence appears to be in China in the Lin Xian county of the Henan Province, where carcinoma of the esophagus occurs at a rate of 130 to 161 per 100,000.[3,4] The incidence is also high in the Caspian littoral of Iran, where the incidence is 93 per 100,000 men and 110 per 100,000 women.[5] The disease also occurs frequently in the Transkei in South Africa[6] and in the regions of Brittany and Normandy of northern France. The incidence of carcinoma of the esophagus is also high in some Moslem Soviet republics.

ETIOLOGY

Surprisingly, the marked geographic differences in the incidence of carcinoma of the esophagus have not yielded more useful information concerning the cause of the disease. A variety of etiologic factors are probably involved. Genetic factors do not seem to play a role except in individuals with the rare condition of keratosis palmaris et plantaris (tylosis), which is inherited as an autosomal dominant trait.[7] Dietary factors may play a role because concentrations of nitrosamines and their precursors (nitrates and nitrites) are high in food and water samples from areas in China with a high incidence of esophageal carcinoma.[8] In these regions, the consumption of moldy and fermented foods that are heavily contaminated by fungi, thus promoting the synthesis of nitrosamines, is high. Nitrosamines and alcoholic beverages have been implicated in the high incidence of this disease among the Bantu in South Africa.[9] Alcohol and tobacco, which have been found to contain nitrosamine compounds, have also been implicated in the occurrence of carcinoma of the esophagus in the northern coastal region of France[10] and in the United States.[11] Apparently ethanol and nicotine act synergistically through an unknown mechanism to produce a higher rate of esophageal cancer than can be caused by either drug alone.[12] A low socioeconomic background and a deficient diet may be factors common to all high incidence areas of this disease.

Although the precise role of various carcinogens in the development of esophageal cancer remains conjectural, the occurrence of certain precancerous lesions has been recognized for a long time. The incidence of carcinoma of the esophagus among patients with achalasia is approximately seven times greater than that of healthy individuals,[13] and the tumor has been shown to occur with increasing frequency in patients with Paterson-Kelley (Plummer-Vinson) syndrome.[14] The incidence of carcinoma of the esophagus in patients with caustic injury of this organ who are observed for 24 years or more has been reported to be a thousand times greater than in the normal population.[15] Studies on the association between adenocarcinoma of the esophagus and Barrett's esophagus have revealed a prevalence ranging from 8.6 per cent to almost 50 per cent, depending on the patient population observed.[16,17]

The risk of carcinoma that develops in patients with Barrett's esophagus is difficult to determine. Incidence rates ranging from 1 per 81 to 1 per 441 patient years of follow-up have been reported.[18, 19] Additional studies are needed to identify the risk of carcinoma developing in patients with Barrett's mucosa.

PATHOLOGY

Malignant lesions can occur at any level of the esophagus. When the esophagogastric junctional area is included, almost 50 per cent of surgically treated malignant lesions occur at this level (Fig. 3–1). Of the remaining tumors, half occur in the upper thoracic and cervical esophagus and half in the lower thoracic esophagus.

Squamous Cell Carcinoma

Squamous cell carcinoma (Fig. 3–2A) is the most common malignant tumor, accounting for approximately two-thirds of all esophageal cancers. These tumors are usually fungating ulcerating lesions that project into the esophageal lumen. Submucosal spread and skip areas of microscopic carcinoma are common. Nodal metastases are present in about three-fourths of the patients who undergo operation. Local extension of the lesion may frequently involve vital intrathoracic structures, which can occasionally lead to catastrophic events such as tracheoesophageal fistula and massive hemor-

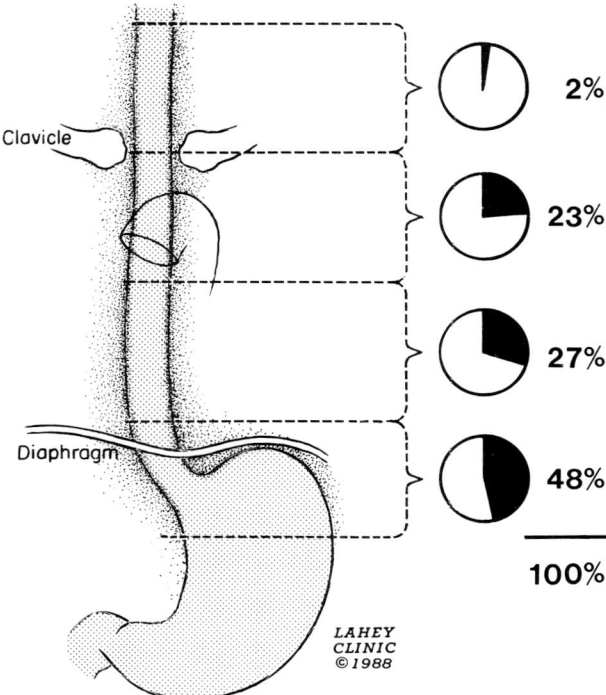

Figure 3–1. Location of surgically treated carcinomas of the esophagus and cardia. (Reprinted with permission of Lahey Clinic.)

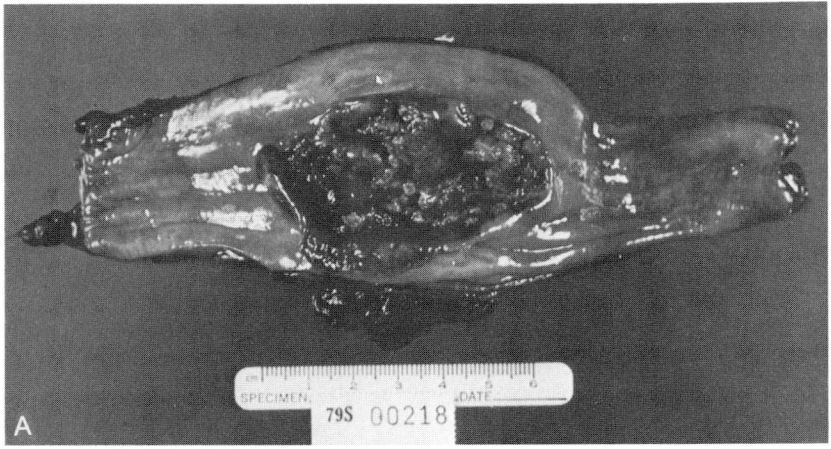
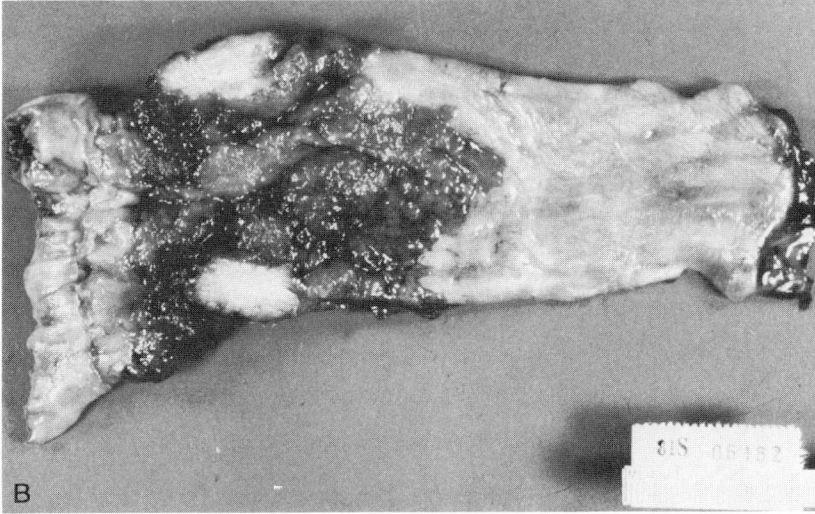

Figure 3–2. A, Macroscopic appearance of squamous cell carcinoma of esophagus. B, Adenocarcinoma in a Barrett's esophagus. (From Ellis, F. H., Jr., and Shahian, D. M.: Tumors of the esophagus. In Glenn, W. L. W., Baue, A. E., Geha, A. S., et al. (Eds.): Thoracic and Cardiovascular Surgery, 4th ed. Norwalk, CT, Appleton-Century-Crofts, 1983, p. 562.)

rhage. The liver and lungs are the most common sites of systemic spread; bone, kidneys, and adrenal glands are less commonly involved. The association of carcinoma of the esophagus with similar tumors in other portions of the respiratory tract, such as the mouth, larynx, and pharynx, is well known.

Adenocarcinoma

Adenocarcinoma (Fig. 3–2B), which is currently seen more frequently than in the past, is the next most common malignant lesion of the esophagus. Although in rare instances esophageal adenocarcinoma may arise from ectopic glandular rests in the upper esophagus,[20] most adenocarcinomas arise from Barrett's mucosa. In one series,[21] such lesions accounted for 86 per cent of all adenocarcinomas of the esophagus. The columnar epithelium of Barrett's esophagus adjacent to and remote from the invasive adenocarcinoma characteristically exhibits a spectrum of abnormalities that range from mild dysplasias to carcinoma in situ.

Carcinosarcoma and Pseudosarcoma

Carcinosarcoma and pseudosarcoma are less common lesions that usually present as bulky intraluminal polypoid growths. Both lesions are slow growing and require an aggressive surgical approach.

Miscellaneous Malignant Tumors

Sarcomas represent less than 1 per cent of all malignant esophageal neoplasms and include histologic diagnoses such as fibrosarcoma, leiomyosarcoma, and rhabdomyosarcoma. Plasmacytomas and lymphosarcomas have also been reported. Another rare esophageal tumor is primary melanoma of the esophagus, which occurs predominantly in the lower portion of the esophagus and tends to appear macroscopically as a bulky polypoid lesion. This tumor metastasizes early and is associated with a poor prognosis.[22]

Tumors that are similar in microscopic appearance to those that arise in the salivary glands account for a very small percentage of glandular tumors of the esophagus; only 27 such tumors had been reported prior to 1980.[23] These tumors are thought to arise from the ducts of the esophageal submucosal glands. Occasionally, an adenocarcinoma of the esophagus occurs in which squamous differentiation is evident—a tumor that has been termed *adenosquamous carcinoma*.

Another rare tumor whose biologic behavior makes it susceptible to cure is verrucous squamous cell carcinoma, which can be recognized macroscopically by its papillary or warty features.[24] Metastatic deposits from this tumor are rare. Oat cell carcinoma of the esophagus has also been reported.[25] These tumors are considered true apudomas that arise from the argyrophilic Kulchitsky's cells of the surface epithelium. Oat cell carcinomas are bulky and obstructive, slightly predominant in men, and usually occur in the lower esophagus. They are highly malignant lesions; no 5-year survivors have been reported.

DIAGNOSIS

Symptoms

Dysphagia is by far the most frequent complaint of patients with esophageal carcinoma and is usually apparent first with the ingestion of bulky foods, later with the ingestion of soft foods, and ultimately with liquids. Weight loss, regurgitation, and aspiration pneumonitis may also be present. Patients without dysphagia or odynophagia (pain on swallowing) may have gastroesophageal reflux symptoms, which are associated in some cases with minor degrees of blood loss. Massive bleeding, however, is uncommon unless the tumor has perforated a major vascular structure such as the aorta. Symptoms that have ominous significance include hoarseness, which is suggestive of recurrent nerve involvement, and coughing or choking after swallowing, which is suggestive of tracheobronchial involvement. Pain, an unusual symptom, may indicate local extension to adjacent structures, raising the issue of resectability.

Roentgenography

Esophageal roentgenography is an essential part of the work-up for a patient who complains of swallowing difficulty. The finding of an irregular, ragged mucosal pattern with luminal narrowing is typical of carcinoma of the esophagus (Fig. 3–3). Unlike benign obstructive lesions, carcinoma is not usually associated with proximal dilatation of the esophagus. Cinefluorography may also be useful in the diagnosis of problem cases. The exact role of computed tomography (CT) remains controversial. It may be helpful in identifying invasion of tissues outside the esophagus, although the accuracy of CT in defining resectability leaves much to be desired.[26]

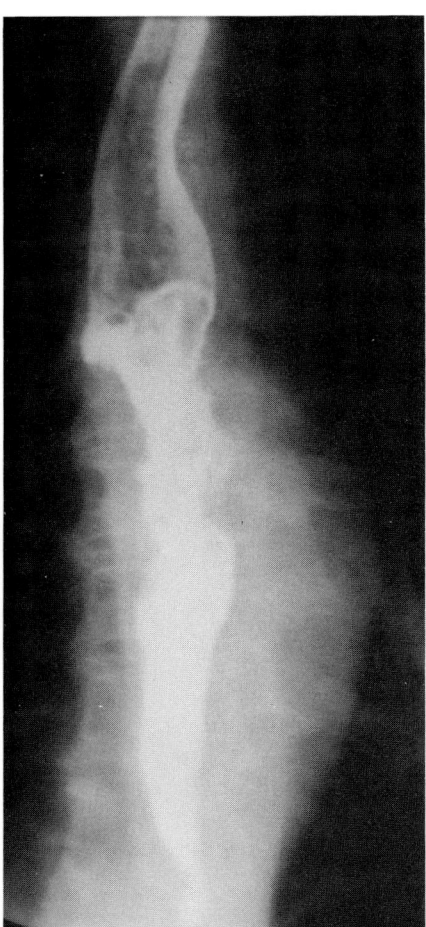

Figure 3–3. Roentgenographic appearance of carcinoma of upper thoracic esophagus.

Endoscopy

Esophagoscopy is required to confirm a clinical suspicion of carcinoma. The use of fiberoptic instruments has simplified the performance of this study, which must be associated with biopsy or brushings or both to provide histologic material for pathologic evaluation. Lesions that involve the upper portion of the thoracic esophagus near the tracheal carina necessitate bronchoscopy in addition to esophagoscopy to determine the presence or absence of involvement of the trachea or bronchial tree.

Screening Techniques

The use of supravital staining techniques as an aid to early diagnosis, with such agents as iodine (Lugol's) toluidine blue or indigo carmine, may help to identify potential biopsy sites during esophagoscopy. The addition of brush biopsy may provide useful material for cytologic study in patients at risk for the development of esophageal carcinoma. Another promising technique is the use of radioisotopes in tumor scanning. Materials preferentially picked up by esophageal cancer cells, such as gallium 67 or bleomycin Co 57, may be useful in early diagnosis.

TREATMENT

Until the diagnosis of esophageal carcinoma can be made earlier than is now possible, the main goal of therapy is palliation of the debilitating symptoms of dysphagia. Treatment can be divided into nonsurgical and surgical methods, the latter being preferred because its benefits far outweigh those of nonsurgical treatment. Accordingly, nonsurgical therapy should be reserved for patients who cannot undergo operative treatment for either medical or other reasons.

Nonsurgical Therapy

Radiotherapy

Squamous cell carcinoma is radiosensitive, and local tumor eradication is frequently obtainable, particularly for lesions above the aortic arch. When no metastatic deposits are detectable and the lesion is still limited to the mediastinum or supraclavicular areas, curative treatment to relieve symptoms and to prolong life may be successful. Occasionally, long-term survival may be obtained. Obstructive symptoms may be relieved in as many as 75 per cent of patients.[27] Furthermore, radiotherapy may provide satisfactory relief of pain in patients with local extension of disease. The usual therapeutic approach is to treat patients daily with fractionated radiotherapy of 9 to 10 Gy per week, the total curative tumor dose being in the range of 60 to 70 Gy. Intracavitary radiation (brachytherapy), using after-loading catheters in which a radioactive source is positioned to provide an intensive dose directly to the tumor, is associated with less danger to surrounding tissues. Preliminary results of this therapy are encouraging.[28]

The unusually good results of radiotherapy reported some 30 years ago and updated 10 years ago, when a 17 per cent 5-year survival rate was obtained using radiotherapy alone,[29] have not been duplicated in the United States. An exhaustive review of the literature by Earlam and Cunha-Melo[30] revealed only a 6 per cent 5-year survival rate using radiotherapy alone. Treatment with radiotherapeutic techniques is not without complications. These complications include radiation myelitis, esophagitis, pneumonitis, and mediastinal fibrosis. However, radiotherapy does provide temporary palliation of dysphagia for a significant number of patients. Unfortunately, the duration of palliation tends to be brief, and, if radiation stricture develops, the palliative effects of radiotherapy may be negated.

Chemotherapy

Chemotherapeutic drugs with activity against squamous cell carcinoma of the esophagus include cisplatin, bleomycin, methotrexate, 5-fluorouracil, Adriamycin, vindesine, mitomycin C, and CCNU (lomustine). Single-drug therapy with any one of these agents plays little role in the management of disease because response rates are low, ranging from 15 to 20 percent.[31] Multidrug therapy is associated with increased response rates of 33 to 63 per cent; however, the duration of the response is again brief, and the treatment is associated with considerable toxicity.[32]

The results of combined radiotherapy and chemotherapy have been somewhat better than with either therapy alone; a median survival of 22 months was reported in one series[33] and was associated with effective palliation of dysphagia. Patients with no clinical evidence of residual tumor after completion of therapy had a median survival of 35 months.

Endoprosthesis

A variety of prosthetic devices are currently available to permit peroral intubation of the area of malignant obstruction (Fig. 3–4). A recent review of the use of one of these devices in 400 patients, most of whom had esophageal cancer, identified a 95 per cent incidence of satisfactory tube function.[34] However, the treatment was not without complications. Bleeding occurred in 1 per cent of the patients, perforation in 7 per cent, migration

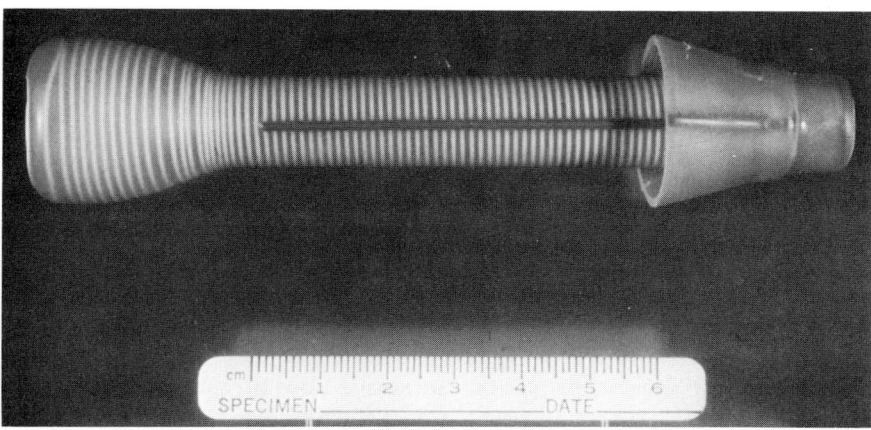

Figure 3–4. Modified Celestin tube for peroral endoscopic placement.

of the tube in 23 per cent, and obstruction of the tube in 6 per cent. The mortality rate was 4 per cent.

Miscellaneous

Dilation of malignant esophageal strictures may provide temporary relief of dysphagia,[35] and in some patients relief may be surprisingly long-lasting. Dilation is especially useful in preparing patients with inoperable disease for more definitive palliative therapy such as peroral pulsion intubation. The use of neodymium:yttrium aluminum garnet (Nd:YAG) laser coagulation as palliative therapy for obstructing esophageal carcinoma has aroused considerable interest among endoscopists. In a recent report on 76 patients, Nd:YAG laser treatment was successful in 86 per cent of the patients and rendered them either asymptomatic or able to ingest most solids.[36] The mortality rate from the procedure was 5 per cent, but the median survival of 19 weeks was no different from that of untreated patients. Another report, however, demonstrated a tripling of the survival interval after laser therapy when compared with that of controls.[37] Whether laser therapy will be preferred over bipolar electrocoagulation of the tumor remains to be determined.[38] Photoirradiation, whereby patients are presensitized with a hematoporphyrin derivative before treatment with light delivered by an argon-pumped dye laser, is also being studied with considerable enthusiasm.[39] Photoirradiation has proved to be an effective alternative to other forms of palliation. Its ultimate role in the therapeutic regimen of physicians caring for patients with esophageal carcinoma remains to be determined.

Surgical Therapy

Resection

Not all physicians agree that resection provides the best treatment for patients with carcinoma of the esophagus. This pessimistic view has been fostered to some extent by some discouraging results reported in the literature. Table 3–1 lists the results of treatment by resection in several large series of patients from different parts of the world during a recent 10-year period. Some of these reports also include data on the surgical treatment of carcinoma of the cardia. A wide variation in operability and hospital mortality rates as well as in 5-year survival rates is evident. The discouraging figures presented in the worldwide review of Earlam and Cunha-Melo[44] are based to some extent on outdated statistics. The figures quoted in the report of Wu and Huang,[41] in my opinion, more accurately reflect current-day practice, with high operability and resectability rates, low hospital mortality rates, and reasonable 5-year survival statistics. As a result of increasing operability and resectability rates as well as a falling hospital mortality rate, more treated patients are candidates for long-term survival than was true in the past.

Discouraged by the reported results after standard resection, some surgeons have elected to enlarge the extent of the operation to a super-radical procedure in highly selected favorable patients.[46, 56] This approach has resulted in higher mortality and morbidity rates and, as yet, has not resulted in any significant improvement in the overall 5-year survival rate.

TABLE 3-1. SURGERY FOR CARCINOMA OF THE ESOPHAGUS*

Author	Year	Country	Operability (%)	No. Cases	Resectability (%)†	Hospital Mortality (%)	5-Year Survival (%)‡
van Andel et al.[40]	1979	Holland	42	328	61	21.0	21
Wu and Huang[41]	1979	China	85	669	69	5.6	25
Griffith and Davis[42]	1980	England	NS	513	41	12.0	15
Giuli and Gignoux[43]	1980	Europe	NS	2400	NS	30.0	14
Earlam and Cunha-Melo[44]	1980	Review	58	83,783	67	33.3	16
Akiyama et al.[45]	1981	Japan	NS	354	59	1.4	35
Skinner[46]	1983	U.S.	66	181	80	11.0	18
Xu et al.[47]	1983	China	NS	850	78	10.0	22
Orringer[48]	1984	U.S.	NS	100	NS	6.0	17§
Ellis et al.[49]	1985	U.S.	80	219	87	2.1	16
Hennessy and O'Connell[50]	1986	Ireland	87	200	100	17.5	20
Bluett et al.[51]	1987	U.S.	46	144	72	10.0	13
Wong[52]	1987	Hong Kong	75	284	82	6.9	24‖
King et al.[53]	1987	U.S.	NS	100	NS	3.0	22.8
Mathisen et al.[54]	1988	U.S.	NS	104	NS	2.9	¶
Mansour and Downey[55]	1989	U.S.	NS	100	NS	3.0	NS

*Modified from Ellis, F. H., Jr.: Treatment of carcinoma of the esophagus or cardia. Mayo Clin. Proc. 64:945–955, 1989, with permission.
†Percentage of patients operated on
‡Percentage of patients surviving resection
§4-Year survival
‖3.5-Year survival
¶33.2 per cent for squamous cell carcinoma, 8 per cent for adenocarcinoma
NS = Not stated

Thus, I continue to support an aggressive surgical approach that employs standard resection for all patients with resectable disease. A brief description follows of my operative technique and a summarization of the results, which have been analyzed recently.[57]

For lesions at the esophagogastric junction and distal lower esophagus, esophagogastrectomy through a left thoracotomy is performed (Fig. 3–5). Access to the upper abdomen is obtained through a semilunar incision bordering the costal arch. The omentum and spleen are not removed unless involved by tumor, nor is the tail of the pancreas. Adequate margins of 5 cm or more on either side of the tumor are desired. After resection, gastrointestinal continuity is restored by an end-to-side two-layer esophagogastrostomy. For lesions in the upper thoracic esophagus, an Ivor-Lewis approach is preferred (Fig. 3–6). An intrathoracic esophagogastrostomy is performed at the level of the azygos vein or above. Only when frozen sections show extensive submucosal spread is it necessary to perform a third incision in the left neck to permit cervical esophagogastrostomy with uninvolved margins. If CT evaluation and exploration suggest that the lesion is confined to the esophagus proper and that it has not extended into surrounding tissue, a transhiatal approach is preferred for lesions at any level of the

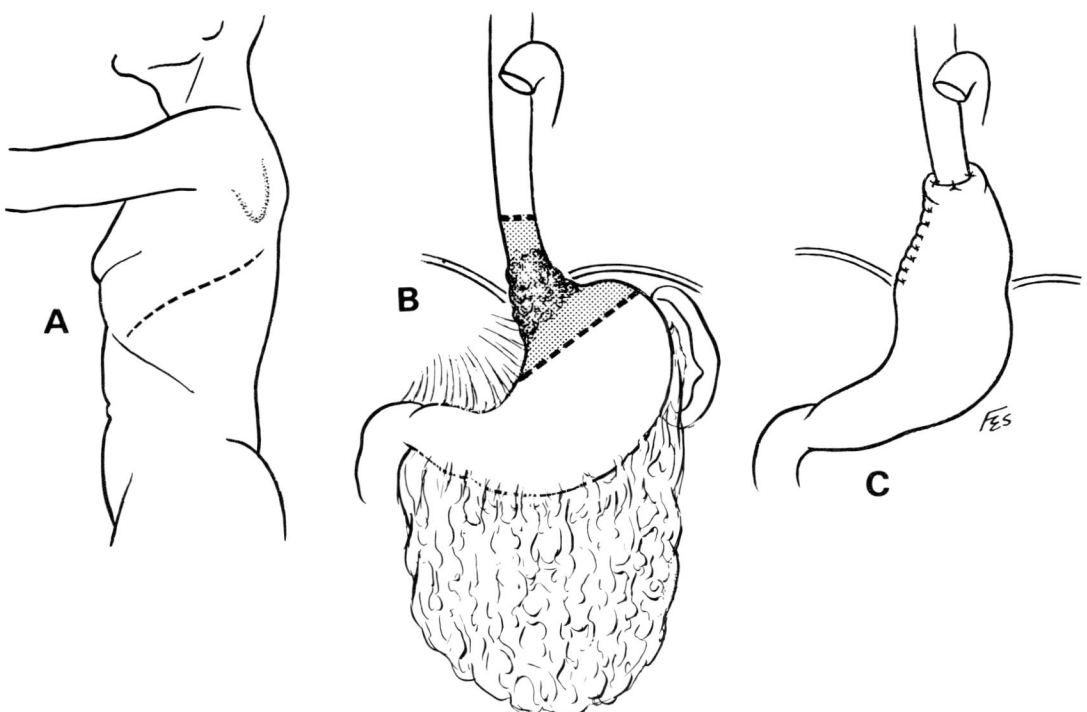

Figure 3–5. Technique of esophagogastrectomy and esophagogastrostomy for carcinoma of the cardia. *A,* Site of incision. *B,* Extent of resection (shaded area). *C,* Completed esophagogastrostomy. (Reproduced with permission from Ellis, F. H., Jr.: Surgical palliation: Esophageal resection—a surgeon's opinion. *In* Delarue, N. C., Wilkins, E. W., and Wong, J. [Eds.]: International Trends in General Thoracic Surgery, vol. 4. St. Louis, C. V. Mosby, 1988, p. 377.)

esophagus, particularly for those at the thoracic inlet and upper thoracic esophagus (Fig. 3–7). A colon interposition procedure is performed only on patients in whom an adequate amount of stomach is not available to function as an esophageal substitute.

Our experience with 366 patients operated on between 1970 and 1990 for carcinoma of the esophagus or cardia, all of whom were followed up, is listed in Table 3–2. Almost half of the lesions were adenocarcinomas of the esophagogastric junction. The overall operability rate was 81.7 per cent. Three hundred twenty-six patients (89.1 per cent) underwent resection. Eight patients died within 30 days, a mortality rate of 2.4 per cent. Postoperative complications developed in 84 patients, which were of major consequence in 43 patients (13.1 per cent) and of minor significance in 41 patients (12.6 per cent). The overall adjusted actuarial 5-year survival rate for patients surviving resection performed before 1989 was 20.8 per cent (Fig. 3–8). When only patients undergoing curative resection were considered, the overall survival was 23.3 per cent (Fig. 3–9). The importance of the stage of the disease on longevity is evident from the fact that nearly 40 per cent of the patients with stage I or stage IIA disease survived 5 years, whereas only about 13.0 per cent of the patients with stage IIB or stage III disease had a similar longevity (Fig. 3–10). No patient with stage IV disease survived more than two and one-half years. There was no statistically significant difference

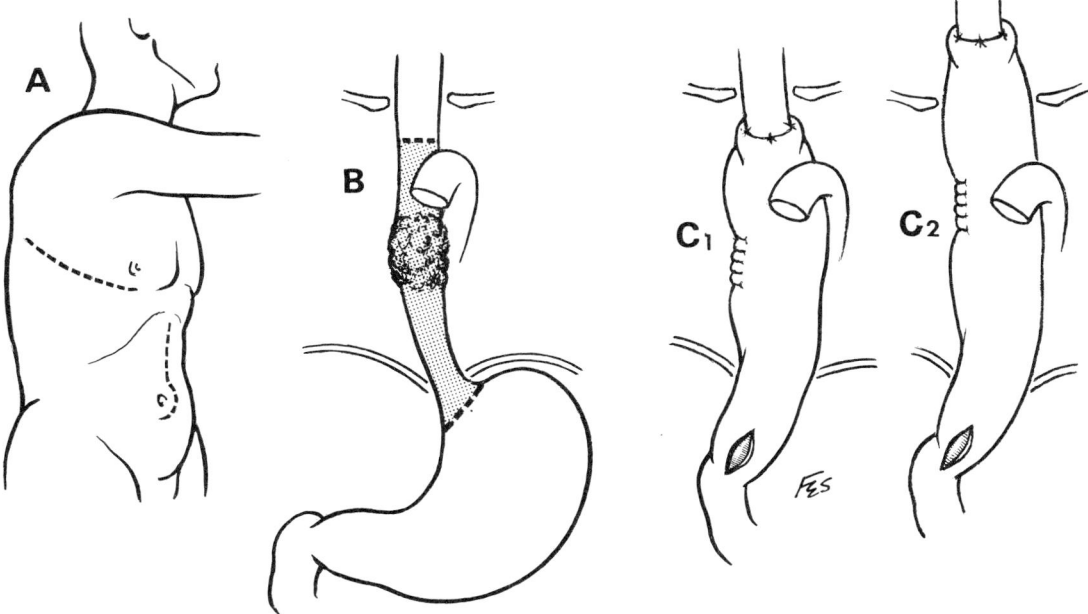

Figure 3–6. Combined abdominal incision and right thoracotomy for lesions of the upper thoracic esophagus. *A*, Site of incisions. *B*, Extent of resection (shaded area). *C*(1), Esophagogastrostomy can be performed within the chest. *C*(2), If submucosal spread is present, cervical anastomosis through a third incision can be made. (From Ellis, F. H., Jr.: Esophagogastrectomy for carcinoma: Technical considerations based on anatomic location of lesion. Surg. Clin. North Am. *60*:273, 1980.)

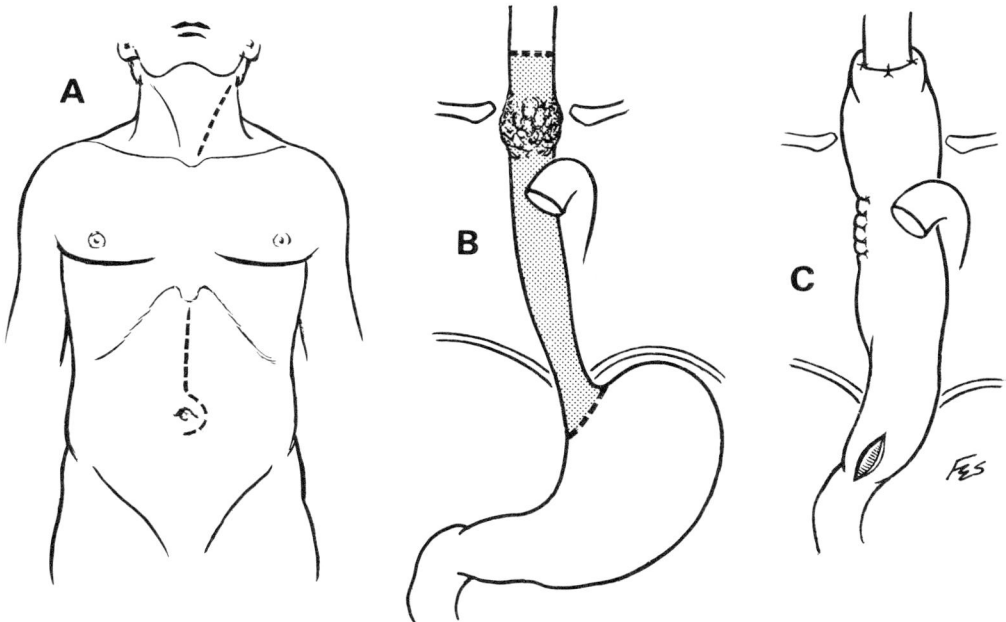

Figure 3–7. For esophagectomy without thoracotomy the patient is in the supine position. *A*, Upper midline and surgical incisions (broken) are made. *B*, Extent of resection (shaded area). *C*, Completed anastomosis. (From Ellis, F. H., Jr.: Esophagogastrectomy for carcinoma: Technical considerations based on anatomic location of lesion. Surg. Clin. North Am. *60*:275, 1980.)

in survival figures when squamous cell carcinoma, adenocarcinoma of the cardia, and adenocarcinoma in Barrett's esophagus were compared. Palliation was achieved in 80 per cent of the patients as demonstrated by the ability to swallow satisfactorily.

Combined Therapy

Adjunctive therapies, such as preoperative radiotherapy, chemotherapy, or chemoradiotherapy, have been used as alternative therapeutic options in an effort to improve the survival statistics after surgical treatment. Two prospective randomized controlled studies comparing operation alone with operation plus preoperative radiotherapy did not identify any advantage of the combined approach.[58, 59] However, evidence exists that, in certain cases, postoperative radiotherapy may have some advantages.[60]

A variety of combinations of drugs have been used preoperatively in an effort to improve overall results. All of these combinations have included cisplatin. Overall drug toxicity appears tolerable, and operative morbidity and mortality remain low. Overall response rates in terms of regression or elimination of the primary tumor have ranged from 40 to 60 per cent.[61, 62] Although the short-term survival of patients undergoing combined therapy appears to have improved over that of historical controls and is better in patients who have exhibited a complete response to chemotherapy, there is as yet no convincing evidence that long-term survival has been beneficially affected.[63]

The same may be said for preoperative chemoradiation.[61, 64, 65] Early encouragement has not been borne out by any meaningful impact on long-term survival. Although protocols vary, in general the duration of treatment is prolonged, with three or four weeks of chemotherapy and radiotherapy followed by a three-week interval before initiating operation. After operation, chemotherapy, radiotherapy, or both may be resumed in selected patients. Thus, treatment may last for two or three months compared with the two weeks or more required for operation alone. Only time will tell whether this form of therapy will prove to have a significant impact on survival rates.

TABLE 3–2. TREATMENT OF CARCINOMA OF THE ESOPHAGUS OR CARDIA: OVERALL OPERABILITY 81.7%

	No.	%
Total operations	366	
Resections	326	89.1
30-Day mortality	8	2.5
Complications	84	
Major	43	13.1
Minor	41	12.6
5-Year survival		
Overall		20.8
Curative resection		23.3
Stage I		40.4 ± 19.4
Stage IIA		37.7 ± 7.0
Stage IIB		13.0 ± 7.9
Stage III		12.4 ± 3.6
Stage IV		0
Palliation of dysphagia		80.0

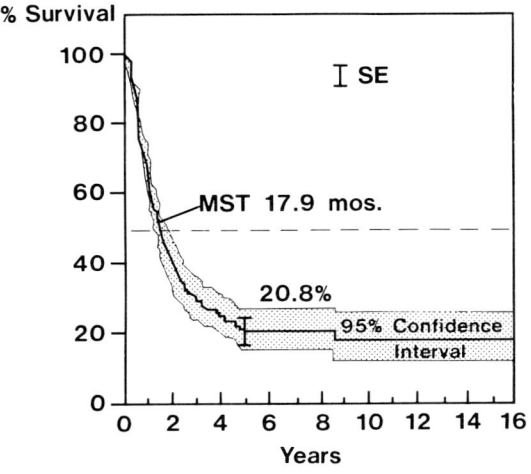

Figure 3–8. Adjusted actuarial survival rates for all patients surviving resection performed before 1989. SEM = Standard error of the mean; MST = Median survival time. (From Ellis, F. H., Jr.: Treatment of carcinoma of the esophagus or cardia. Mayo Clin. Proc. 64:950, 1989.)

Surgical Bypass

When local extension of the tumor prohibits resection, a variety of surgical options remain. For nonresectable lesions at the cardia, side-to-side esophagogastrostomy around the tumor that leaves the carcinoma in situ, as originally proposed by d'Allaines and associates,[66] can provide excellent palliation with a reasonably low mortality rate. When the lesion is located at a higher level in the thoracic esophagus, an operation first proposed by Kirschner[67] provides useful palliation. As modified by Ong,[68] the operation consists of thorough mobilization of the stomach, division and closure of the distal esophagus, and substernal placement of the stomach to facilitate cervical esophagogastrostomy after transection of the cervical esophagus and suture closure of its distal end. This procedure is particularly applicable to patients with a malignant tracheoesophageal fistula but is not without risk and should be used only when the patient's condition permits because the reported mortality rate has been high.[69]

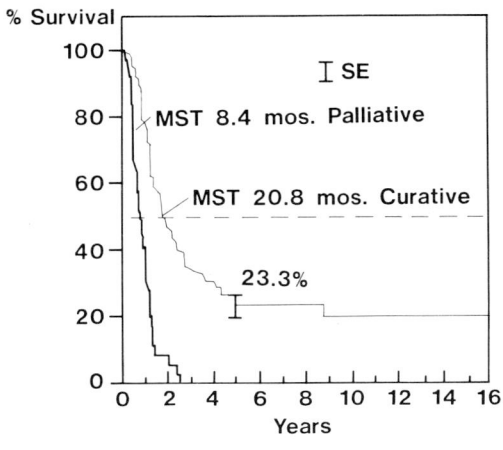

Figure 3–9. Adjusted actuarial survival rate for palliative resection compared with curative resection performed before 1989. (From Ellis, F. H., Jr.: Treatment of carcinoma of the esophagus or cardia. Mayo Clin. Proc. 64:951, 1989.)

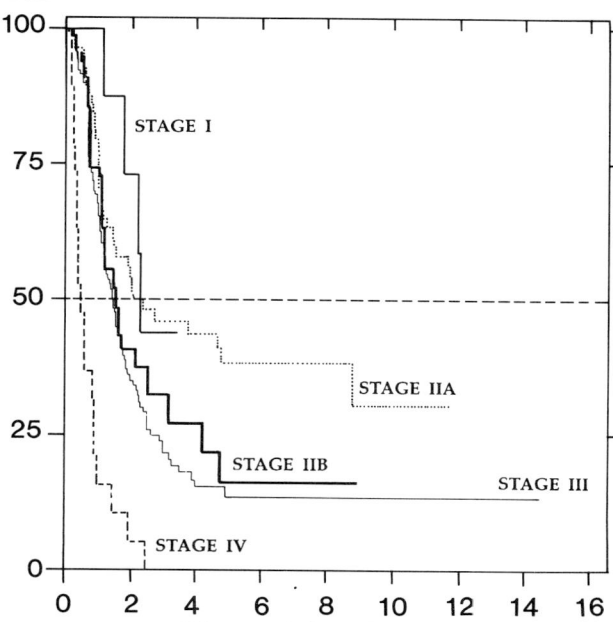

Figure 3–10. Adjusted actuarial survival rates after resection performed before 1989 according to stage of disease.

Traction Intubation

When the lesion proves to be nonresectable, another treatment alternative is intraoperative placement of a plastic prosthesis across the obstruction. This approach is not without risk. Complications, such as dislodgment, hemorrhage, and perforation, are all potential hazards of this technique, which was associated with a hospital mortality rate of 18 per cent in one series.[70] Some favor endoscopic intubation over surgical intubation for this reason.[71] Both techniques may provide satisfactory palliation; yet patients must restrict themselves to a mechanically soft diet, and the longevity is not different from that for untreated patients.

Gastrostomy

A feeding gastrostomy or jejunostomy as a palliative procedure is mentioned only to be condemned. These procedures provide no palliation because they do not restore the swallowing mechanism and are not without risk. Occasionally, such procedures may be justified as a temporizing measure between the stages of a reconstructive procedure, such as a colon interposition operation, or to maintain adequate nutrition in a patient undergoing chemotherapy or radiotherapy in anticipation of normal alimentation.

REFERENCES

1. Bomag, C.C., Squires, T.S. and Tong, T.: Cancer statistics, 1991. CA *41*:19–30, 1991.
2. Garfinkel, L., Poindexter, C.E., and Silverberg, E.: Cancer in black Americans. CA *30*:39–44, 1980.
3. Day, N.E.: Some aspects of the epidemiology of esophageal cancer. Cancer Res. *35*(11 Pt. 2):3304–3307, 1975.

4. Qui, S., and Yang, G.: Precursor lesions of esophageal cancer in high-risk populations in Henan Province, China. Cancer 62:551–557, 1988.
5. Mahboubi, E.O., and Aramesh, B.: Epidemiology of esophageal cancer in Iran, with special reference to nutritional and cultural aspects. Prev. Med. 9:613–621, 1980.
6. Rose, E.F.: Cancer of the esophagus. S. Afr. J. Hosp. Med. 4:110–112, 1978.
7. Lynch, H.T., and Lynch, P.M.: Heredity and gastrointestinal tract cancer. In Litkin, M., and Good, R.A. (Eds.): Gastrointestinal Tract Cancer. New York, Plenum Publishing Co., 1978, pp. 241–274.
8. Yang, C.S.: Research on esophageal cancer in China: A review. Cancer Res. 40:2633–2644, 1980.
9. McGlashan, N.D., Walters, C.L., and McLean, A.E.: Nitrosamines in African alcoholic spirits and oesophageal cancer. Lancet 2:1017, 1968.
10. Tuyns, A.J., Péquignot, G., and Jensen, D.M.: Role of diet, alcohol, and tobacco in oesophageal cancer as illustrated by two contrasting high-incidence areas in the north of Iran and west of France. Front. Gastrointest. Res. 4:101–110, 1979.
11. Wynder, E.L., and Bross, I.J.: A study of etiological factors in cancer of the esophagus. Cancer 14:389–413, 1961.
12. Fielding, J.E.: Smoking: Health effects and control (1). N. Engl. J. Med. 313:491–498, 1985.
13. Wychulis, A.R., Woolam, G.L., Andersen, H.A., and Ellis, F.H., Jr.: Achalasia and carcinoma of the esophagus. JAMA 215:1638–1641, 1971.
14. Larsson, L.G., Sandström, A., and Westling, P.: Relationship of Plummer-Vinson disease to cancer of the upper alimentary tract in Sweden. Cancer Res. 35(11 Pt. 2):3308–3316, 1975.
15. Kiviranta, U.K.: Corrosion carcinoma of the esophagus: 381 cases of corrosion and 9 cases of corrosion carcinoma. Acta Otolaryngol. 42:89–95, 1952.
16. Naef, A.P., Savary, M., and Ozzello, L.: Columnar-lined lower esophagus: An acquired lesion with malignant predisposition. Report on 140 cases of Barrett's esophagus with 12 adenocarcinomas. J. Thorac. Cardiovasc. Surg. 70:826–835, 1975.
17. Skinner, D.B., Walther, B.C., Riddell, R.H., et al.: Barrett's esophagus: Comparison of benign and malignant cases. Ann. Surg. 198:554–565, 1983.
18. Sprung, J., Ellis, F.H., Jr., and Gibb, S.P.: Incidence of adenocarcinoma in Barrett's esophagus. Am. J. Gastroenterol. (abstr). 79:817, 1984.
19. Cameron, A.J., Ott, B.J., and Payne, W.S.: The incidence of adenocarcinoma in columnar-lined (Barrett's) esophagus. N. Engl. J. Med. 313:857–859, 1985.
20. Carrie, A.: Adenocarcinoma of upper end of the oesophagus arising from ectopic gastric epithelium. Br. J. Surg. 37:474, 1950.
21. Haggitt, R.C., Tryzelaar, J., Ellis, F.H., Jr., and Colcher, H.: Adenocarcinoma complicating columnar epithelium-lined (Barrett's) esophagus. Am. J. Clin. Pathol. 70:1–5, 1978.
22. Sabanathan, S., Eng, J., and Pradhan, G.N.: Primary malignant melanoma of the esophagus. Am. J. Gastroenterol. 84:1475–1481, 1989.
23. Bell-Thomson, J., Haggitt, R.C., and Ellis, F.H., Jr.: Mucoepidermoid and adenoid cystic carcinomas of the esophagus. J. Thorac. Cardiovasc. Surg. 79:438–446, 1980.
24. Meyerowitz, B.R., and Shea, L.T.: The natural history of squamous verrucose carcinoma of the esophagus. J. Thorac. Cardiovasc. Surg. 61:646–649, 1971.
25. McFadden, D.W., Rudnicki, M., and Talamini, M.A.: Primary small cell carcinoma of the esophagus. Ann. Thorac. Surg. 47:477–480, 1989.
26. Duignan, J.P., McEntee, G.P., O'Connell, D.J., et al.: The role of CT in the management of carcinoma of the oesophagus and cardia. Ann. R. Coll. Surg. Engl. 69:286–288, 1987.
27. Wara, W.M., Mauch, P.M., Thomas, A.N., and Phillips, T.L.: Palliation for carcinoma of the esophagus. Radiology 121(3 Pt. 1):717–720, 1976.
28. Rowland, C.G., and Pagliero, K.M.: Intracavitary irradiation in palliation of carcinoma of oesophagus and cardia. Lancet 2:981–983, 1985.
29. Pearson, J.G.: The present status and future potential of radiotherapy in the management of esophageal cancer. Cancer 39(suppl. 2):882–890, 1977.
30. Earlam, R., and Cunha-Melo, J.R.: Oesophageal squamous cell carcinoma: II. A critical review of radiotherapy. Br. J. Surg. 67:457–461, 1980.
31. Kelsen, D.: Chemotherapy of esophageal cancer. Semin. Oncol. 11:159–168, 1984.
32. Kelsen, D., Hilaris, B., Coonley, C., et al.: Cisplatin, vindesine, and bleomycin chemotherapy of local-regional and advanced esophageal carcinoma. Am. J. Med. 75:645–652, 1983.
33. Coia, L.R., Engstrom, D.F., and Paul, A.: Nonsurgical management of esophageal cancer: Report of a study of combined radiotherapy and chemotherapy. J. Clin. Oncol. 5:1783–1790, 1987.
34. Van der Brandt-Grädel, V., den Hartog Jager, F.C.A., and Tytgat, G.N.J.: Palliative intubation of malignant esophagogastric obstruction. J. Clin. Gastroenterol. 9:290–297, 1987.
35. Lundell, L., Leth, R., Lind, T., et al.: Palliative endoscopic dilatation in carcinoma of the esophagus and esophagogastric junction. Acta Chir. Scand. 155:179–184, 1989.

36. Krasner, N., Barr, H., Skidmore, C., and Morris, A.I.: Palliative laser therapy for malignant dysphagia. Gut 28:792–798, 1987.
37. Karlin, D.A., Fisher, R.S., and Krevsky, B.: Prolonged survival and effective palliation in patients with squamous cell carcinoma of the esophagus following endoscopic laser therapy. Cancer 59:1969–1972, 1987.
38. Jensen, D.M., Machicado, G., Randall, G., et al.: Comparison of low-power YAG laser and BICAP tumor probe for palliation of esophageal cancer strictures. Gastroenterology 94:1263–1270, 1988.
39. Thomas, R.J., Abbott, M., Bhathal, P.S., et al.: High-dose photoirradiation of esophageal cancer. Ann. Surg. 206:193–199, 1987.
40. van Andel, J.G., Dees, J., Dijkhuis, C.M., et al.: Carcinoma of the esophagus: Results of treatment. Ann. Surg. 190:684–689, 1979.
41. Wu, Y.K., and Huang, K.C.: Chinese experience in the surgical treatment of carcinoma of the esophagus. Ann. Surg. 190:361–365, 1979.
42. Griffith, J.L., and Davis, J.T.: A twenty-year experience with surgical management of carcinoma of the esophagus and gastric cardia. J. Thorac. Cardiovasc. Surg. 79:447–452, 1980.
43. Giuli, R., and Gignoux, M.: Treatment of carcinoma of the esophagus: Retrospective study of 2,400 patients. Ann. Surg. 192:44–52, 1980.
44. Earlam, R., and Cunha-Melo, J.R.: Oesophageal squamous cell carcinoma: I. A critical review of surgery. Br. J. Surg. 67:381–390, 1980.
45. Akiyama, H., Tsurumaru, M., Kawamura, T., and Ono, Y.: Principles of surgical treatment for carcinoma of the esophagus: Analysis of lymph node involvement. Ann. Surg. 194:438–446, 1981.
46. Skinner, D.B.: En bloc resection for neoplasms of the esophagus and cardia. J. Thorac. Cardiovasc. Surg. 85:59–71, 1983.
47. Xu, L.T., Sun, Z.F., Li, Z.J., and Wu, L.H.: Surgical treatment of carcinoma of the esophagus and cardiac portion of the stomach in 850 patients. Ann. Thorac. Surg. 35:542–547, 1983.
48. Orringer, M.B.: Transhiatal esophagectomy without thoracotomy for carcinoma of the thoracic esophagus. Ann. Surg. 200:282–288, 1984.
49. Ellis, F.H., Jr., Gibb, S.P., and Watkins, E., Jr.: Overview of the current management of carcinoma of the esophagus and cardia. Can. J. Surg. 28:493–496, 1985.
50. Hennessy, T.P., and O'Connell, R.: Carcinoma of the hypopharynx, esophagus and cardia. Surg. Gynecol. Obstet. 162:243–247, 1986.
51. Bluett, M.K., Sawyers, J.L., and Healy, D.: Esophageal carcinoma: Improved quality of survival with resection. Am. Surg. 53:126–132, 1987.
52. Wong, J.: Esophageal resection for cancer: The rationale of current practice. Am. J. Surg. 153:18–24, 1987.
53. King, R.M., Pairolero, P.C., Trastek, V.F., et al.: Ivor Lewis esophagogastrectomy for carcinoma of the esophagus: Early and late functional results. Ann. Thorac. Surg. 44:119–122, 1987.
54. Mathisen, D.J., Grillo, H.C., Wilkins, E.W., Jr., et al.: Transthoracic esophagectomy: A safe approach to carcinoma of the esophagus. Ann. Thorac. Surg. 45:137–143, 1988.
55. Mansour, K.A., and Downey, R.S.: Esophageal carcinoma: Surgery without perioperative adjuvant chemotherapy. Ann. Thorac. Surg. 48:201–205, 1989.
56. DeMeester, T.R., Zaninotto, G., and Johansson, K.E.: Selective therapeutic approaches to cancer of the lower esophagus and cardia. J. Thorac. Cardiovasc. Surg. 95:42–54, 1988.
57. Ellis, F.H., Jr.: Treatment of carcinoma of the esophagus or cardia. Mayo Clin. Proc. 64:945–955, 1989.
58. Launois, B., Delarue, D., Campion, J.P., and Kerbaol, M.: Preoperative radiotherapy for carcinoma of the esophagus. Surg. Gynecol. Obstet 153:690–692, 1981.
59. Gignoux, M., Roussel, A., Paillot, B., et al.: The value of preoperative radiotherapy in esophageal cancer: Results of a study of the E.O.R.T.C. World J. Surg. 11:426–432, 1987.
60. Kasai, M., Mori, S., and Watanabe, T.: Follow-up results after resection of thoracic esophageal carcinoma. World J. Surg. 2:543–551, 1978.
61. Kelsen, D.P.: Preoperative chemotherapy in esophageal carcinoma. World J. Surg. 11:433–438, 1987.
62. Hilgenberg, A.D., Carey, R.W., Wilkins, E.W., Jr., et al.: Preoperative chemotherapy, surgical resection, and selective postoperative therapy for squamous cell carcinoma of the esophagus. Ann. Thorac. Surg. 45:357–363, 1988.
63. Andersen, A.P., Berdal, P., Edsmyr, F., et al.: Irradiation, chemotherapy and surgery in esophageal cancer: A randomized clinical study. The first Scandinavian trial in esophageal cancer. Radiother. Oncol. 2:179–188, 1984.
64. Orringer, M.B., Forastiere, A.A., Perez-Tamayo, C., et al.: Chemotherapy and radiation therapy before transhiatal esophagectomy for esophageal carcinoma. Ann. Thorac. Surg. 49:348–355, 1990.

65. MacFarlane, S.D., Hill, L.D., Jolly, D.C., et al.: Improved results of surgical treatment for esophageal and gastroesophageal junction carcinomas after preoperative combined chemotherapy and radiation. J. Thorac. Cardiovasc. Surg. 95:415–422, 1988.
66. d'Allaines, F., DuBost, C., and Galley, J.J.: Oesophagogastrostomies palliatives sans résection dans les cancers de l'oesophage et du cardia. J. Chir. 65:289–301, 1949.
67. Kirschner, M.A.: Ein neues Verfahren der Oesophagoplastik. Arch. klin. Chir. 114:606–663, 1920.
68. Ong, G.B.: The Kirschner operation—a forgotten procedure. Br. J. Surg. 60:221–227, 1973.
69. Orringer, M.B.: Substernal gastric bypass of the excluded esophagus—results of an ill-advised operation. Surgery 96:467–470, 1984.
70. Saunders, N.R.: The Celestin tube in the palliation of carcinoma of the oesophagus and cardia. Br. J. Surg. 66:419–421, 1979.
71. Watson, A.: A study of the quality and duration of survival following resection, endoscopic intubation and surgical intubation in oesophageal carcinoma. Br. J. Surg. 69:585–588, 1982.

Discussion

by Sidney Levitsky, M.D.

This scholarly chapter, written by a senior thoracic surgeon with a personal operative experience for cancer of the esophagus and cardia exceeding 310 patients, places Dr. Ellis in the forefront of surgeons who believe that aggressive intervention by means of esophagogastrectomy is the best therapy for this disease for both extended survival and palliation (relief of dysphagia). Thus, operative intervention is advised, within limits, even in the presence of metastatic disease. While Ellis states that the current pessimism for treatment of carcinoma of the esophagus is overstated, the 5-year survival rate has remained relatively constant at below 8 per cent since 1950.[1, 2] However, he does present selected reports, including his own experience, that indicate 5-year survival rates to be up to the 20 to 25 per cent range following aggressive surgery.

While Ellis advocates an activist approach, others with similar impressive personal experiences argue against performing radical or palliative resection except in patients who have a favorable prognosis.[3, 4] Many of the differences debated by Ellis and other authors regarding resectional therapy could be resolved if a uniformly acceptable and relatively reproducible method of preoperative staging was available. Ellis, using the TMN system adopted in 1988 by the American Joint Committee on Cancer Staging and End Results Reporting,[5] demonstrates a stratification in 5-year survival between stages I and IIA compared with stages IIB, III, and IV. However, criteria for preoperative staging are not provided. Similarly, Skinner et al. suggest a variant of the TMN system, which has an added focus of measuring the number of lymph nodes involved and suffers from the same problem requiring intraoperative and postoperative analysis to achieve accurate staging.[6] DeMeester et al. suggest an intraoperative algorithm for both staging and decision-making to avoid "unhelpful" en bloc dissections of the esophagus.[3] Others stress that mediastinoscopy, celiotomy,[7] and laparoscopy[8] are useful in preoperative staging as a means of avoiding resectional therapy. In the future, the development of new technologies, such as endoscopic ultrasonography[9] and respiratory-gated magnetic resonance imaging,[10, 11] may allow precise staging to limit esophageal resectional therapy to a selected group of patients with the best possibility for extended survival.

Ellis exhibits little enthusiasm for multimodal therapy that consists of preoperative chemotherapy administered concurrently with radiotherapy prior to esophageal resection. In a discussion of a report by Orringer et al.,[12] Ellis argues that it is the responders, namely those patients (about 30 per cent in most series) treated with chemotherapy and/or radiotherapy, who appear to benefit the most from multimodal therapy. It is obvious that a prospective randomized study is required to settle this issue. In addition, the tumor biology of the responsive patient requires extensive study to determine which patients may benefit from this form of therapy.

REFERENCES

1. National Cancer Institute: End Results in Cancer. Bethesda, MD, Department of Health, Education and Welfare. Publication no. 4. 73:272, 1972.
2. Earlam, R., and Cunha-Melo, J.R.: Esophageal squamous cell carcinoma: I. A critical review of surgery. Br. J. Surg. 67:381, 1980.
3. DeMeester, T.R., Zaninotto, G., and Johansson, K-E.: Selective therapeutic approach to cancer of the lower esophagus and cardia. J. Thorac. Cardiovasc. Surg. 95:42, 1988.
4. Lund, O., Kimose, H.H., Aagaard, M.T., et al.: Risk stratification and long-term results after surgical treatment of carcinomas of the thoracic esophagus and cardia. A 25-year retrospective study. J. Thorac. Cardiovasc. Surg. 99:200, 1990.
5. American Joint Committee on Cancer: Manual for Staging of Cancer. Philadelphia, J.B. Lippincott, 1988.
6. Skinner, D.B., Ferguson, M.K., Soriano, A., et al.: Selection of operation for esophageal cancer based on staging. Ann. Surg. 204:391, 1986.
7. Murray, G.F., Wilcox, B.R., and Starek, P.J.K.: The assessment of operability of esophageal carcinoma. Ann. Thorac. Surg. 23:393, 1977.
8. Dagnini, G., Caldironi, M.W., Moren, G., et al.: Laparoscopy in abdominal staging of esophageal carcinoma. Gastrointest. Endosc. 32:400, 1986.
9. Takemoto, T., Ito, T., Aibe, T., et al.: Endoscopic ultrasonography in the diagnosis of esophageal carcinoma, with particular regard to staging it for operability. Endoscopy 18(suppl. 3):22, 1986.
10. Weiber, H.F., Lange, R., and Feussner, H.: How can one diagnose the early stage of esophageal cancer? Endoscopy 18(suppl. 3):2, 1986.
11. Hyman, R., Rehn, S., Glimolius, B., et al.: Magnetic resonance imaging, chest radiography, computed tomography and ultrasonography in malignant lymphoma. Acta Radiol. 28:253, 1987.
12. Orringer, M.B., Forastiere, A.A., Perez-Tamayo, C., et al.: Chemotherapy and radiation therapy before transhiatal esophagectomy for esophageal carcinoma. Ann. Thorac. Surg. 49:348, 1990.

4

PRIMARY LUNG CANCER

by Wilford B. Neptune, M.D.

INTRODUCTION

At the time of writing, the projected deaths from lung cancer for 1990 in the United States was to be more than 142,000 victims.[1] This is now the leading cause of death from cancer in men and women. The cure rate more than a decade ago was estimated at five per cent by the American Cancer Society; currently this has increased to 12 per cent.[2] This slight improvement, however, is undoubtedly due to earlier diagnosis and management, because the results of therapy, stage for stage, have been no different over the past four decades.[3, 4]

In spite of this grim outlook, primary carcinoma of the lung is selectively curable. Regardless of the stage of disease, it cannot be predicted which patients may be long-term survivors. In the absence of cure, most patients can be offered an improvement in the quality of life with a reasonable cost in terms of morbidity and mortality. Finally, there is every reason to believe, through published data, that if cigarette smoking were to be discontinued, primary lung cancer would virtually disappear.

This chapter represents a single philosophy in management of primary lung cancer based on observations made through thoracic surgery practice in an office with over 59 years of experience, dating back to Dr. Richard H. Overholt's first published report of a lobectomy for lung cancer in 1932.[5] In a series of more than 5000 patients with lung cancer, 48 per cent had undergone a surgical resection. When favorable, 48 per cent survived more than five years; when unfavorable, only 12 per cent survived more than five years.[6] The terms favorable and unfavorable were originally used to designate prognosis. Favorable referred to an operation where all tumor was satisfactorily removed, and there was no evidence of metastases to regional lymph nodes. Based on current staging criteria, most of these cases would now be classified as stage I with T_1 or T_2N_0 lesions (see Tables 4–1 to 4–7). Unfavorable meant that all tumor could not be removed, or that there were histologically verified lymph node metastasis. Most of these would now be

TABLE 4–1. DEFINITIONS OF THE CATEGORIES FOR CARCINOMA OF THE LUNG[7]

Category*	Definition
Primary Tumors (T)	
T_0	No evidence of primary tumor.
T_x	Tumor proved by the presence of malignant cells in bronchopulmonary secretions but not visualized radiographically or bronchoscopically; any tumor that cannot be assessed.
T_{IS}	Carcinoma in situ.
T_1	Tumor that is 3.0 cm or less in greatest diameter and without evidence of invasion proximal to a lobar bronchus at bronchoscopy.
T_2	Tumor more than 3.0 cm in greatest diameter or tumor of any size that invades the visceral pleura or has associated atelectasis or obstructive pneumonitis extending to the hilar region. At bronchoscopy, the proximal extent of demonstrable tumor must be within a lobar bronchus or at least 2.0 distal to the carina. Any associated atelectasis or obstructive pneumonitis must involve less than an entire lung, and there must be no pleural effusion.
T_3	Tumor of any size with direct extension into adjacent structure, such as parietal pleura or chest wall, diaphragm, or mediastinum and its contents, or tumor demonstrable bronchoscopically to involve a main bronchus less than 2.0 cm distal to the carina, or any tumor associated with atelectasis or obstructive pneumonitis of an entire lung or pleural effusion.
Nodal Involvement (N)	
N_0	No demonstrable metastasis to regional lymph nodes.
N_1	Metastasis to lymph nodes in peribronchial or ipsilateral hilar region or both, including direct extension.
N_2	Metastasis to lymph nodes in mediastinum.
Distant Metastasis (M)	
M_x	Not assessed.
M_0	No known distant metastasis.
M_1	Distant metastasis as in scalene, supraclavicular, cervical, or contralateral hilar lymph nodes, brain, bones, liver, or contralateral lung.

*Each case must be assigned the highest category of T, N, or M that describes the full extent of disease in that case.

classified as stage III with T_2 or T_3N_2 disease. Of the patients who did not have surgical removal of the tumor, being considered inoperable or nonresectable after exploration, only five per cent survived more than one year; of those who had removal of the tumor, regardless of the assessment concerning favorable or unfavorable, 40 per cent survived more than one year. These general statistics have been presented in numerous studies and will serve as reference points for all subsequent statistics that are based on personal cases unless noted otherwise.

RESULTS IN STAGE I DISEASE

There is little or no controversy in the management of stage I lung cancer. Surgical removal is the treatment of choice if at all feasible; and with

TABLE 4–2. STAGE GROUPING IN CARCINOMA OF THE LUNG

Occult Stage

$T_xN_0M_0$ — Occult carcinoma with bronchopulmonary secretions containing malignant cells but without other evidence of metastasis to regional lymph nodes or distant metastasis.

Stage I

$T_{IS}N_0M_0$ — Carcinoma in situ.

$T_1N_0M_0$ — Tumor that can be classified T_1 without any metastasis or with metastasis to the lymph nodes in the peribronchial or ipsilateral hilar region or tumor that can be classified T_2 without any metastasis to nodes or distant metastasis.
NOTE: $T_xN_1M_0$ and $T_0N_1M_0$ are also theoretically possible, but such a clinical diagnosis would be difficult if not impossible to make. If such a diagnosis is made it should be included in stage I.

Stage II

$T_2N_1M_0$ — Tumor classified as T_2 with metastasis to lymph nodes in peribronchial or ipsilateral hilar region only.

Stage III

T_3 with any N or M
N_2 with any T or M
M_1 with any T or N

Any tumor more extensive than T_2; any tumor with metastasis to lymph nodes in mediastinum; any tumor with distant metastasis.

TABLE 4–3. THE NEW INTERNATIONAL STAGING SYSTEM FOR LUNG CANCER[8]*

T_x Tumor proven by the presence of malignant cells in bronchopulmonary secretions but not visualized roentgenographically or bronchoscopically, or any tumor that cannot be assessed as in a retreatment staging.

T_0 No evidence of primary tumor.

T_{IS} Carcinoma in situ.

T_1 A tumor that is 3.0 cm or less in greatest dimension, surrounded by lung or visceral pleura, and without evidence of invasion proximal to a lobar bronchus at bronchoscopy.†

T_2 A tumor more than 3.0 cm in greatest dimension, or a tumor of any size that either invades the visceral pleura or has associated atelectasis or obstructive pneumonitis extending to the hilar region. At bronchoscopy, the proximal extent of demonstrable tumor must be within a lobar bronchus or at least 2.0 cm distal to the carina. Any associated atelectasis or obstructive pneumonitis must involve less than an entire lung.

T_3 A tumor of any size with direct extension into the chest wall (including superior sulcus tumors), diaphragm, or the mediastinal pleura or pericardium without involving the heart, great vessels, trachea, esophagus, or vertebral body, or a tumor in the main bronchus within 2 cm of the carina without involving the carina.

T_4 A tumor of any size with invasion of the mediastinum or involving heart, great vessels, trachea, esophagus, vertebral body or carcinoma, or presence of malignant pleural effusion.*

*This staging system has not been used in this presentation.
†See Table 4–6.

T_1 or $T_2N_0M_0$ disease, a 50 per cent five-year survival should be expected.[9] From a technical viewpoint, most stage I lesions are resectable; however, there are a few such patient cases with comorbid complications in which lesions are inoperable. In an even more favorable subset (T_1N_0), diagnosed by survey radiography of the chest while asymptomatic, the five-year survival approaches 80 per cent.[10-12] These are not isolated results but represent what can be achieved with early recognition and an aggressive approach to the problem. For these reasons, many clinicians disagree with the recent recommendation of the American Cancer Society to stop survey chest films.[13] This advice, essentially based on studies in the 1950s, is flawed because even though lesions were identified early, they were usually not definitively managed until they had progressed and became symptomatic or larger on subsequent chest films.[14] I believe that everyone past the age of 40 years should have a yearly chest x-ray; if the patient has any history of smoking, this should be increased to twice a year.

The favorable results that can be obtained in stage I lung cancer, however, accentuate the need for an effective adjuvant therapy for cases in which treatment fails due to unrecognized visceral metastases.

Seldom are patients with stage I disease symptomatic. Unfortunately, the majority of patients with symptoms, as well as many with new-found lesions on survey chest films, are in an advanced stage of disease. In any program of therapy, it is this large group of patients, with a guarded prognosis, that must also be addressed. I must admit to a bias in favor of surgery as the best form of therapy in terms of comfort and an increased survival as well as a chance for cure. Because of this prejudice, most of my assessment is focused on cardiopulmonary function and the physiologic status of the patient. In the age group involved, with a smoker's disease, coronary artery heart disease and chronic obstructive lung disease are common. Regardless of how favorable a prognosis a cancer might have, the patient must be able to functionally tolerate the proposed treatment.

OPERABILITY

Recently I reviewed my own cases over a five-year period and found that 30 per cent were considered inoperable.[15] A few of these patients showed such severe pulmonary insufficiency as to preclude a thoracotomy. There were a few cases involving such severe cardiac disease that they were consequently considered inoperable. I have performed a few operations with the concomitant use of an intra-aortic balloon, and a few have had a preliminary coronary artery bypass procedure followed by a pulmonary resection. I also have done pulmonary resection in conjunction with a coronary bypass procedure. The majority of patients considered inoperable, however, had documented visceral metastases, malignant pleural effusions, superior vena caval obstruction, or such extensive mediastinal involvement to technically preclude a pulmonary resection.

I have never seen a patient with a malignant pleural effusion due to primary lung cancer who improved with surgical removal of the tumor. One must, however, make sure of the diagnosis, since there may be more than one cause of fluid with an associated lung cancer. In our hospital laboratory we have observed that pleural fluid is one of the more difficult specimens to evaluate for malignant cells. In the presence of documented pleural metastases with an effusion, cytology and cell block studies have been positive in only 37 per cent of the cases. Thus it is most important that someone with a presumed lung cancer and pleural fluid malignancy be completely staged so as not to miss an opportunity at effective therapy (see Case 14).

Visceral metastases, in general, are contraindications to major thoracic surgery. This advice must be tempered with the knowledge that there are exceptional situations when surgery for the primary and the metastatic deposit may be the best form of treatment and may even be followed by long-term survival (see Cases 11 and 12).

In the assessment of operability, a number of diagnostic procedures are available. However, these all need not be applied in a standard manner to every patient with a suspicion of lung cancer. One soon learns that as symptoms increase, the operability and cure rate decreases.

Routine sputum cytology examination has been proven impractical.[13] Simple chest x-rays are currently the best way to pick up a pulmonary abnormality. Computed tomography (CT) scanning should be done for all abnormal chest films since it offers the best means of evaluating the chest and its contents. In any screening program, chest x-ray has been the most sensitive method in finding lung cancer; 40 per cent of those cancers detected will be stage I when the results of treatment are most beneficial.[16]

In the absence of pain, anemia, or specifically abnormal blood chemistries, bone scans are seldom productive; however, I have observed abnormality due to metastatic involvement as much as two months prior to the onset of pain. Among patients being evaluated for advanced disease, however, bone scans probably should be advised, since metastases to bone occurs in at least 30 per cent of patients dying of lung cancer.

In the absence of abnormal liver function tests, liver-spleen scans have been of little value. CT scanning of the upper abdomen, as an extension of the lower thorax imaging, should be done on all patients being evaluated for lung cancer to include the liver and adrenals. Among patients dying from lung cancer, liver is the site for metastases in another 30 per cent, and the adrenals are second only to the triumvirate of bone, liver, and brain for metastatic involvement.

Because of the propensity for metastases to the brain, all patients being evaluated should have CT scanning of the brain even in the absence of symptoms.

Bronchoscopy is an excellent means of evaluating operability for central lesions. However, it is not a good initial diagnostic tool due to the fact that in our experience only about 35 per cent of lung cancers have a positive bronchoscopic finding. I do not use bronchoscopy on all patients during the period of evaluation. In more than four decades of studying a large number of patients, I have not encountered any with peripheral parenchymal nodules and concomitant mainstem bronchial or tracheal lesions, although I have heard of it as one of the reasons for advising bronchoscopy on all patients suspected of lung cancer. For determination of operability, however, it may be indispensable in demonstrating carinal or tracheal involvement.

Mediastinoscopy is advocated by many authors as part of any preoperative staging. I believe this can play an important role in assessment of the patient. One can, under selected circumstances, use the positive or negative findings as an indication for or against surgery. If on CT imaging of the

TABLE 4–4. TNM DEFINITIONS

Nodal Involvement (N)

N_0 No demonstrable metastasis to regional lymph nodes.

N_1 Metastasis to lymph nodes in the peribronchial or the ipsilateral hilar region, or both, including direct extension.

N_2 Metastasis to ipsilateral mediastinal lymph nodes and subcarinal lymph nodes.

N_3 Metastasis to contralateral mediastinal lymph nodes, contralateral hilar lymph nodes, ipsilateral or contralateral scalene, or supraclavicular lymph nodes.

---

mediastinum there appears to be nodal involvement in the upper or middle mediastinum, then I will perform mediastinoscopy as part of the preliminary evaluation. In the absence of small cell undifferentiated lung cancer, with what otherwise appears to be technically operable disease, I may proceed with an exploratory thoracotomy regardless of the findings on mediastinoscopy, since I believe that removal of the tumor offers the most for comfort, survival time, and chance of cure even in the presence of verified N_2 disease (see Case 15).

Of the 70 per cent coming to exploration, 90 per cent (63 per cent of the original group) have had a pulmonary resection. This aggressive approach to operability will be discussed later in terms of the conservative extent of resection (Table 4–7).

Mediastinotomy, or open exploration of the anterior, middle and posterior mediastinum, is an extension of mediastinoscopy for evaluating node-bearing areas. The same usage and implications hold true for both procedures.

Needle biopsy, especially with CT scan guidance, is invaluable. I do not, however, believe it must be used on all patients. Under the best of circumstances, about one in four patients will develop a complicating pneumothorax and about half of these will require insertion of a chest tube. There are also the rare instances of serious bleeding or spread of infection or tumor along needle tracks. One must realize that a needle biopsy must obtain sufficient, representative tissue to offer a definitive diagnosis. We have seen instances of a biopsy diagnosis of small cell undifferentiated carcinoma changed to non–small cell on the surgical specimen (see Case 6). Moreover, if the biopsy is not representative of the lesion and is reported as negative for tumor cells, one is usually left with an undiagnosed pulmonary nodule that still needs excisional biopsy for diagnosis and management. In our laboratory it is estimated that a needle biopsy will be about 90 per cent accurate.

TABLE 4–5. TNM DEFINITIONS

Distant Metastasis (M)

M_0 No (known) distant metastasis.

M_1 Distant metastasis present—Specify site(s).

TABLE 4–6. TNM DEFINITIONS

Footnote to TNM Definitions

T_1 The uncommon superficial tumor of any size with its invasive component limited to the bronchial wall, which may extend proximal to the main bronchus, is classified as T_1.

T_4 Most pleural effusions associated with lung cancer are due to tumor. There are, however, some few patients in whom cytopathological examination of pleural fluid (on more than one specimen) is negative for tumor, the fluid is nonbloody, and is not an exudate. In such cases where these elements and clinical judgment dictate that the effusion is not related to the tumor, the patients should be staged T_1, T_2, or T_3, excluding effusion as a staging element.

RISK OF UNDIAGNOSED PULMONARY NODULE

Selective use of needle biopsy has been influenced by the risk of the undiagnosed pulmonary abnormality. In the 1950s, the accepted risk of an undiagnosed pulmonary shadow in an individual past the age of 40 years and without an acute history of recent pulmonary infection was about a 50 per cent chance of malignancy.[17] In that period of time the nonmalignant problems were frequently due to tuberculosis. Today, in the northeastern United States, that is no longer the case.

I have recently reviewed 100 consecutive patients who had an exploratory thoracotomy for an undiagnosed pulmonary shadow and found that 86 per cent were malignant[18, 19] (see Table 4–8).

Since needle biopsy is only 90 per cent accurate and the risk of the abnormal shadow being malignant is 86 per cent, if there are no other contraindications to surgery, I believe that direct exploration is the best approach to arrive at a correct diagnosis and to definitively manage the problem.

SURGICAL THERAPY

Limited Resection

In a recent personal consecutive patient series, 90 per cent of those explored had resection of the tumor. Only 16 patients underwent pneumo-

TABLE 4–7. OPERABILITY FOR LUNG CANCER

Operability for Lung Cancer

- 30% Inoperable
- 70% Explored
  - 10% Nonresectable
  - 90% (63% of original) Resected

TABLE 4–8. RISK OF UNDIAGNOSED PULMONARY NODULE IN 100 CONSECUTIVE ASYMPTOMATIC PATIENTS PAST THE AGE OF 40

Malignant Tumor	86%
Benign	14%
Hamartoma	
Organizing pneumonia	
Lung abscess	
Granuloma	
Tuberculosis	
Pseudotumor	
Aspergilloma	
Pulmonary infarct	
Pleural plaque	
Intrapulmonary lymph node	

nectomy, 30 underwent lobectomy, and 54 underwent limited resection such as a wedge, bilobe segmentectomy, or segmentectomy (Tables 4–9, 4–10, and 4–11).

The first segmental resection for lung cancer in our office was done by Overholt in 1949. At that time, segmental resection was primarily used in elderly patients or those with limited pulmonary reserve. However, in recent years it has become my procedure of choice if the tumor can be completely removed with an adequate margin. In my opinion, there is nothing to indicate that removing more lung tissue, e.g., lobectomy over segmentectomy or pneumonectomy over lobectomy, increases the likelihood of cure once the primary tumor is excised. Lymph nodes should be sampled for staging; however, extensive node dissection does not increase the chance for cure.

Review of 100 consecutive patients with lung cancer managed by a limited resection revealed 20 that were performed for metastatic malignancy. Survival in this subset was identical to a similar group having a more extensive pulmonary resection with five, or 25 per cent, surviving more than five years. Of the 80 with primary lung cancer managed by a limited resection, 48 (60 per cent) had T_1 or T_2N_0 lesions; 18 were T_3N_0; 2 were T_1 or T_2N_1; 10 were T_1 or T_2N_2; and 2 were T_3N_2. The follow-up on each subset was comparable to those patients having a more extensive pulmonary resection (Table 4–12).

One must be sure of an adequate margin, in doing a limited pulmonary resection for lung cancer. Of the group reviewed, two patients developed evidence of recurrence in the surgical field within one year of follow-up that

TABLE 4–9. 100 CONSECUTIVE PATIENTS WITH MALIGNANCY

Primary Lung Cancer		82
Bronchial Adenoma		4
Sarcoma		1
Metastatic Malignancy		13
Colon	4	
Breast	2	
Melanoma	2	
Osteogenic sarcoma	2	
Renal	1	
Endometrium	1	
Hodgkin's	1	

TABLE 4–10. CELL TYPE IN 82 PATIENTS WITH PRIMARY LUNG CANCER

Adenocarcinoma	39
Epidermoid	25
Large cell undifferentiated	13
Adenosquamous	2
Adenosquamous—large cell	1
Small cell (oat cell)	2

was thought to be due to inadequate initial margin of resection. Both patients had a second operation with completion of the lobectomy. Both are alive and well more than five years later. Although one must be careful with regard to the margins, I still believe that a limited resection is indicated when technically feasible, since the follow-up results are comparable and in this group of patients there has been no hospital mortality and no major morbidity. Defining an adequate margin is difficult and depends, to a large extent, on experience. I like to see a minimum of one centimeter of lung parenchyma surrounding the gross margins of tumor in the fresh specimen and always have the margins checked by frozen section examination by the pathologist for freedom from tumor. If the possibility of obtaining a satisfactory margin is questionable during the segmentectomy, it is better to proceed with a lobectomy. With experience, however, based upon visual inspection and palpation of the tumor, one can usually decide initially if a limited resection will be feasible and adequate.

Stage II and Stage III Disease

Although the treatment of stage I lung cancer may have a uniform consensus as to its best management, this is not the case in stage II and stage III disease. The perception of many medical oncologists, radiotherapists, and thoracic surgeons is that surgery has little to offer (Table 4–13). In an effort to demonstrate the influence of surgery on this group of patients, I have reviewed 100 operations on 95 consecutive patients with stage II (n = 7) and stage III (n = 88) disease with a minimum follow-up of two years.[15] There were 62 men and 33 women in the study group with an average age of 61 years. In contrast to those encountered during routine surgery for lung cancer, where only 16 per cent underwent pneumonectomy, 30 per cent lobectomy, and 54 per cent limited resection, the group with stage II or stage III disease required pneumonectomy in 44 per cent and lobectomy in 33 per cent. Limited resection was possible in only 23 per cent and was

TABLE 4–11. EXTENT OF PULMONARY RESECTION IN 100 CONSECUTIVE PATIENTS WITH LUNG CANCER

Pneumonectomy		16
Lobectomy		30
Limited		54
Segmentectomy	34	
Wedge	16	
Bilobe segmentectomy	4	

TABLE 4–12. 100 CONSECUTIVE LIMITED RESECTIONS FOR LUNG CANCER

Metastatic malignancy		20%
Primary lung cancer		80%
T_1 or T_2N_0	48	
T_3N_0	18	
T_1 or T_2N_1	2	
T_1 or T_2N_2	10	
T_3N_2	2	

performed only in instances such as superior sulcus tumor, or T_1 or T_2 disease with nodal involvement.

The cell types in this group of stage II and stage III tumors concurred with our general office statistics in recent years with adenocarcinoma as the predominant histology.[5] The five-year survival was 50 per cent for epidermoid (n=34), 32 per cent for large cell undifferentiated carcinoma (n=14), and 25 per cent for adenocarcinoma (n=42).

Nodal involvement was a serious prognostic finding as evidenced by a five-year survival of 41 per cent for epidermoid (n=22), 26 per cent for adenocarcinoma (n=26), and none for large cell undifferentiated carcinoma (n=6). There were no five-year survivors in patients with small cell carcinoma and nodal involvement. Although the cases studied were small in number, these figures are interesting because, in contrast to several reports in the literature, a significant number of patients with adenocarcinoma and nodal disease are long-term survivors[20] (see Cases 11 and 15). Unfortunately, none of only six patients with large cell undifferentiated carcinoma and nodal disease survived for five years.

Among the 95 consecutive patients managed with surgery for stage II or stage III disease, 34 per cent survived for five years and the median survival was 32 months (Table 4–14). Of 12 patients with N_1 disease, 58 per cent survived for five years; 21 per cent of 50 with N_2 involvement survived five years. The five-year survival was 47 per cent for 33 with T_3N_0, 60 per cent for 5 with T_3N_1, 29 per cent for 21 with T_3N_2, 12 per cent for 27 with T_1 or T_2N_2, and 57 per cent for 7 with $T_{1-2}N_1$. The survival for 13 with superior sulcus tumors or chest wall involvement was 75 per cent at 12 months, 50 per cent at 49 months, and 40 per cent at 10 years.

TABLE 4–13. INFLUENCE OF SURGERY IN STAGE II AND III DISEASE 100 OPERATIONS ON 95 CONSECUTIVE PATIENTS

Cell Type	Number	Projected Five-Year Survival
Epidermoid	34	50%
Large Cell Undifferentiated	14	32%
Adenocarcinoma	42	25%
With Node Involvement		
Epidermoid	22	41%
Large Cell Undifferentiated	6	0
Adenocarcinoma	26	26%

TABLE 4–14. 100 OPERATIONS ON 95 CONSECUTIVE PATIENTS, STAGE II AND III DISEASE

Disease	Number	5-year Survival
N_1	12	58%
N_2	50	21%
T_3N_0	33	47%
T_3N_1	5	60%
T_3N_2	21	29%
$T_{1-2}N_1$	7	57%
$T_{1-2}N_2$	29	12%
	95	34%

Preoperative Radiotherapy

Among our group of patients with stage II or stage III disease, 40 per cent received preoperative radiotherapy in the hope of improved likelihood of subsequently successful pulmonary resection.[21] These patients either had extensive primary tumors, documented nodal involvement, chest wall involvement, or a chest x-ray, which in my opinion represented the type of situation that most likely would present technical problems for a resection. Some of this is subjective and impossible to specifically describe. I believe, however, that the subsequent 90 per cent success in resection of those explored, with such extensive disease, has justified this approach. Although resectability may be improved with the use of preoperative radiotherapy, to date all randomized trials have failed to demonstrate any increase in survival.[22] Since my goal has been to resect the primary, when technically feasible, I have used this technique in a consecutive series of 64 such patients and believe that the following data justify such an approach. During the course of preoperative radiotherapy, seven cases (11 per cent) became inoperable due to visceral metastases; five of 57 cases explored remained unresectable; and 52 cases (91 per cent of those explored) were resected. Not all of these cases had pretherapy verification of carcinoma and three of those resected had no evidence of tumor in the surgical specimen. These have been judged errors in diagnosis. However, it might well be that tumors in these cases were destroyed by the preoperative radiotherapy, since they had all of the characteristics of carcinoma. Furthermore, most importantly, among pretherapy histologically verified cases in this small series, 26 per cent had no demonstrable tumor in the surgical specimen. These findings are consistent with those in the literature.[22]

Of the 49 patients who had a pulmonary resection for histologically verified cancer, who were managed with preoperative radiotherapy, 26 subsequently died of tumor; 10 died from other causes; and 13 are alive and well without tumor. There was no postoperative mortality. Of the 26 who died from tumor, all had T_3, eleven had N_2, two had N_1, and one had M_1 due to scalene node involvement. Of the 10 who died without evidence of tumor, nine were T_3, one was T_1, and one was N_2. The patient with T_1 disease had a bilateral synchronous carcinoma and received radiotherapy as a "holding procedure" following a resection for stage I disease on the contralateral side. This patient died three years later from acute pulmonary tuberculosis. Among the 13 patients still alive without tumor, all had T_3, six had N_2, one had N_1, and two had M_1 involvement. In the life table and survival analysis, 75 per cent survived 7.3 months; 50 per cent for 19.3 months; 34 per cent for five years; 25 per cent for 93 months; and 16 per cent for 12 years (see Case 3).

Postoperative Radiotherapy

In most cases with documented nodal involvement, radiotherapy will be advised as part of the treatment plan. Among those patients who receive preoperative radiotherapy, with demonstration of nodal metastases, or in most instances of superior sulcus tumors, completion of the radiotherapy will be given in the postoperative period (see Case 8). Following pneumonectomy, radiotherapy will usually be delayed for at least four to six weeks following surgery until the patient has made a satisfactory recovery and is free of any obvious problems related to the recent surgery.

Currently, in the postoperative period, if radiotherapy is advised because of nodal metastases, infusion chemotherapy will be used concomitantly. For those who do not receive preoperative radiotherapy, the majority of patients found to have nodal metastases during resection of the primary tumor will be advised to receive a full course of radiotherapy following satisfactory recovery from surgery.

Postoperative Chemotherapy

I have not used chemotherapy in the preoperative preparation of any patient for lung cancer. I have been satisfied with the benefits of preoperative radiotherapy for improving the likelihood of a subsequently successful resection in the presence of an unfavorable technical problem for advanced disease.

We have, however, been evaluating the use of infusion chemotherapy in the postoperative period. This is given in conjunction with radiotherapy, either completion of that started preoperatively or that deemed advisable due to documentation of nodal involvement during a surgical exploration, in the assumption that chemotherapy may sensitize tumor cells and make them more vulnerable to the effects of radiotherapy. Although no randomized trials have demonstrated any increased five-year survivals following the use of chemotherapy in lung cancer, there is reason to believe that the combination of chemotherapy, together with radiotherapy, may increase local control as well as the tumor-free interval.[23] If this proves to be correct, then the beneficial effects for palliation will be worthwhile, since infusion chemotherapy has had little toxicity (see Case 15).

Currently, we are using an infusion of 5-fluorouracil, at a dosage rate of 300 mg/m²/day, on a continuous basis by means of a portable infusion pump. The delivery of chemotherapy is through a central-venous access, and usually is started one week prior to initiation of radiotherapy and maintained for one week following termination of radiotherapy. Dosage adjustments are made as necessary depending on patient tolerance.

Cost: Morbidity and Mortality

In evaluating the results of treatment in a group of patients where the majority will eventually die of their disease, one must look at the cost in morbidity and mortality. Among those patients having a limited resection, there has not been a death or major complication. There were no deaths in the group of 64 unfavorable cases in which preoperative radiotherapy was used in an effort to make a subsequent pulmonary resection more successful. Among the 95 patients with stage II and stage III disease who had 100 operations, there was one patient who died from a myocardial infarction 30 days following a pneumonectomy. One patient who had a lobectomy two years previously for stage III disease ($T_2N_2M_0$) died from a pulmonary embolus two days following a curative lobectomy for a second primary carcinoma of the lung classified as stage I with $T_2N_0M_0$ disease. As noted in Case 10, there was one bronchopleural fistula and that patient was a long-term survivor. There has been no other major morbidity.

This is not to imply that one can do extensive surgery in this age group with compromised cardiac and pulmonary function, stage III disease, and following radiotherapy without risk. With attention to details, however, those risks should be at an absolute minimum. Since the risk of morbidity and mortality has been so low, surgery, when feasible, appears to offer a favorable means of producing palliation, possibly improving the survival time, and giving the most reasonable chance for cure. The criticism is frequently made that unless one is specifically relieving pain, bleeding, or infection, palliation is not justified as an indication for surgery. In following the natural course of disease, over a long period of time, one learns that these findings occur too often as part of the progression of tumor locally. If the primary tumor can be safely removed and local control obtained, then the natural course of the disease may be altered; I believe this constitutes palliation—particularly so if it is accompanied by an increased survival and an improved chance for cure.

Technical Considerations in Surgery

Diagnostic Bronchoscopy

I have always performed bronchoscopy under topical anesthesia—previously with the rigid bronchoscope, and currently with the flexible, fiberoptic bronchoscope. These examinations are frequently done on an outpatient basis in the office. When determining operability, I do the bronchoscopy as a separate procedure, but if operability is not in doubt I will do it under anesthesia prior to thoracotomy.

Anesthesia

Although I have used double lumen tubes for control of ventilation, I do not like this technique and believe it is unnecessary. I have competent anesthetists available, and they use this technique for other surgeons, but since I am aware of recurring technical problems with placement or use of the double lumen tubes and find they are not needed, I continue to do all cases with a simple, single lumen endotracheal tube.

Position

Proper exposure for all surgery is important. For cancer surgery it is imperative. Various incisions and positions are useful and have their place.

The supine position, with a midline sternal splitting incision, offers access to bilateral problems when indicated and has the added feature of producing the least physiologic derangement of any thoracic incision.

Anterior thoracotomy in the supine or oblique position is of value for lesions in the middle lobe or anterior segment of the upper lobe when one is relatively sure only a limited procedure will be necessary.

Axillary incision in the lateral position is tempting since there is minimal cutting of muscles and the postoperative period is presumed to be easier. I doubt if this is true and find the exposure to be less than ideal, so I use it only for simple diagnostic procedures or, on occasion, for management of recurrent pneumothorax.

Lateral thoracotomy in the lateral position has universal acceptance by most thoracic surgeons. Any type of unilateral problem involving the lung can be managed by this approach.

The posterolateral thoracotomy in the prone position is the procedure of choice in most cancer cases since it allows excellent exposure; it is second only to the supine position for physiologic stability and it is the most comfortable when managing a technically difficult dissection.

Use of the Stapler

Use of the stapler has markedly improved the management of peripheral lung tissue when doing wedge excisions, segmentectomies and developing incomplete fissurae. Under no circumstance, however, do I ever close the bronchus with staples.

Bronchial Closure

I still believe that bronchopleural fistulae are essentially technical. I believe there should be minimal dissection of the bronchus so as not to make it ischemic. Closure should be done with fine sutures and with as few as possible so as not to further damage the blood supply. With rare exceptions, most bronchi, including main-stem divisions, can be adequately closed with only three sutures. I am using a technique that was first described by Overholt in 1949 and have yet to find one superior.[24] No effort is made to have a short stump as so often is reported as being desirable, and, in fact, a fairly long stump is necessary for proper closure of a main-stem bronchus by the infolding technique with three sutures. No effort is ever made to cover any bronchus during a subtotal resection since I believe expansion of residual lung and obliteration of the pleural space is the best protection against a fistula. In cases of pneumonectomy I may cover the bronchus but only with well-vascularized tissue. On the right, this tissue may be within the circle of the azygous vein, or frequently a portion of mobilized esophagus is used, which leaves the closed bronchus buried in the mediastinum. On the left, the bronchus usually retracts within the circle of the aortic window and can be closed with periaortic tissue. Closure of the main-stem bronchus may be of value in postirradiation therapy or in the presence of a high risk for pleural infection.

Chest Tubes

Following any pulmonary resection, chest tubes are needed for drainage and evacuation of postoperative fluid and air. Two large tubes are routinely used. Usually the intrapleural end is anchored in place by using an absorbable suture to make certain the tube position of choice is maintained. The tubes should be tunneled subcutaneously and brought out separately from the thoracotomy incision. The tube site should have a mattress suture in place so that when the tube is removed the wound can be closed rather than being allowed to heal as an open wound. There will be minimal risk of developing a pneumothorax on removal by tunneling the tubes. The subsequent risk of wound complications is reduced by bringing them out separately from the incision. Furthermore, if a pleural complication develops, it is relatively simple to manage compared with the involvement of large thoracotomy incisions and the extrapleural space.

In the case of a pneumonectomy, I use a single tube placed anteriorly and superiorly. This tube is clamped and opened several times every day to allow for releasing a buildup in intrapleural pressure during the accumulation of fluid in the pleural space. With its location anterior and superior it will be in an air pocket until the pleural space is completely filled with fluid. The tube is removed on the third postoperative day. Many thoracic surgeons do not use a tube, but adjustment of the intrapleural pressure postoperatively may be required and the tube is a convenient means of doing this. Some surgeons use a tube connected to balanced suction drainage that may be of value in the occasional patient with an infected pleural space; otherwise the fluid is drained off and merely depletes the patient, since the space will eventually fill.

EXAMPLES IN MANAGEMENT

Examples are frequently criticized as being selected and anecdotal, and of course that is true. Nothing, however, can compare with specific examples to demonstrate philosophy and details in management.

Case 1. F.D., a 56-year-old man with a history of smoking, had a survey lesion found on a routine chest radiograph. Bronchoscopy showed a lesion in the right upper lobe bronchus with involvement of the mainstem bronchus laterally up to the level of the carina. A right pneumonectomy was done on December 10, 1962. The final staging (retrospectively) was $T_3N_0M_0$ adenocarcinoma. No other therapy was used. He is alive and well at the time of this writing.

Comment: This case is used as the introduction because it represents my longest-surviving patient following a pulmonary resection for primary lung cancer. Considering the age group involved with this disease, even when cured, there are few patients who will subsequently survive for more than 25 years. This represents a T_3 lesion. It was considered favorable, however, since nodes were negative and it was discovered by survey chest film while the patient was free of symptoms. In my experience, T_3 lesions of this type without nodal involvement carry no more risk than T_1 or T_2 lesions, and one should expect a 50 per cent or better likelihood of five-year survival with surgery. Although this patient has done well, one must realize that 50 per cent of such cases may fail, usually due to unrecognized visceral metastases at the time of surgery and, as such, some type of effective adjuvant therapy is needed.

Case 2. G.H., a 66-year-old woman with a history of smoking, developed acute left chest pain and had a chest radiograph the next day that showed a right lung nodule. A bone scan was done, which showed positive uptake in a rib on the left side. The left sixth rib was removed for biopsy on July 15, 1974 and the pathology report was metastatic tumor in bone. The patient was initially started on chemotherapy using Cytoxan; arrangements were made for radiotherapy for palliation of pain from the presumed area of bony metastases. Some time later, the department of pathology reported that it had been concerned over the original diagnosis and after further study had changed the diagnosis to hyperplastic callus in a fracture.

Upon further questioning of the patient, a history of trauma to the left chest about one month prior to the onset of pain was determined. The patient was readmitted and had a right upper lobectomy on September 11, 1974. The final staging was $T_1N_0M_0$ epidermoid carcinoma of the lung. She did well until 1981 when she developed a primary adenocarcinoma of the duodenum and died four months following surgery. There was no recurrence of her pulmonary tumor in the seven-year period.

Comment: Findings of a single focus of abnormality on a bone scan are well recognized as frequently being the result of many things other than metastatic malignancy. In this instance, with acute pain and the abnormal bone scan, biopsy was indicated. Although the patient came close to missing her opportunity for preferred therapy, thanks to a conscientious department of pathology, the problem was pursued and ultimately the proper management took place.

Case 3. M.C., a 52-year-old man with a history of smoking, complained of fatigue and weight loss. On physical examination he had wheezing on the right side. Chest radiography revealed an extensive lesion with presumed hilar involvement (Fig. 4–1). He was treated with 3000 rad (30 cGy) of preoperative radiotherapy without a histologic diagnosis. On January 4, 1971, a radical right pneumonectomy was performed with removal of a portion of pericardium, the phrenic nerve, and dissection of a group of involved nodes from the mediastinum behind the azygous vein and along the superior vena cava. The final pathology showed

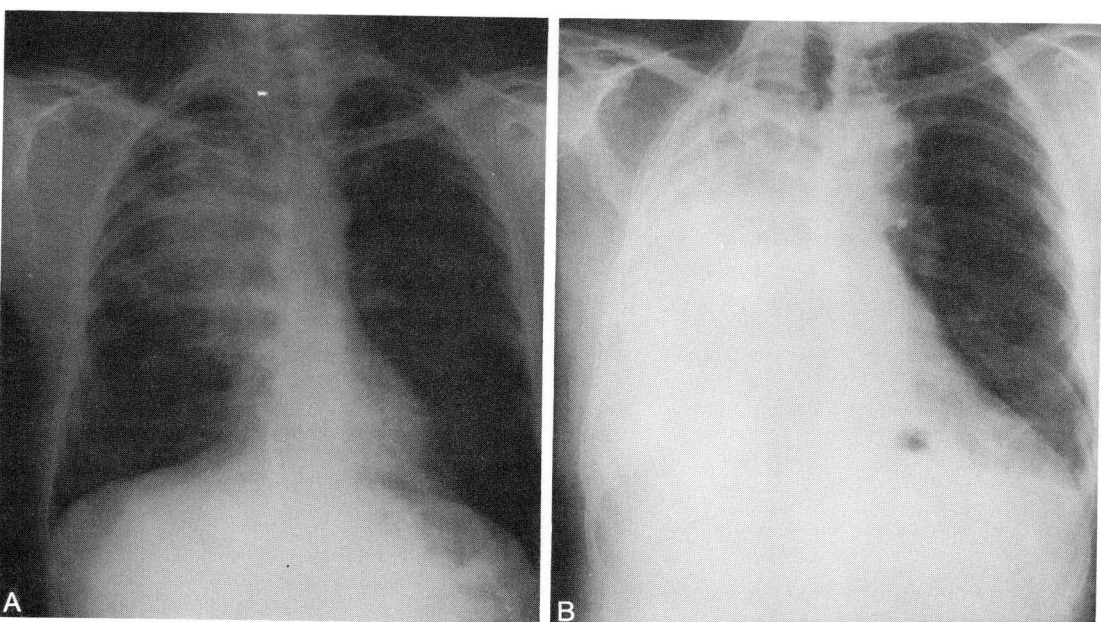

Figure 4–1. Case 3—$T_xN_2M_0$ epidermoid carcinoma. *A*, PA view showing extensive right upper lobe lesion. *B*, Chest radiograph 17 years after treatment.

abscess formation but no recognizable tumor in the lung. Nodes from behind the vena cava were positive for metastatic tumor. Final staging was $T_xN_2M_0$ epidermoid carcinoma. He received no follow-up therapy and was alive and well at the time of this writing.

Comment: This patient's prognosis was considered unfavorable from the beginning. He was symptomatic with wheezing and systematic complaints of fatigue and weight loss. It was my goal to offer palliation; however, after improvement following 3000 rad of radiotherapy, an exploration was deemed advisable. Although I rarely believe definitive therapy should be given without a verifying histologic diagnosis, I originally planned after preoperative radiotherapy to do either an exploratory thoracotomy or a biopsy. As it turned out, a resection was possible, although all evidence of tumor in the lung was destroyed by the 3000 rad of radiotherapy. This is not unusual. Nodes were positive in the upper mediastinum and in my experience are little different from positive nodes in the lower mediastinum in terms of prognosis. In this particular patient no additional therapy was used and he has done well. Today, however, I would advise completion of radiotherapy in the postoperative period and would now add infusion chemotherapy to increase the likelihood of local control and the tumor-free interval, realizing that neither, as of this time, has been shown to improve five-year survival chances.

Case 4. J.M., a 46-year-old man with a history of smoking, was known to have a pulmonary cyst in the right upper lobe since 1953. He had experienced pain in the right upper anterior chest since 1963. A chest radiograph revealed thickening of the outer wall of the cyst in 1969. On February 24, 1970, a right exploratory thoracotomy was done with plication of blebs and bullae in the lower lobe, extraperiosteal mobilization of adherent right upper lobe, and removal of the posterior segment of the right upper lobe. Final pathology showed adenocarcinoma with blood vessel invasion, tumor in pleura, and extra pleural fat, but submitted nodes were negative for tumor. Final staging was $T_3N_0M_0$. The mobilized area had been marked with clips and postoperatively he received 5500 rad to this area.

He did well until April 1981, when a contralateral pulmonary nodule was found on routine follow-up. He was then 78 years of age, in good clinical condition, and free of symptoms. A left exploratory thoracotomy was done on July 20, 1981, more than 11 years after his previous pulmonary resection. A left upper lobectomy was required for a $T_1N_0M_0$ adenocarcinoma, which was thought to be a second primary. The patient was well with a satisfactory chest radiograph in December 1982. Unfortunately, he died suddenly following some type of cerebral complication on July 20, 1982, exactly two years following his last pulmonary resection. No autopsy was obtained and it was assumed that death was due to cerebral metastases, although at his age and with an originally favorable lesion this is not necessarily true.

Comment: This patient was originally explored because of a questioned change in a follow-up chest radiograph, which had been known to be abnormal for 16 years. A tumor was ultimately found in the wall of a cyst. Although this finding is not unusual, it was not suspected initially and simple extraperiosteal mobilization was used rather than resection of the involved chest wall, which would have been the procedure of choice. Fortunately the combination of surgery and postoperative radiotherapy was effective for control of this tumor. The second primary is in keeping with our finding of 12 per cent of patients developing a new tumor among those surviving pulmonary resection for lung cancer.[25] For this reason, we believe that after a resection for lung cancer the patient should be carefully followed for life. In most instances when a second primary is found, it will be in an asymptomatic stage, usually stage I, and usually a favorable reoperation can be offered unless the patient has developed some type of additional morbid disease.

Case 5. L.P., a 52-year-old man with a history of smoking, was found to have an abnormal shadow on a survey chest film. On May 29, 1973, he had a right upper lobectomy for what proved to be a limited stage lesion due to small cell (oat cell) undifferentiated carcinoma. No other treatment was given. He is alive and well at the time of this writing. In small cell carcinoma, TNM staging is not used.

Comment: With a diagnosis of small cell cancer, the prognosis changes considerably. In this setting, however, resection of the tumor in a limited stage has been frequently followed by long-term survival.

Case 6. C.L., a 61-year-old woman, with a history of smoking, had an abnormal pulmonary nodule found on a routine chest radiograph. She was seen elsewhere and a needle biopsy revealed an oat cell tumor. Because of this, surgery was thought to be contraindicated and she was referred for chemotherapy. The medical oncologist thought the lesion was still most likely in a limited stage and referred her for another opinion. A mediastinoscopy revealed a large lymph node in the right paratracheal region but was negative for tumor on microscopic examination. A right lower lobectomy was done on June 29, 1979, and the final pathology showed a large cell undifferentiated carcinoma. She was finally staged as $T_1N_0M_0$. She is alive and well at the time of this writing.

Comment: This patient demonstrates several points. She was asymptomatic, relatively young, and in excellent clinical condition. In my opinion with a small, new-found pulmonary nodule, she had an indication for surgery for definitive diagnosis and proper management. I do not believe that needle biopsy should be used in this type of situation since, as demonstrated here, one may not be able to make an accurate diagnosis either as to malignancy or specific cell type. Furthermore, as shown in Case 5, even with an oat cell carcinoma, I believe surgery is the best form of therapy while the tumor is in a limited stage.

Case 7. J.L., a 68-year-old physician who had a history of smoking, noticed wheezing for one year with recent hoarseness. He was found to have a vocal cord polyp and was admitted to the hospital for removal. Preoperative chest radiography was abnormal (Fig. 4–2). Bronchoscopy was positive for epidermoid carcinoma in the left main-stem bronchus. An anterior mediastinotomy was considered negative. He was initially turned down for surgery and was referred to me by his son who was also a physician. The patient was treated with 3000 rad of preoperative radiotherapy and on April 8, 1976 had a left pneumonectomy. Tumor was surrounding the main pulmonary artery and the superior pulmonary vein and the final pathology showed blood vessel invasion with five of 11 nodes from the upper posterior mediastinum containing metastatic epidermoid carcinoma. This was staged as $T_3N_2M_0$. Radiotherapy was completed to 5500 rad in the postoperative period. He is alive and well at the time of this writing.

Comment: This was a stage III patient with a known unfavorable situation. Again, however, I do not believe one can predict the outcome for any individual and do believe that removal of the primary offers the best palliation and the most reasonable chance of cure.

Case 8. S.W., a 47-year-old woman with a history of smoking, had a hysterectomy for epidermoid carcinoma of the cervix. She now gave a seven-month history of left shoulder pain and for four months had been hospitalized and treated for tuberculosis. She was referred because all sputum studies were negative for tubercle bacilli. When first seen in July 1972, a diagnosis of a superior sulcus tumor was made and she was referred for 3000 rad of preoperative radiotherapy (Fig. 4–3). On July 27, 1972, a left pneumonectomy was performed together with resection

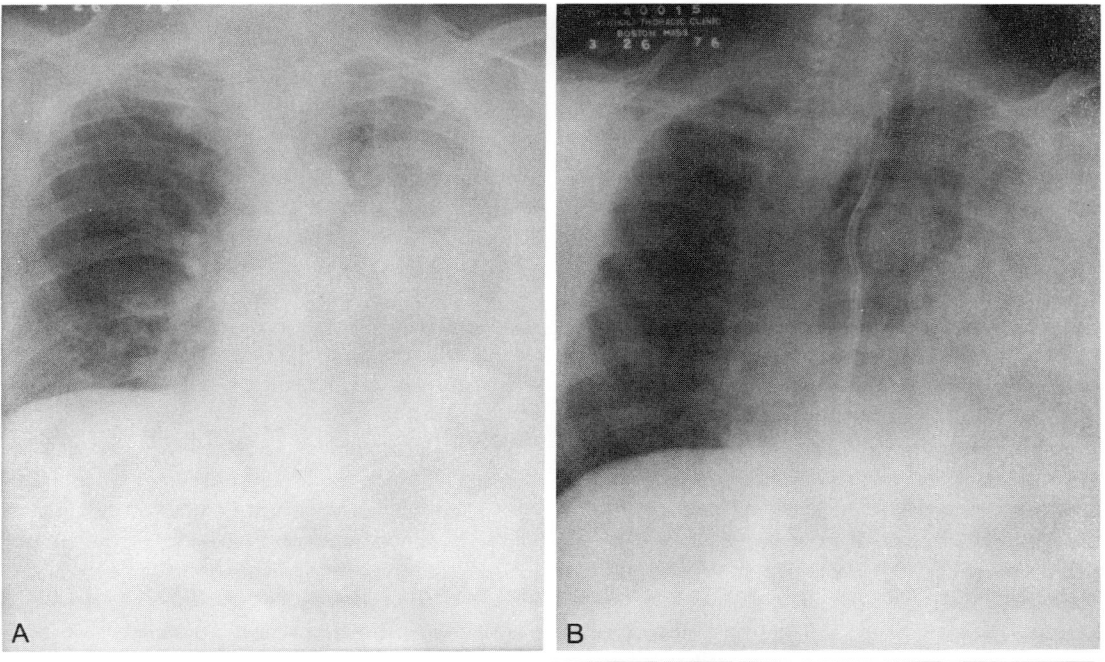

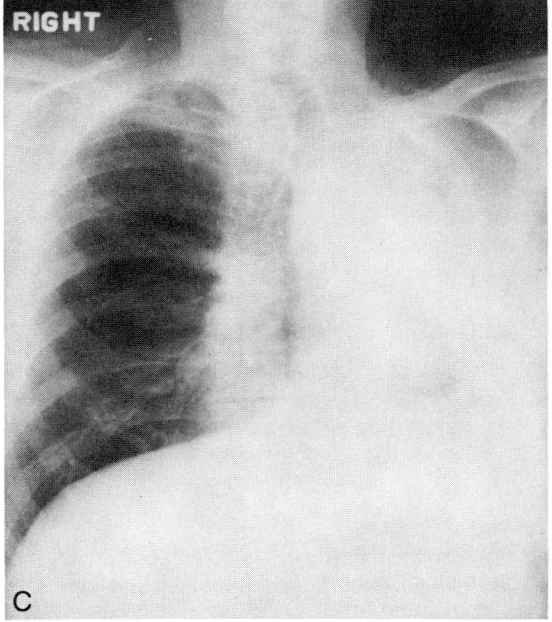

Figure 4–2. Case 7—$T_xN_2M_0$ epidermoid carcinoma. *A,* PA view after mediastinotomy, preradiotherapy. *B,* RAO view. *C,* Chest view more than 11 years after treatment.

of ribs one, two, and three, the inferior root of the brachial plexus, sacrifice of the phrenic nerve, the vagus nerve during dissection of involved nodes in the aortic window, and the superior portion of the pericardium.

Final pathology showed epidermoid carcinoma with involvement of periosteum, pericardium, all nodes from the aortic window, as well as one node from above the first rib. The patient was staged as $T_3N_2M_1$—supraclavicular lymph node. Postoperatively she had dyspnea but this improved, and three months later she was well with good accommodation

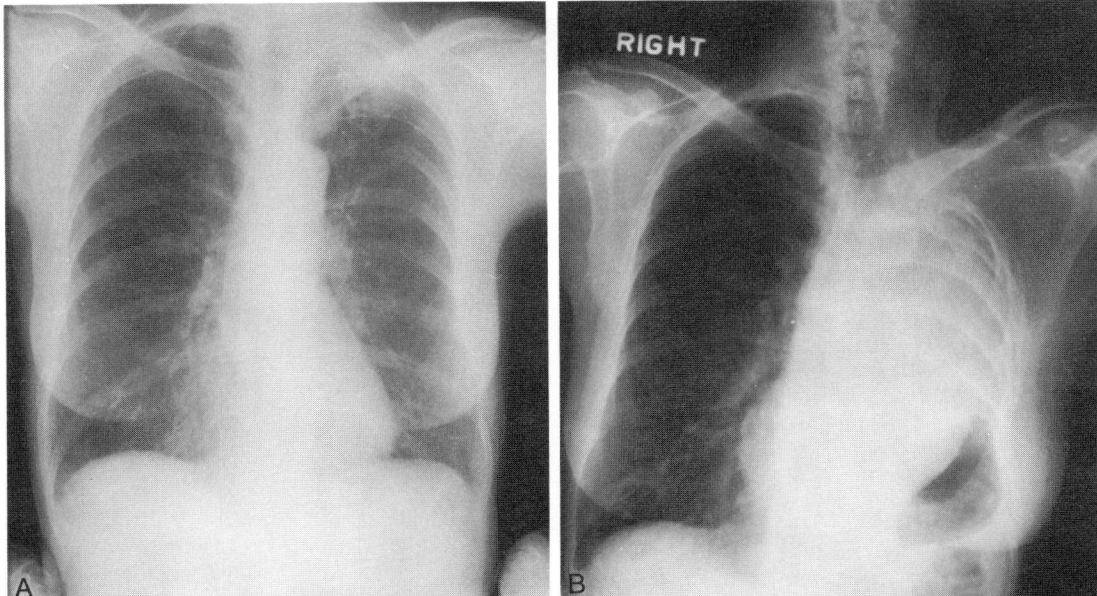

Figure 4–3. Case 8—$T_3N_2M_1$ epidermoid carcinoma. *A,* PA view showing typical appearance of a left superior sulcus tumor. *B,* PA view 15 years after treatment.

in her voice. She then had an additional 3000 rad of radiotherapy with an estimated dosage of 4000 rad delivered to the spinal cord. She was alive and well at the time of this writing.

Comment: Prior to the use of preoperative radiotherapy in superior sulcus tumors, as first reported by Shaw and Paulson in 1961, we had never had a five-year survivor by any form of therapy.[26] Since then, the results have been satisfactory and our survival data are presented above. This patient also had a positive node above the first rib and thus became M_1 by definition. She was also important for our subsequent cases since she was given radiotherapy in a porta advocated by Shaw and Paulson. At surgery she was found to have positive nodes in the aortic window and, when the postoperative radiotherapy was completed, in order to cover this area, she required a total dosage of 4000 rad to the spinal cord. Since then, all of our sulcus tumors have received radiotherapy preoperatively through a porta that includes the mediastinum as well as the primary and supraclavicular areas.

Case 9. V.B., a 61-year-old man with a history of smoking, was found to have an abnormal chest radiograph and subsequent normal bronchoscopy (Fig. 4–4). Because he was considered to have an unfavorable situation, he was treated with 3000 rad of preoperative radiotherapy and, on March 16, 1979, had a radical right pneumonectomy. Final pathology showed this to be an epidermoid carcinoma with one out of three lymph nodes in the hilum and one out of 20 nodes in the mediastinum to be positive for metastatic tumor. He was staged as $T_3N_2M_0$ with a stage III lesion. He was discharged on the thirteenth postoperative day but returned seven days later with a bronchopleural fistula. The immediate problem was managed with insertion of a chest tube and, on the following day, a rib resection was performed for adequate, dependent drainage. On May 25, 1979, 49 days later, a Shede thoracoplasty, together with closure of the fistula and coverage with a subscapularis muscle flap, was performed. Following this, he required prolonged ventilator support and eventually a tracheostomy. On August 3, 1979, 120 days following readmission, he

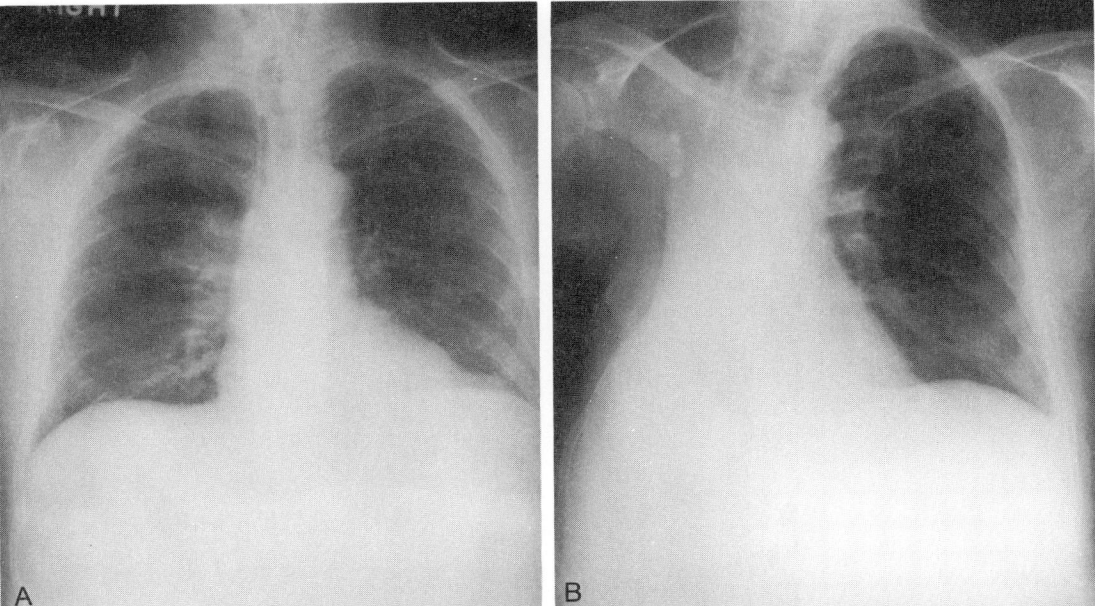

Figure 4–4. Case 9—$T_3N_2M_0$ epidermoid carcinoma. *A*, PA view. *B*, PA view more than eight years after treatment.

was discharged with all wounds healed. Because of this complication, he did not receive subsequent completion of his radiotherapy. He remained free of tumor for more than 10 years and died on January 30, 1990 from other causes.

Comment: I still believe that bronchopleural fistulae are technical in origin. This complication is unusual in my experience and may well be related to the use of preoperative radiotherapy, although I have not considered 3000 rad to adversely affect the subsequent healing of tissues. Completion of radiotherapy was never done due to this complication. However, in spite of documented nodal involvement, the patient remained well more than ten years later.

Case 10. T.C., a 60-year-old man with a history of smoking, had pain in his right shoulder for three months. When first seen, a diagnosis of lung cancer with chest wall involvement was made and he was referred for preoperative radiotherapy (Fig. 4–5). On January 22, 1979, he had surgery. The apical segment of the right upper lobe was removed together with a block of ribs two, three, and four. Irradiated gold seeds were implanted into the bed of enucleated tumor and, based on the calculated irradiation, 3000 rad preoperatively by means of 8 MEV and 2000 rad intraoperatively by means of 2.11 mCi, no added therapy was deemed necessary in the postoperative period. The final pathology was epidermoid carcinoma and he was staged as $T_3N_0M_0$. He was alive and well at the time of this writing.

Comment: This patient was not analyzed in our group of patients with superior sulcus or Pancoast tumors since the circle of the first rib was not involved. He did have documented chest-wall involvement and, when recognized preoperatively, such lesions are managed the same as superior sulcus tumors.

Case 11. D.D., a 45-year-old man with a history of smoking, was found to have a lesion in the brain, after having several seizures four years

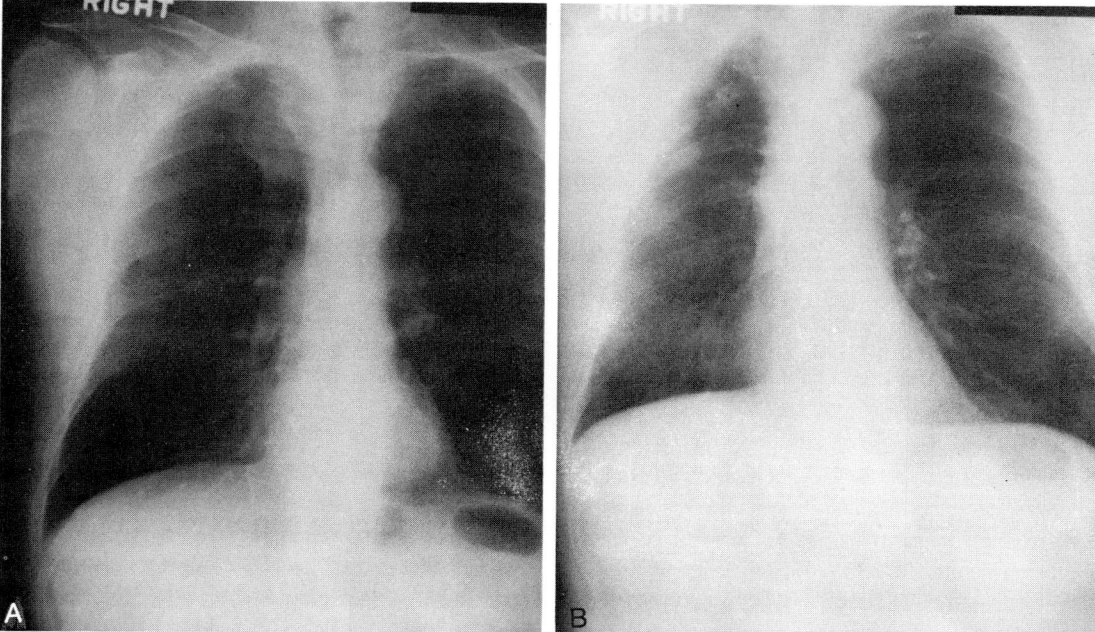

Figure 4–5. Case 10—$T_3N_0M_0$ epidermoid carcinoma. *A,* PA view showing right upper lobe tumor with chest wall involvement. *B,* PA view more than eight years after treatment. Note markers of irradiated Gold seeds.

previously. The lesion was removed and proved to be a metastatic focus of adenocarcinoma. Further evaluation revealed a nodule in the apex of the right lung and a needle biopsy confirmed this to be adenocarcinoma. This area was treated with 4000 rad of radiotherapy. Afterwards he complained of right shoulder pain and a chest radiograph showed a mass in the superior sulcus of the right hemithorax. Under CT scan guidance, a needle biopsy confirmed a diagnosis of adenocarcinoma. Further evaluation was noncontributory other than a bone scan showing involvement of ribs two, three, and five. The initial thoracic surgeon did not believe surgery was indicated. The patient was referred to me by his medical oncologist who wished for a surgical excision if at all possible. On June 22, 1983, the apical and posterior segments of the right upper lobe, together with a block of ribs one through five as well as the inferior root of the brachial plexus, were removed. Nine iridium loading tubes were sutured in place in the bed of enucleated tumor, and in the postoperative period iridium was introduced for delivery of 4000 rad to a limited bed. He received an additional 2000 rad of external beam in the postoperative period with the total calculated dosage to the spinal cord being no more than 5000 rad. The final pathology showed adenocarcinoma with blood vessel invasion, extension through the pleura into soft tissues of the chest wall, and with metastases to one submitted mediastinal lymph node. He was staged as $T_3N_2M_1$—brain. This patient was alive and well at the time of this writing.

Comment: This case serves as an example of the value of nondogmatic thinking. I usually consider visceral metastases as a contraindication to major surgery. I believe, in hindsight, that this patient would have been better served if he had had a resection of the small pulmonary nodule after the metastatic brain deposit was removed. His physicians elected to treat the pulmonary lesion with a modality known to be less effective, which may be understandable in view of documented visceral metastases.

Unfortunately, that metastasis apparently was a single focus and was cured, but subsequent growth of the primary tumor produced superior sulcus involvement when eventually recognized. With his previous radiotherapy the patient was not a suitable candidate for preoperative radiation and the case became even more unfavorable in terms of long-term control. The use of induction tubes was a good maneuver suggested by the radiotherapist and allowed for near ideal radiation focused in the area of questionable margins.

Case 12. A.S., a 64-year-old man with a history of smoking, was found to have an abnormal shadow on roentgenographic examination of the chest. Bronchoscopy was negative, but cytology of washings was positive for malignancy. He was referred for surgery and a wedge excision of a small lesion in the lingula was performed on August 18, 1982. The final pathology revealed this to be an epidermoid carcinoma and he was staged as $T_1N_0M_0$. He did well until August 1985, three years after his pulmonary resection, when he developed headaches and a visual field defect in the left eye. Evaluation revealed a single abnormal lesion in the right occipital lobe. On August 28, 1985, a metastatic deposit of epidermoid carcinoma was removed from the right occipital region. The patient made a good recovery and was alive and well, with only the expected homonymous hemianopsia, as of this writing. Final staging was $T_1N_0M_1$—brain.

Comment: This patient demonstrates the need for effective adjuvant therapy since he obviously had an unrecognized visceral metastasis at the time of what appeared to be a very favorable resection of an asymptomatic, survey lesion that was only $T_1N_0M_0$. The recognition three years after the pulmonary resection is in keeping with the usual course of the disease in contrast to the previous example, Case 11, where the presenting symptom was due to central neurologic involvement. Probably 30 per cent of all patients who die from lung cancer have brain involvement. An occasional patient will have what appears to be a single focus of disease and removal may well result in long-term control.

Case 13. L.D., a 56-year-old woman with a history of smoking, had voice changes and anemia and during evaluation was found to have a left superior mediastinal mass on chest radiography (Fig. 4–6). She was evaluated by a thoracic surgeon who considered her lesion inoperable. I first saw her in November, 1982 and noted marked clubbing of the distal phalanges. CT examination revealed a large mass in the posterior lung with the mass extending from the subclavian artery down to the carina, filling the aortic window. A bronchoscopy was noncontributory. Needle biopsy revealed epidermoid carcinoma. At that time her lesion was considered nonresectable and was tentatively staged as T_3N_2. She was referred for radiotherapy and after 3000 rad showed improvement but was still considered unfavorable. After a rest period, she had completion of her therapy to 5500 rad. Radiotherapy was given from November 30, 1982, until February 23, 1983. By May she still had a parahilar mass on plain roentgenogram and CT revealed a mass in the aortic window. Clubbing was unchanged and she now complained of tingling and some pain in all fingers. At times she was hoarse and other times her voice was normal. After considerable discussion, surgery was performed on May 11, 1983, and an extended left pneumonectomy by means of an intrapericaridal dissection was performed. A mass of tissue was removed from the aortic window and nodes were sampled from the contralateral bronchus. In removing the mass in the aortic window, mobilization was done by means of dissection in the periaortic tissue, which was markedly thickened. The vagus nerve proximal to the take-off of the recurrent laryngeal nerve was involved with the mass and was sacrificed. Final pathology showed a residual mass of only 1.5 × 1.0 × 0.8 centimeters in the anterior segment of the upper lobe, which extended to the pleural surface. Microscopy revealed this to be mixed epidermoid and adenocar-

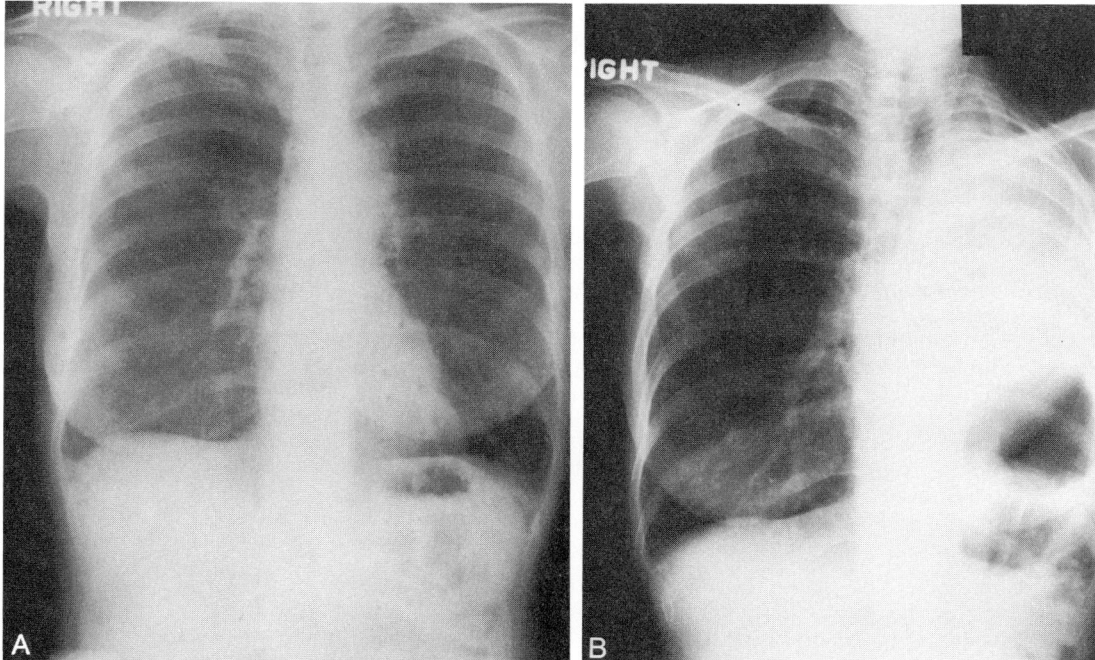

Figure 4–6. Case 13—$T_3N_2M_0$ on medical staging, final staging $T_1N_xM_0$ mixed adenoepidermoid carcinoma. *A*, PA view showing left hilar mass filling aortopulmonary window. *B*, PA view 52 months after treatment. The patient was free of tumor more than seven years after surgery.

cinoma with extensive necrosis. The submitted periaortic tissue and all lymph nodes, including the mass from the aortic window, revealed necrosis and dense fibrosis but no recognizable tumor. She was alive and well seven years after surgery. Because of her hoarseness she has had Teflon injection into her paralyzed vocal cord and had a near normal voice.

Comment: The patient had a relative contraindication to surgery with early involvement of the recurrent laryngeal nerve. I now have treated a number of long-term survivors with this type of involvement. Although they need careful evaluation, the condition in all such patients should not necessarily be considered inoperable. Final staging on this patient is impossible. Originally she was considered T_3N_2; however, based on absolute data, postoperatively, one could consider her T_1N_0. Most likely the radiotherapy destroyed recognizable tumor in lymph nodes. Although this is known to occur, it is conjecture. She was doing well after her case was considered inoperable with an unfavorable tumor, demonstrating that patients must be serially re-evaluated during therapy, and one must have an open mind with regard to changes in management.

Case 14. V.D., a 59-year-old man with a history of smoking, developed acute onset of left chest pain and three weeks later had a radiograph that showed an opacity of the left chest (Fig. 4–7). Bronchoscopy showed a tumor in the left main bronchus just beyond the carina, which was histologically an epidermoid carcinoma. A thoracentesis showed serous fluid, but cytologic examination was negative for tumor cells. He was considered inoperable due to a combination of bronchoscopic findings plus pleural fluid, which was thought most likely to be on a basis of malignancy. He was referred for another opinion. Since he had not had documentation of a malignant pleural effusion, I elected to explore the

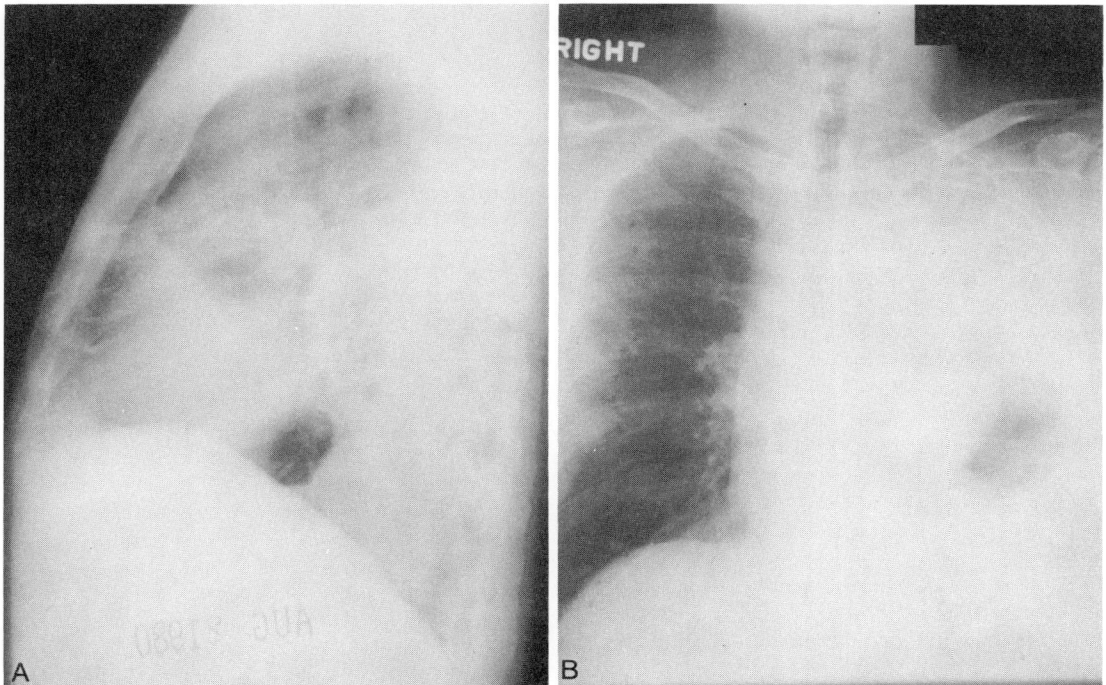

Figure 4–7. Case 14—$T_3N_1M_0$ epidermoid carcinoma. *A*, Left lateral view showing densities representing loculated fluid. *B*, PA view seven years after treatment.

left thorax. On August 4, 1980, a small lateral incision was made and a thick parietal peel was encountered. During operation, a pocket of thick, creamy pus was found. Culture of this later demonstrated the presence of *Staphylococcus aureus*. No tumor was found in the pleura. An extrapleural pneumonectomy was done; during removal over the dome of the diaphragm, a second pleural space containing serous fluid was encountered, but no evidence of tumor was found. The final pathology report revealed an epidermoid carcinoma with blood vessel invasion, involvement of one hilar node, and no tumor in 16 submitted mediastinal nodes. He was staged as $T_3N_1M_0$, stage III. Postoperatively antibiotics were used parenterally and intrapleurally and he was discharged after 10 days. Because of N_1 involvement he received 5000 rad of radiotherapy in the postoperative period. He was alive and well ten years later.

Comment: This patient was erroneously considered inoperable because of presumed pleural involvement with tumor. Although I consider a malignant pleural effusion to be an absolute contraindication to major thoracic surgery, one must document the diagnosis. Although this was a stage III by virtue of T_3 due to involvement in the main bronchus near the carina, this carries no significant difference in prognosis from T_1 or T_2. Survival of resected epidermoid carcinoma for nodal involvement in the hilum (N_1) in contrast to the mediastinum (N_2) is not much different statistically than in patients without nodal disease. This patient's pleural fluid undoubtedly was secondary to pulmonary infection distal to an obstructing tumor; in addition he had developed secondary infection of one isolated pocket of fluid with an empyema. In hindsight, after pursuing a correct evaluation of the etiology of the pleural effusion, he turned out to have a reasonably favorable situation and was a long-term survivor.

Case 15 H.L., a 67-year-old man with a former history of smoking, stopped 12 years previously because of cough and wheezing. He recently developed a new cough and increasing dyspnea. He had limitation in breathing reserve and ventilatory studies revealed an FVC of 2.03 L and an FEV_1 of .79 L. Roentgenographic examination of the chest showed a nodule in the right upper lobe (Fig. 4–8). CT scan demonstrated a soft tissue mass that measured 5 centimeters anteroposteriorly and 4 centimeters transversely. The mass blended in with the superior vena cava and passed posteriorly and medially to the vena cava and extended to the lateral wall of the trachea. There was a rounded mass of lymph nodes 2.5 centimeters in maximal dimension in the precarinal area. Mediastinoscopy showed a group of nodes in the right paratracheal region above the upper lobe bronchus and biopsy proved that they contained metastatic adenocarcinoma. This patient was treated with 3000 rad of radiotherapy

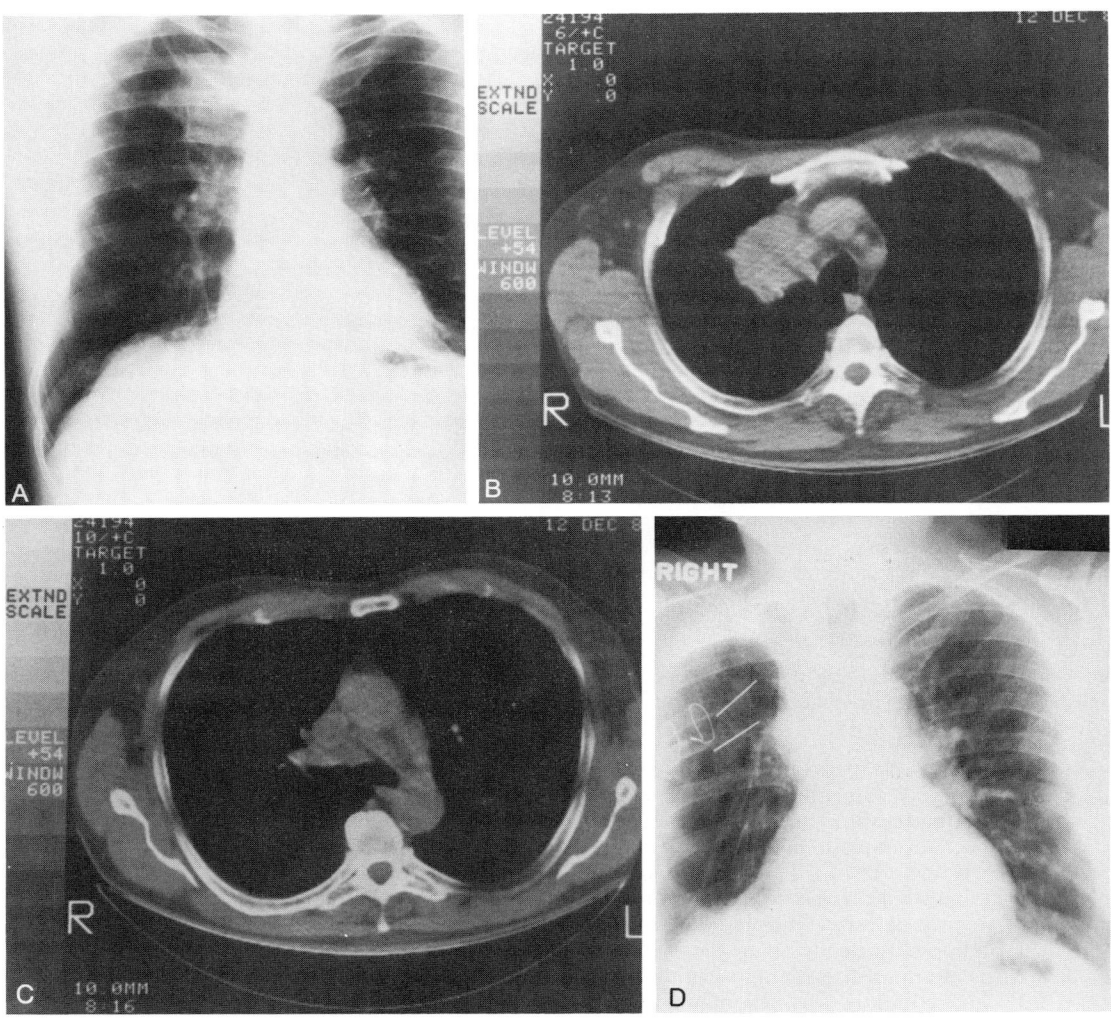

Figure 4–8. Case 15—$T_2N_2M_0$ adenocarcinoma. *A*, PA view showing mass in right upper lobe. *B*, CT image showing right upper lobe mass blending in with mediastinum. *C*, CT image above PA, showing enlarged nodes behind aorta and cava and in front of trachea. They were positive on mediastinoscopy. *D*, PA view 22 months after treatment. The patient was free of tumor 52 months after surgery.

with marked diminution in size of the parenchymal mass and no abnormality could then be demonstrated in the mediastinum by CT scan. On February 10, 1986, a right upper lobectomy was performed, at which time no demonstrable lymph nodes could be found in the mediastinum for sampling. He was staged as $T_2N_2M_0$ adenocarcinoma. Postoperatively, he received an additional 3200 rad of radiotherapy together with continuous infusion chemotherapy over a two-week course. He was alive and well with a satisfactory radiograph and CT evaluation of the chest 52 months later.

Comment: This case is included to demonstrate current management of documented nodal involvement—namely, the use of preoperative and postoperative radiotherapy together with continuous infusion chemotherapy. Although only about a year had passed following surgery at this writing, this patient had received excellent palliation; it is hoped that he will be a long-term survivor.[23]

CONCLUSIONS

For the uninformed patient who has a verified diagnosis of primary lung cancer, the outlook in terms of general statistics is grim. Fortunately, individual outcomes are variable and, based on subsets, the prognosis may be favorable. Asymptomatic patients found to have a lung cancer on survey roentgenographic examination of the chest which is still stage I, with $T_1N_0M_0$, may have up to an 80 per cent likelihood of five-year survival with surgical therapy. Stage I, with T_1 or $T_2N_0M_0$, indicates a 50 per cent five-year survival with surgery. Among patients with stage III disease, probably as many as 35 per cent may survive more than five years, with specific subsets doing even better.

Even with an aggressive approach to surgical management, as many as 30 per cent of patients will present with inoperable disease. Most of these, as well as those in whom surgery fails, can be offered an attempt at improvement of quality of life as well as the possibility of increased survival. Currently, there is a need for effective adjuvant therapy for unrecognized metastases. Simultaneous chemotherapy and radiotherapy appear to be of distinct benefit in improving resectability in unfavorable cases, improving local control, and perhaps extending the period of the tumor-free interval. Neither appears to change the five-year survival. To justify our aggressive approach, surgery must be done with low cost to the patient in terms of morbidity and mortality. When technically feasible, and in the absence of clear-cut contraindications, surgical removal of the primary lung cancer appears to offer the most comfort, survival time, and chance for cure.

REFERENCES

1. Incidence estimates based on rates of National Cancer Institutes surveillance, epidemiology and end results program, 1984–1986.
2. Bailer, J.C., and Smith, E.M.: Progress against cancer: N. Engl. J. Med. *314:*1226–1232, 1986.
3. Pearson, F.G.: Lung cancer, the past twenty-five years. Chest *89*(suppl.):200S–205S, 1986.
4. Feinstein, A.R., Sosin, D.M., and Wells, C.K.: The Will Rogers phenomenon. N. Engl. Med. *312:*1604–1608, 1985.
5. Overholt, R.H.: Primary carcinoma of the lung: Surgical extirpation. Am. J. Surg. *22:*181–186, 1933.

6. Overholt, R.H., Neptune, W.B., and Ashraf, M.M.: Primary cancer of the lung. Ann. Thorac. Surg. *20*:511–519, 1975.
7. American Joint Committee for Cancer Staging and End-Result Reporting: Task Force on the Lung. Manual for Staging of Cancer. Chicago, 1977, pp. 59–61.
8. Mountain, C.F.: A new international staging system for lung cancer. Chest *89*:225S–233S, 1986.
9. The Lung Cancer Study Group. Prepared by Thomas, P.A., and Piantadosi, S.: Postoperative T_1N_0 non-small cell lung cancer. J. Thorac. Cardiovasc. Surg. *94*:349–354, 1987.
10. The Lung Cancer Study Group. Prepared by Gail, M.H., Eagan, R.T., Feld, R., et al.: Prognostic factor in patients with resected stage I non-small cell lung cancer. Cancer *54*:1802–1813, 1984.
11. Overholt, R.H., Bougas, J.A., and Woods, F.M.: Surgical treatment of lung cancer found on x-ray survey. N. Engl. J. Med. *252*:429–432, 1955.
12. Rheinlander, H.: Personal communication, 1989.
13. IV World Conference on Lung Cancer. Screening Chairman, Miller, A.B.: Chest *89*(suppl.):324S–326S, 1986.
14. Boucot, K.R., Horie, U., and Sokoloff, M.J.: Lung cancer detected by survey methods. Am. J. Public Health *49*:793–799, 1959.
15. Neptune, W.B.: Primary lung cancer—Influence of surgery in stage II and stage III disease. Arch. Surg. *123*:583–585, 1988.
16. Early lung cancer detection: Summary and conclusions. Am. Rev. Respir. Dis. *130*:565–570, 1984.
17. Davis, E.W., Katz, S., and Peabody, J.W., Jr.: Coin lesions: Surgical implications of solitary tumors of lung. Am. J. Surg. *89*:402–407, 1955.
18. Szeluga, D.J.: Consulting statistician, 1988.
19. Kaplan, E.L., and Meir, P.: Nonparametric estimation from incomplete observations. J. Am. Stat. Assoc. *53*:457–481, 1958.
20. Kirsh, M.V., and Sloan, H.: Mediastinal metastases in bronchogenic carcinoma: Influence of postoperative irradiation in cell type and location. Ann. Thorac. Surg. *5*:459–463, 1982.
21. Sherman, D.M., Neptune, W.B., Weichaelbaum, R., et al.: An aggressive approach to marginally resectable lung cancer. Cancer *41*:2040–2045, 1978.
22. Shields, T.W., Higgins, G.A., Lawton, R., et al.: Preoperative x-ray therapy as an adjuvant in the treatment of bronchogenic carcinoma. J. Thorac. Cardiovasc. Surg. *59*:49–61, 1970.
23. The Lung Cancer Study Group. Prepared by Holmes, E.C., Hill, L.C., and Gail, M.: A randomized comparison of the effects of adjuvant therapy on resected stages II and III non-small cell carcinoma of the lung. Ann. Surg. *202*:335–341, 1985.
24. Overholt, R.H., and Langer, L.: The Technique of Pulmonary Resection. Springfield, IL, Charles C Thomas, 1949.
25. Neptune, W.B., Woods, F.M., and Overholt, R.H.: Reoperation for bronchogenic carcinoma. J. Thorac. Cardiovasc. Surg. *52*:342–350, 1966.
26. Shaw, R.R., Paulson, D.L., and Kee, J.L.: Treatment of the superior sulcus tumor by irradiation followed by resection. Ann. Surg. *154*:29–40, 1961.

Discussion

by Sidney Levitsky, M.D.

This informative chapter by Wilford B. Neptune, M.D., reflects his and his associate Dr. Richard H. Overholt's 55 years of experience with pulmonary resection for the treatment of lung cancer. This work begins with the important admonition that despite almost five decades of surgical treatment for this disease, the possibility of extended survival for unselected patients more than five years postoperative is essentially unchanged and ranges from approximately 8 to 12 per cent.

Before staging became fashionable, Neptune classified operative resections into favorable (no evidence of regional node metastases, e.g., N_0), which resulted in a 48 per cent five-year survival and unfavorable with a 12 per cent five-year survival. These data are similar to the Lung Cancer Study Group report on T_1N_0 non-small cell lung cancer.[1] Contrary to the recommendation by the American Cancer Society to eliminate survey chest films, Neptune favors annual chest films in patients over 40 years of age and particularly in smokers, to enhance early pickup of lesions favorable for surgical therapy. However, large public expenditures for healthcare surveys are decreasing in our society with the advent of medical rationing and "cost-benefit" analysis.

It is in the realm of indications for operative intervention that Neptune proves to be a contrarian. He does not believe in the usefulness of routine sputum cytology, routine bone scans in the absence of pain, anemia, or abnormal blood chemistries, or liver and spleen scans in the absence of abnormal liver function studies and routine bronchoscopy for diagnosis (but agrees to its usefulness in determining operability for central lesions). However, he is a strong advocate of CT imaging of the chest, upper abdomen, and head. As far as mediastinoscopy is concerned, Neptune's thoughts are most controversial, since he favors the procedure only when enlarged mediastinal nodes are demonstrated on CT imaging. In the absence of small cell undifferentiated lung cancer, he believes that both the presence of ipsilateral and contralateral nodes are not contraindications to operative intervention. Much of his belief is based on personal experience indicating that the removal of a tumor offers the patient the greatest comfort and possibility of extended survival.

It is difficult to critique a single surgeon's experience with a disease entity as variable as cancer of the lung. Nevertheless, most authorities agree that preoperative and intraoperative staging is essential to evaluate effectiveness of the various therapeutic modalities applied for the treatment of lung cancer. While CT and magnetic resonance imaging (MRI) are highly accurate in assessing the hilum and mediastinum for adenopathy, neither method is capable of detecting mediastinal invasion or differentiating hyperplastic from metastatic nodes.[2] Similarly, mediastinoscopy is commonly used both for staging as well as to determine which patients are candidates for surgical intervention.[3] Others believe that "mediastinoscopy positive" patients may be managed by resection and adjuvant radiotherapy provided that the positive mediastinal nodes are ipsilateral, the nodal masses are neither fixed to the trachea or aortic arch, and oat cell carcinoma is not present.[4] Since Neptune proceeds with thoracotomy "regardless of the findings on mediastinoscopy" (except for small cell undifferentiated cancer), it is difficult to understand why he performs mediastinoscopy at all. Nevertheless, prospective studies indicate that mediastinoscopy is the most accurate method of preoperatively assessing mediastinal node status when staging a patient with lung cancer.[5]

Neptune and Overholt have argued since 1949 that segmental resection for lung cancer is a valid operation for extended survival and should not be limited to elderly patients or those with marginal pulmonary reserve. When first suggested, this idea seemed radical, since either pneumonectomy or lobectomy was the treatment of choice for primary bronchogenic carcinoma; however, recent reports indicate that there may be merit in this approach. Neptune carries this concept one step further by stating that extensive node dissection does not increase the potential for extended survival and supports this argument by presenting data on stage II and stage III disease suggesting significant five-year survival for this group of patients. However, Neptune's publication, involving a review of 95 consecutive patients, indicates a T_3N_1 five-year survival of 60 per cent and a T_1 or T_2N_2 five-year survival of 12 per cent, which is contrary to expectations. Those data demonstrate the necessity for statistical comparison between carefully staged treatment groups and the dangers of basing clinical therapeutic decisions on small numbers of patients. The issue of whether to perform unilateral radical mediastinal node dissection in N_2M_0 disease or even to extend the dissection to include positive contralateral mediastinal nodes is presently unsettled.[6] Some investigators even argue that systematic dissection of draining nodes may not be superior to node sampling for staging purposes.[7] Because of the lack of standardization in what constitutes a hilar and mediastinal lymphadenectomy, it is difficult to obtain equivalent data to reach statistically valid conclusions.

In the realm of preoperative and postoperative radiotherapy, Neptune again takes an alternative stance. While admitting that randomized trials have failed to demonstrate an increase in survival in patients undergoing preoperative radiotherapy, he again argues that resectability is the goal and that preoperative radiotherapy improves resectability. To support this concept, he presents a series of 64 subjectively staged patients undergoing preoperative radiation and reports a 34 per cent five-year survival rate. Similarly, Neptune advises postoperative radiotherapy in patients with documented nodal involvement and further suggests that this should be accompanied by postoperative chemotherapy, e.g., 5-fluorouracil. Again, the data presented involve small groups of patients rendering statistical validation impossible. Neptune continues his contrarian position in describing the specific details of his operative technique. He prefers a posterolateral thoracotomy with the patient in the prone position as described by Overholt; he never closes a bronchus with staples, leaves long bronchial stumps, and uses only three sutures to close even a main-stem bronchus.

To support his thinking, Neptune describes 15 clinical cases, fully accepting the criticism that these examples are preselected and the results anecdotal. In conclusion, it is difficult to refute the arguments of a technically superb thoracic surgeon who has devoted a lifetime to the treatment of cancer of the lung. While the modes of therapy detailed in this chapter are controversial and may not gibe with accepted wisdom, they reflect the unvarnished thinking of a caring, devoted, and successful thoracic surgeon.

REFERENCES

1. Thomas, P.A., Piantadosi, S., and the Lung Cancer Study Group: Postoperative T_1N_0 non-small cell lung cancer. Squamous versus nonsquamous recurrences. J. Thorac. Cardiovasc. Surg. *94:*349, 1987.
2. Martini, N., Heelan, R., and Westcott, J.: Comparative merits of conventional, computed tomographic, and magnetic resonance imaging in assessing mediastinal involvement in surgically confirmed lung carcinoma. J. Thorac. Cardiovasc. Surg. *90:*639, 1985.
3. Ashraf, M.H., Milsom, P.L., and Walesby, R.K.: Selection by mediastinoscopy and long-term survival in bronchial carcinoma. Ann. Thorac. Surg. *30:*208, 1980.
4. Pearson, F.G.: Use of mediastinoscopy in selection of patients for lung cancer operations. Ann. Thorac. Surg. *30:*205, 1980.
5. Patterson, G.A., Ginsberg, R.J., and Poon, P.Y.: A prospective evaluation of magnetic resonance imaging, computed tomography, and mediastinoscopy in the preoperative assessment of mediastinal node status in bronchogenic carcinoma. J. Thorac. Cardiovasc. Surg. *94:*679, 1987.
6. Naruke, T., Goya, T., and Tsuchiya, R.: The importance of surgery to non-small cell carcinoma of lung with mediastinal lymph node metastasis. Ann. Thorac. Surg. *46.*603, 1988.
7. McKneally, M.F.: Invited comment. *In* Naruke, T., Goya, T., and Tsuchiya, R.: The importance of surgery to non-small cell carcinoma of lung with mediastinal lymph node metastasis. Ann. Thorac. Surg. *46:*609, 1988.

5

GASTRIC CANCER

by Blake Cady, M.D.

Gastric cancer, despite its rapidly falling incidence throughout the past 50 years, remains a significant oncologic problem and results in almost 15,000 deaths per year. Gastric cancer is of particular interest because of the changing patterns and types of disease that have occurred within the stomach over the last five decades.[1-4] The large decrease in overall incidence has been accompanied by a proportional shift in the location of the cancer from the distal stomach to the proximal stomach. Before 1950 only a small proportion of gastric adenocarcinomas arose in the upper stomach or the gastric cardia area. Now, over one-third of all gastric cancers originate in that proximal location. Furthermore, the histologic appearance of the cancers has changed so that a more anaplastic undifferentiated form now predominates in contrast to the better-differentiated varieties that constituted the majority of cases in previous decades.[5]

Another trend in clinical presentation of gastric cancer is the larger proportion of superficial gastric carcinomas; these are extremely early lesions that are totally curable by surgery and occur in between 5 and 10 per cent of cases reported in the United States. These superficial gastric cancers have comprised over 30 per cent of Japanese cases in recent years because of the Japanese experience of extensive public health screening by routine endoscopic examination of the stomach (Table 5–1).

Screening is cost effective in Japan because of the extremely high incidence of gastric carcinoma in contrast to that in the United States, in which population screening would be impractical.

Gastric cancer otherwise occurs clinically either as linitis plastica with diffuse gastric wall involvement in about 15 per cent of cases or as the usual focal lesions that are either ulcerated or polypoid and constitute approximately 75 to 80 per cent of cases.

In addition, gastric lymphoma is now proportionally more common among patients with gastric malignancies because of the marked decrease of

TABLE 5-1. GASTRIC CANCER—NIIGATA, JAPAN

	Time Period			
	1961–1970	1971–1975	1976–1980	1981–1985
# Cases	698	300	344	347
% Early Gastric Cancer	15%	27%	36%	47%
% Transmural Cancers	49%	41%	36%	31%
% Curative Operations	76%	72%	72%	79%
% with + nodes	62%	58%	49%	38%
# nodes per case	30	31	34	38
% of nodes +	16%	14%	9%	6%
5-year survival:				
Node −		76%	87%	92%
Node +		35%	42%	50%

From Soga, J., Ohyama, S., Miyashita, K., et al.: A statistical evaluation of advancement in gastric cancer surgery with special reference to the significance of lymphadenectomy for cure. World J. Surg. *12*:398–405, 1988.

adenocarcinoma. Gastric lymphomas now constitute between 5 and 10 per cent of all cases of gastric malignancy, a much higher proportion than the 1 or 2 per cent reported in previous decades.[6,7]

The epidemiology of gastric adenocarcinoma has been more thoroughly defined in recent years and is at present clearly related to defined dietary constituents in the usual distal gastric adenocarcinoma. The ingestion of large quantities of pickled and salted foods and certain carbohydrates that are converted to nitrates in the stomach are associated with a high incidence of gastric cancer. In contrast, the presence of larger quantities of fresh fruits and vegetables in the diet and the absence of more traditional preservation techniques replaced by freezing, drying, or canning is associated with a low risk of gastric adenocarcinoma. The discrepancy between the rapidly disappearing distal gastric cancers (related to these defined dietary constituents) and the relatively stable absolute incidence but increasing relative proportion of proximal cancers clearly indicates different epidemiologic aspects of these two types. The exact epidemiology of the proximal gastric cancers has not yet been established. Migrant studies indicate that people coming to the United States from areas of high gastric cancer incidence lose the high gastric cancer risk within two or three generations and develop an incidence of gastric cancer much like that of the remainder of the population in the United States. This rapid shift that results from migration and changing lifestyle clearly indicates that the vast majority of gastric adenocarcinoma worldwide is environmental (dietary) in origin. Clearer definition of these dietary features is still required, but the circumstantial data about dietary features are compelling enough to accept as proven.

The diagnostic evaluation of gastric carcinoma has been much simplified in recent years with the advent of endoscopic gastroscopy and computed tomography. Flexible endoscopic inspection of the stomach has enabled accurate biopsies to be obtained from lesions that appeared as abnormalities on gastrointestinal contrast studies. Indeed many patients now are first evaluated for gastric symptoms by primary endoscopic inspection of the stomach even without contrast x-rays of the usual type. Thus, the preoperative diagnosis of gastric cancer is almost always obtained, virtually eliminating the necessity of abdominal explorations with unknown preoperative gastric pathology. Furthermore, patients with obvious unresectable or inoperative gastric carcinoma, demonstrated through the presence of a rectal shelf, ascites, or extensive liver metastases, can be spared diagnostic exploration because of the reliable endoscopic biopsies that can be obtained. Preoperative computed tomography (CT) scanning or magnetic resonance imaging (MRI) of patients with known gastric carcinoma can provide useful information for the surgeon by demonstrating involvement of adjacent organs and the extent of involvement of the stomach as well as the presence of liver metastases, bulky celiac lymph node metastases, and small quantities of ascites.

The major therapeutic controversy in the treatment of gastric adenocarcinoma today is the conflict between proponents of a radical approach to gastric cancer by the routine use of total gastrectomy or extensive lymph node resections of the upper abdomen with sacrifice of adjacent organs, or both, in a high percentage of cases and the conservative viewpoint, which advocates a subtotal gastrectomy with preservation of the uninvolved stomach after achieving a reasonable local margin around the cancer, with avoidance of total gastrectomy if at all possible, and limited perigastric lymph node resection.[8–12]

The cure rate with conservative surgery is as high as that with the more extensive resections and is accompanied by far lower rates of operative mortality and postoperative morbidity. The radical general approach to gastric cancer is advocated more by Japanese and European surgeons, while a conservative approach is more widely advocated in the United States. Currently, a randomized prospective therapeutic trial comparing radical and conservative gastric surgery for gastric adenocarcinoma is under way in Japan and Europe.[13–15] The results will not be available for several years but obviously will provide the definitive answers regarding the possible advantages of one approach over the other or the lack of effectiveness of very radical surgery. A small randomized study in South Africa confirmed the higher morbidity of extensive resection and the lack of advantage in outcome (Table 5–2). Retrospective studies are unable to answer the question because of the less accurate lymph node staging if only a few nodes are removed as well as the rapidly improving clinical presentation. At a time of marked decrease in advanced disease, with fewer node metastases and smaller cancers, a change in therapy cannot be credited with the improved outcome (see Table 5–1). It may well be that the seeming advantage of more radical surgery has only to do with more accurate staging, referred to as the "Will Rogers effect." More accurate staging may make the results in each presumed stage seem better by dropping more advanced (but previously unrecognized) cases out of less advanced stages, thus artificially increasing cure rates. Such an interpretation can be presumed by examining data from some recent Japanese studies (Table 5–3). Tables 5–1 and 5–2 indicate several factors. Even in the Japanese programs that advocate super-radical resections with extensive nodal removal, only a very small proportion of patients actually undergoes such surgery. These tables also illustrate the rapid improvement in clinical presentation of gastric cancer and present the assumption of the classic fallacy that a change in therapy has produced better results that occur solely as a result of improved stage, as well as improved cases or earlier disease even within stages.[16–18] This fallacious reasoning has occurred in

TABLE 5–2. R1 VS R2 GASTRIC CANCER RESECTION[14]

Randomized Trial

Total Patients	608	Eligibility for Protocol 43 (7%)	
Total Operations	403 (66%)	Eligibility for Protocol 43 (11%)	
		R1	*R2*
Cases		22	21
Operating time, hours		1.7 +0.6	2.3 +0.7
Transfusions		4	25
Postoperative stay days		9.3 +4.7	13.9 +9.7
Re-operations		0	4
Survival			
DOD		4	5
LWD		1	0
NED		16	15
Probability of 3-year survival		78%	76%

From Dent, D.M., Madden, M.V. and Price, S.K.: Randomized comparison of R1 and R2 gastrectomy for gastric carcinoma. Br. J. Surg. 75:110–112, 1988.

areas of surgery in which more radical or less radical approaches have been advanced at times of improving disease presentation; such reason reemphasizes the absolute necessity of concurrent controls to illustrate the changed natural history. Until clear advantages can be proven to result from radical surgery, it would be wisest to practice a more conservative safer approach with less mortality and morbidity.

Adenocarcinoma that originates in the body or antrum of the stomach can be approached in a traditional manner with removal of the proximal duodenum, lesser omentum, and gastrocolic omentum and sacrifice of the distal stomach such that a 3 or 4 cm margin of normal stomach is achieved

TABLE 5–3. 1906 GASTRIC CANCER CASES 1966–1986 YONAGOTA, JAPAN
367 (19%) CURATIVE RESECTIONS, SCEROSAL INVOLVEMENT 8 (2.2%) OPERATIVE MORTALITY[10]

	5-Year Survival			
	"R2" Dissection 188 cases		"R3" Dissection 165 cases	
Operative Mortality	3	1.6%	5	3.0%
Survival: Overall	49%	NS	50%	
N_0	49%	NS	84%	
N_1	71%	NS	56%	
N_2	42%	NS	35%	
N_3	31%	NS	26%	
Hepatoduodenal N_3	—		31%	

R2 operations earlier years; R3 operations later years
R3 = R2 + hepatoduodenal, retropancreatic, colon, mesenteric nodes
NS = not significant

Data from Kaibara, N., Sumi, K., Yonekawa, M., et al.: Does extensive dissection of lymph nodes improve the results of surgical treatment of gastric cancer? Am. J. Surg. 159:218–221, 1990.

above the cancer. This usually necessitates sacrifice of three-quarters or more of the stomach with a Billroth II gastrojejunostomy utilized for reconstruction of the gastrointestinal tract. If the gastric adenocarcinoma by direct extension involves the transverse colon, the left lobe of the liver, or the pancreas or spleen, a complete removal of incontinuity disease can still be achieved by sacrifice of these organs.

Proximal gastric carcinomas warrant a proximal gastrectomy of greater or lesser extent, the crucial feature that determines the operative approach being the extent of involvement of the distal esophagus, the esophageal hiatus, and the celiac lymph node area. A smaller proportion of proximal gastric adenocarcinomas is resectable because extensive involvement of adjacent unremovable areas occurs relatively early in the disease course. While many proximal gastric carcinomas can be resected from below the diaphragm transabdominally when there is minimal esophageal involvement, any significant upward spread in the esophagus requires a concurrent thoracotomy for wider exposure of the distal esophagus. While a left thoracotomy was at one time the most widely practiced thoracoabdominal approach, there are limitations in resecting extensive amounts of esophagus because of the location of the heart.[19] Thus, the most satisfactory contemporary approach to lesions involving a significant portion of the distal esophagus is by a right thoracotomy after the entire stomach has been freed up abdominally. The abdominal portion of the procedure is completed, the wound closed, and the patient repositioned for a right lateral thoracotomy. The gastroesophageal anastomosis is performed at an appropriate level without tension.

In our recent report of gastric adenocarcinoma,[1] 85 per cent of all lesions were operable and 60 per cent of all lesions were resectable. Roughly 60 per cent of the resections were performed for cure, while 40 per cent were strictly palliative in that gross disease was left behind at the end of the operative procedure. Initial exploration of the abdomen, when surgery was performed for gastric adenocarcinoma, should include the inspection of the peritoneal surfaces, the pelvic cul-de-sac, the gastrocolic and the greater omentum, the duodenum, and the splenic hilum and a search for evidence of lymph node enlargement in the peripancreatic and porta hepatis area, and for the presence of hepatic metastases. The celiac axis area is also examined for the extent of local and regional disease around the stomach to evaluate resectability. Because of ulceration, bleeding, obstruction, and pain, the primary cancer in the stomach should be removed if at all possible for palliation even if grossly involved lymph nodes are left behind. While this can generally be achieved, in a proportion of patients the removal of the stomach itself is impossible because of the extensive involvement of surrounding lymph nodes or the massive direct spread of the primary cancer. Removal of the stomach is certainly justified even if gross disease is left behind; only when the technical performance of a gastrectomy and anastomosis seems impossible should the malignancy be declared unresectable.

Traditionally, the radical surgical approach to gastric carcinoma has included resection of the greater omentum, the spleen, lymph nodes of the celiac axis and peripancreatic area that are adjacent to the stomach, and any adjacent organs such as the tail of the pancreas and the left lateral segment of the liver that are adherent. There is little evidence, however, that arbitrary removal of these other organs or extensive lymph node regions in a doctrinaire, routine manner improves survival, since disease that is so extensive as to involve those organs is generally not curable. There is evidence that the routine removal of the spleen, for instance, or the greater omentum contributes nothing to overall survival. The omental removal is done because of the occasional transserosal metastases that lodge; however, if that is to occur, the malignancy is incurable (disease at a distance), and therefore omental sacrifice provides no added increment of cure. Similarly, the possibility of cure in gastric adenocarcinoma if lymph node metastases occur at regions farther from the stomach than the perigastric lymph nodes is extremely low. Therefore, extensive lymphatic resections of the celiac, peripancreatic, and entire upper abdominal areas can produce little in terms of incremental increases in survival. In previous studies we have demonstrated only a 10 per cent survival if more than three nodal metastases in the perigastric area lymph nodes occur, while the survival is only 20 per cent if one to three perigastric lymph node metastases are present. Japanese series advocating more extensive lymphatic resections suggest that significant survival gains can be obtained by removing large numbers of negative lymph nodes. Our recent report of generally conservative resections without extensive lymphatic removal or routine sacrifice of the spleen, the omentum, or the total stomach produced survival rates that are actually improved over previous reports from our own institution, where a more radical general approach had been undertaken (Table 5–4). These improved, more recent results occur because of the decreased rate of operative mortality and the earlier appearance of the disease, not because of the more conservative resection. However, earlier disease allows the more conservative, safer surgery.

A further aspect of the Japanese experience advocating super-radical surgery is that gastric cancer in Japan is of the distal, diet-related variety and histology is usually of the intestinal type, and both features are associated with a better overall prognosis. We have shown that patients with lymph node metastases from the intestinal type histology have a far greater likelihood of survival than patients with lymph node metastases from the diffuse histologic type more common in the United States. Since Japanese experience

TABLE 5–4. GASTRIC CANCER CHANGING PATTERNS OF SURGERY AND SURVIVAL LAHEY CLINIC FOUNDATION

	1932–1939	1940–1949	1950–1958	1957–1966	1967–1982
Total cases	308	981	641	403	211
Laparotomy			83%	94%	84%
Operative mortality	23%	9%	7%	6%	2.8%
Palliative resections	7%	11%	18%	14%	24%
Curative resections	39%	37%	41%	44%	34%
Total resection rate	46%	47%	59%	58%	58%
5-year survival as a proportion of:					
All cases	3%	7%	11%	11%	21%
All cases resected	7%	15%	19%	19%	36%
All curative resections	11%	24%	25%	23%	58%

From Cady, B., Rossi, R., Silverman, M.L., et al.: Gastric adenocarcinoma: A disease in transition. Arch. Surg. *124*:303–308, 1989.

with lymph node metastases is overwhelmingly of intestinal type histology while American experience involves diffuse histology in over 50 per cent of cases, extensive lymph node removal may have completely different implications and results in Japan than it would in the United States.[20]

Use of routine total gastrectomy to improve local control rates in gastric carcinoma has continued to be advocated. Linitis plastica of the stomach almost always requires total gastrectomy for removal because of the extensive involvement of the entire gastric wall with relative sparing of the mucosa and delayed evidence of obstruction and bleeding. However, in our experience this clinical presentation of gastric cancer is totally incurable despite extensive resections. Occasionally total gastrectomy is required to remove the entire cancer, even in the absence of a linitis plastica clinical presentation. If required to remove the primary gastric disease, total gastrectomy is certainly appropriate. However, removal of large portions of uninvolved stomach in either proximal or distal carcinomas has not been demonstrated to improve the cure rate and does increase the rates of operative mortality and postoperative morbidity. Nutrition tends to be less satisfactory following total gastrectomy, and the routine construction of intestinal pouches to increase the ability to take foods by mouth has largely been abandoned because of the lack of apparent success and technical difficulty of pouch creation. Thus, even a small residual gastric pouch, either proximal or distal, is better than esophagojejunostomy.

Postoperative follow-up of gastric adenocarcinoma should focus on evidence of recurrence that causes obstruction or metastatic disease that can be treated for symptom relief. Occasionally malignancy will recur at the anastomotic site and obstruction will result. Minimal other metastatic disease that is present may justify re-resection for palliation. Recurrence at the duodenal stump is not uncommon in distal gastric cancers and accounts for the recommendation of Billroth II reconstructions after gastric cancer resection. Billroth I reconstructions more frequently require re-exploration for local recurrence than Billroth II reanastomoses.

Patients undergoing gastric resection for benign ulcer disease in the past have been shown to be at a high risk of proximal gastric cancer at follow-up. This risk increases in each succeeding decade after resection.[21, 22] These resulting cancers are typical proximal type gastric adenocarcinomas with striking male predominance, lower resection rate, and lower cure rate and require more difficult surgery. The risk is high enough so that patients with subtotal gastrectomies for ulcer disease should be screened periodically by endoscopy and undergo biopsy, even if no cancer is seen, to examine for dysplasia and atypical gastritis. Animal models that develop such postgastrectomy cancers illustrate the risk of such patients, although the exact cause is unclear.

Superficial gastric carcinoma is almost 100 per cent curable because of its early presentation and lack of full thickness penetration of the gastric wall. Superficial gastric cancer may initially occur with wide areas of gastric mucosa involvement. Thus, the postoperative management of patients with superficial gastric carcinoma should involve yearly gastroscopy and biopsy of suspicious lesions since malignancy occasionally will recur in the mucosa and still be treatable and curable by re-resection.

OPERATIVE DECISION-MAKING

Following removal of the gastric specimen, the surgeon should have it opened and displayed so that estimations can be made of proximal and distal surgical margins. If there are concerns about adequacy of margins, frozen sections may be obtained. However, in the usual gastric adenocarcinoma the palpably normal area of esophagus or proximal stomach that is several centimeters from the edge of the discernible tumor should provide adequate protection from local recurrence in the suture line.[23] The finding of wide areas of submucosal lymphatic involvement with adenocarcinoma cells indicates a nearly hopeless long-term prognosis and therefore does not in itself justify a re-resection of a palpably normal esophagus to obtain a clear margin. Similarly, if a cuff of duodenum that is found to be adequate by palpation and observed distance from the primary cancer has been resected initially and the margin is positive microscopically, little else can be done that would improve the overall prognosis of such a gastric adenocarcinoma. Further resection of duodenum will not provide a cure. Therefore, frozen sections of margins to confirm that they are not affected are of limited use when a grossly adequate portion of the stomach, duodenum, and esophagus has been obtained.

ADJUVANT TREATMENTS

Recent reports advocate the use of either intraoperative radiation therapy or newer combined chemotherapy for adjuvant therapy of gastric cancer. In Japanese experience with the use of intraoperative radiation therapy, a pentagonal cone has been utilized that radiates the area of the lesser sac and the gastric bed; significant gains have been reported in the survival for advanced stage gastric carcinoma. Such results need to be verified since they are from a nonrandomized experience and seem illogical, given the risk of serosal penetration by gastric adenocarcinoma to the entire peritoneal cavity as well as the high propensity for dissemination systemically or transserosally. While local recurrence in the gastric bed, local lymph nodes, duodenum, or residual stomach may occur, local recurrence is seldom the isolated cause of failure in gastric adenocarcinoma: therefore, more radical local therapy either by radiation or resection would not be expected to improve cure rates. Further developments in this field will be watched with interest but are not expected to contribute to overall survival in advanced gastric carcinoma. Randomized trials are essential to demonstrate whether there is any effect.

Numerous chemotherapeutic programs have been reported in the past for treating gastric adenocarcinoma with limited success. Recently a program of Adriamycin-platinum-etopocide has been reported with impressive partial and complete response rates in recurrent or metastatic gastric adenocarcinoma in early reports. This therapeutic regimen has also been used in a neoadjuvant setting in which unresectable gastric carcinoma was treated and then patients underwent further exploration; roughly half the lesions were then resectable because of the marked shrinkage of the original unresectable carcinoma. Such exciting progress in the chemotherapy of this previously resistant cancer would be a major achievement. However, our own experience and that of others does not support the results reported. As a matter of fact, our response rate has been lower than that achieved with more traditional 5-fluorouracil–based programs (<20 per cent).

SELECTED READINGS

1. Cady, B., Rossi, R., Silverman, M.L., et al.: Gastric adenocarcinoma: A disease in transition. Arch. Surg. *124*:303–308, 1989.
2. Cady, B., and Choe, D.S.: Changing patterns in gastric cancer. *In* Neiburgs, H.E. (Ed.): Prevention & Detection of Cancer. New York, Marcel Dekker, 1982, pp. 2041–2049.
3. Cady, B.: Lymph node metastases. Indicators, but not governors of survival. Arch. Surg. *119*:1067–1072, 1984.
4. Carter, K.J., Schaffer, H.A., and Ritchie, W.P.: Early gastric cancer. Ann. Surg. *199*:604–609, 1984.
5. Correa, P.: Clinical implications of recent developments in gastric cancer pathology and epidemiology. Semin. Oncol. *1*:2–10, 1985.
6. Hayes, J., and Dunn, E.: Has the incidence of primary gastric lymphoma increased? Cancer *63*:2073–2076, 1989.
7. Lim, F.E., Hartman, A.S., Tan, E.G.C., et al.: Factors in the prognosis of gastric lymphoma. Cancer *39*:1715–1720, 1977.
8. Haugsveldt, T., Viste, A., Eide, E.G., et al.: The survival benefit of resection in patients with advanced stomach cancer: The Norwegian multicentre experience. World J. Surg. *13*:617–622, 1989.
9. Herberer, G., Rechimann, R.K., Kramling, H.-J., and Gunther, B.: Results of gastric resection for carcinoma of the stomach: The European experience. World J. Surg. *12*:374–381, 1988.
10. Kaibara, N., Sumi, K., Yonekawa, M., et al.: Does extensive dissection of lymph nodes improve the results of surgical treatment of gastric cancer? Am. J. Surg. *159*:218–221, 1990.
11. Moreaux, J., and Msika, S.: Carcinoma of the gastric cardia: Surgical management and long-term survival. World J. Surg. *12*:229–235, 1988.
12. Noguchi, Y., Imada, T., Matsumoto, A., et al.: Radical surgery for gastric cancer, a review of the Japanese experience. Cancer *64*:2053–2062, 1989.
13. Diggory, R.T., and Cushieri, A.: R2/3 gastrectomy for gastric carcinoma: An audited experience of a consecutive series. Br. J. Surg. *72*:146–148, 1985.
14. Dent, D.M., Madden, M.V., and Price, S.K.: Randomized comparison of R1 and R2 gastrectomy for gastric carcinoma. Br. J. Surg. *75*:110–112, 1988.
15. Gouzi, J.L., Huguier, M., Fagniez, P.L., et al.: Total versus subtotal gastrectomy for adenocarcinoma of the gastric antrum: A French prospective controlled study. Ann. Surg. *209*:162–165, 1989.
16. Msika, S., Chastang, C., Houry, S., et al.: Lymph node involvement as the only prognostic factor in curative resected gastric carcinoma: A multivariate analysis. World J. Surg. *13*:118–123, 1989.
17. Okusa, T., Nakane, Y., Roky, T., et al.: Quantitative analysis of nodal involvement with respect to survival rate after curative gastrectomy for carcinoma. Surg. Gynecol. Obstet. *170*:488–494, 1990.
18. Rohde, H., Gebbensleben, B., Bauer, P., et al.: Has there been any improvement in the staging of gastric cancer? Findings from the German gastric cancer TNM study group. Cancer *64*:2465–2481, 1989.
19. Ellis, H.J.: Esophagogastrectomy for carcinoma: Technical considerations based on anatomic location of lesion. SCNA *60*:265–279, 1980.
20. Lauren, P.: The two histologic main types of gastric carcinoma: Diffuse and so-called intestinal type carcinoma. An attempt at a histo-clinical classification. Acta Pathol. Microbiol. Scand. *64*:31–49, 1965.
21. Greene, F.L.: Early detection of gastric remnant carcinoma: The role of gastroscopic screening. Arch. Surg. *122*:300–303, 1987.
22. Lundegardh, G., Hans-Olov, A., Jelmick, C., et al.: Stomach cancer after partial gastrectomy for benign ulcer disease. N. Engl. J. Med. *319*:195–200, 1988.
23. Papachristou, D.N., Agnanti, N., D'Agostino, H., and Fortner, J.G.: Histologically positive esophageal margin in the surgical treatment of gastric cancer. Am. J. Surg. *139*:711–713, 1980.

6
COLON CANCER

by T.S. Ravikumar, M.D., and Glenn Steele, Jr., M.D.

INTRODUCTION

About 110,000 new cases of colon cancer were diagnosed in 1990 and roughly half of these patients will succumb to the disease. Colon cancer represents the second leading cause of cancer mortality in the United States, superseded only by lung cancer in men and lung and breast cancer in women. Colon cancer accounts for 12 per cent of cancer-related deaths in the United States.[1] The mortality rate has changed very little during the last 25 years. Against this dismal backdrop, three new developments have taken place during the 1980s that have provided an optimistic outlook for the 1990s. The most intriguing area of advance is our understanding of the genetic and molecular basis of colon carcinogenesis, with the delineation of specific molecular events in human colon cancer development from normal epithelium through proliferative and adenomatous changes to overt carcinoma. The second advance is in the clinical correlation of this concept by defining the polyp/cancer sequence and the effect of surveillance and polypectomy in prevention of colon cancer. The third and most recent area of exciting studies in colon cancer involves adjuvant therapy that incidently raises more questions than it provides answers. Thus, the treatment of large bowel cancer, although historically surgical, now integrates physicians of disparate disciplines, including gastroenterology, medical oncology, immunology, family practice, pathology, radiation therapy, and basic science with concentration in genetics and molecular biology.

ANATOMIC CONSIDERATIONS

Acceptable colon cancer operations are based on principles of spread of colon cancer. These have remained unchanged over many decades and will not be described in detail in this discussion. The boundaries for resecting colon cancer are based on the vascular anatomy, the lymphatic drainage of the bowel, and intramural spread. Unlike rectal cancer, the margin of safety in resection (both mural as well as radial) may be easier to obtain in most colon cancer resections, without as much functional or psychologic debility (i.e., no permanent colostomy). While the surgical technique of colon cancer resection is standard, there have been variations in the cure rate and the local/regional recurrence between institutions and between surgeons.[2, 3] Although patient selection is presumed to be important in explaining these differences, surgical technique must be deemed to make a crucial difference in the outcome. Particularly in patients with sigmoid colon cancer, inappropriate limited surgical resection is often performed without adhering to anatomic and biologic tenets of cancer cure. This is unfortunate, since colon cancer occurs most commonly in the sigmoid colon. We believe that it is imperative that ligation and division of the inferior mesenteric artery be performed at its origin and that the colon be taken down at the splenic flexura to achieve adequate margins of resection and anastomosis without undue tension.

While the cecum, the transverse colon, and the sigmoid colon are mobile structures with visceral peritoneal lining on all sides, the dorsal aspect of ascending and descending colon and frequently both flexurae lack a true serosal lining. Tumor spread from these sites may involve retroperitoneal soft tissues, kidney, ureter, and pancreas. Hence, the pattern of recurrence of tumors at these sites may be different, i.e., tumors arising from the anterior surface may fail and result in peritoneal carcinomatosis, while the failure of tumors from the posterior and lateral aspect may present as regional recurrences[4, 5] Such anatomic considerations explain patterns of recurrence and can be used to justify adjuvant regional therapy such as combined chemotherapy/radiotherapy after surgery in such subsets of colon cancer patients.

The depth of bowel wall penetration and presence or absence of lymph node involvement form an anatomic basis for staging of colon cancer. Paracolic nodes along the marginal vascular arcades are the most numerous and important sites of tumor metastasis. These nodes are especially numerous in the rectosigmoid area.[6] Some intramural lymphatics bypass these nodes, passing directly to the intermediate or central nodes, which explains the occasional finding of skip metastasis. Nonetheless, standard resections (as noted further on) provide optimal surgical clearance and pathologic staging of all colon cancers that are not fixed to adjacent organs.

It should be noted that colon cancer is a changing disease with a trend toward more proximal colon cancer that is probably not simply a function of increased diagnosis of proximal bowel tumors by increased access of proximal bowel to colonoscopic screening. Currently, only about 55 to 60 per cent of the cases are diagnosable with rigid proctosigmoidoscopy.[3, 6] This has definite implications for designing screening protocols and may imply differences in biology as well.

ETIOLOGY OF COLON CANCER

It has not yet been possible to identify a specific cause of colon cancer. Epidemiologic studies of nutritional habits and migration patterns of populations have incriminated environmental and dietary factors in colon cancer.

Colorectal cancer is associated with animal tissue, low fiber, and seems to be a disease predominantly of western civilization.[7] Studies of colon cancer epidemiology among immigrants (Japanese in the United States and immigrants in Europe, Israel, Australia, and Puerto Rico) demonstrate a general two-generation assumption of risk of these host countries.

Currently, several etiologic postulates are being tested in preclinical settings with occasional unwieldy attempts at chemoprevention in some clinical trials:

1. Lower intake of calcium in the diet has been associated with colon cancer.[8] Calcium supplementation may modulate the damage by reducing the concentration of free bile acids.[9]

2. Fecapentaenes are potent mutagens found in feces caused by gut microflora. An attempt to lower the intraluminal levels of fecapentaenes has been made by high-fiber supplement and vitamins C and E intake.[10,11]

3. 3-keto steroids and pyrolysis products have been present in higher concentrations in the population at high risk for colon cancer.[7]

4. Free bile acid concentration has been postulated to be crucial in the genesis of colon cancer.[7]

5. Epidemiologic studies comparing South Africa with the United States reveal a higher incidence of colon cancer in subjects with higher stool pH.[12]

6. Serum cholesterol and β-lipoprotein levels have been related to colon cancer in case-controlled studies. It seems that while this issue is far from settled, the individuals in whom colon cancer develops share the same level of serum cholesterol as the general population initially; however, during the 10 years preceding the cancer, these individuals demonstrate a decline in serum cholesterol level that is the opposite to the rising level seen with age in the general population.[13]

Current studies addressing diet and behavior modification are extremely complex, and meaningful conclusions will probably only occur in the unlikely setting of a "home run" positive result. More probably such studies will produce useful results if they are designed with precise biologic postulates that can be measured with precise biologic or chemical assays as end points, such as the effect of various dietary modifications on crypt cell turnover in patients with familial polyposis coli.

RISK FACTORS AND THE GENETICS OF COLON CANCER

While most etiologic factors previously mentioned have been gleaned from population cohort studies and epidemiologic observations, it is possible to identify individual patients at high risk for the development of colon cancer. In fact, a large body of evidence for colorectal carcinogenesis comes from the genetic analyses of such high-risk subjects and their kindred, and surveillance data on the target organ at risk including the serial removal of neoplastic and preneoplastic polyps.

Despite the progressive increase in incidence of colorectal cancer from 1973 to 1986, the adjusted rate of colorectal cancer deaths has declined by 7 per cent.[6] This has been primarily attributed to careful surveillance of high-risk groups and removal of neoplastic and preneoplastic polyps in the non-predisposed individual. Colon cancer is primarily a disease of the older population; median age at diagnosis is 71 years. Risk increases with age. While the incidence rate for 30- to 34-year-olds is 3 per 100,000, it rises to 530 per 100,000 for individuals aged 85 years and older.

What are the risk groups for colon cancer and how can this information be used to determine rational but admittedly empiric screening criteria? Men and women 40 years of age and older are considered at average risk for developing colon cancer. Although no age group is immune, populations under this age group are in the low-risk category. This is the basis for general recommendations by various medical and surgical societies to perform annual rectal digital examination and stool guaiac at age 40 and beyond. At present, those having the following are categorized at high risk for developing colon cancer:

1. family pattern of colon cancers: polyposis and nonpolyposis syndromes;
2. prior colon carcinoma or adenomatous or villous polyp;
3. first-degree relative of an individual with colon cancer;
4. inflammatory bowel disease, most notably ulcerative colitis but also Crohn's colitis;
5. prior pelvic irradiation.

Overall, 94 per cent of colon cancers diagnosed currently fall into the "sporadic" cancer category. Familial polyposis coli accounts for 1 per cent of all colon cancers and the remaining 5 per cent are a part of one or another of the cancer family syndromes. Screening recommendations of known genetic and "garden variety" colon cancers and opportunities for intervention are summarized in Table 6–1.

Familial Polyposis Syndromes

Although rare, familial adenomatous polyposis syndrome has attracted great attention, not only because of its genetic propensity, but more because of the fact that virtually all affected individuals can develop colon cancer that is preventable by early intervention. This is an autosomal dominant trait with greater than 90 per cent penetrance. In adolescence, patients have characteristic multiple polyps, often as many as 1000. If the polyposis is left untreated, the risk of colorectal cancer rises progressively with age until almost 100 per cent will go on to develop cancer. The median age for colon cancer development is in the third decade. In 1987, Bodmer and colleagues identified a locus for the familial adenomatous polyposis gene (FAP locus) and the putative gene responsible for this syndrome on chromosome 5 near the Fq 21–22 band.[14] Subsequent studies have identified allele loss on chromosome 5 in sporadic noninherited colon cancers also.[15] This gene is purported to endow the colonic mucosa with a hyperproliferative signal.

Familial Cancer Syndromes

The most common among the syndromes is Gardner's syndrome, also inherited as an autosomal dominant trait. The entire large and small bowel

TABLE 6–1. RISK FACTORS FOR COLON CANCER

Category	Intervention
Environmental and dietary	Limit total dietary fat and cholesterol. Add fiber, vitamin C, vitamin E, calcium
Genetic	
Familial polyposis coli	Early colonoscopy (adolescence). Total proctocolectomy
Familial cancer syndrome (Gardner, Lynch, Oldfield, Turcot)	Early and yearly screening and surveillance, polypectomy
Family history of colon cancer and familial colorectal cancer syndrome	Early and yearly screening and surveillance, polypectomy
Predisposing colon diseases	
Previous colorectal cancer and/or nonhyperplastic polyps	Postoperative follow-up for metachronous cancers and polyps
Neoplastic polyps	Polypectomy and endoscopic follow-up
Inflammatory bowel disease	Yearly surveillance, benefit difficult to prove
Pelvic irradiation	Proctosigmoidoscopy yearly
Average risk:	
All men and women over age 40	Yearly digital rectal examination and stool blood test. Screening sigmoidoscopy every 3–5 years, over 50 years of age

may be affected by adenomatous changes. Characteristically, other mesenchymal abnormalities may exist (desmoid tumors of mesentery and abdominal wall, lipomas, sebaceous cysts, osteomas, and fibromas).[16] Because the syndrome is not fully expressed in every individual, a thorough evaluation of all family members for both epithelial and mesenchymal features is mandatory.[16] Oldfield syndrome consists of polyposis and adenocarcinoma of the colorectum associated with multiple sebaceous cysts.[17] Turcot syndrome is an autosomal recessive condition as yet ill-defined genetically; it is associated with malignant tumors of the central nervous system and large bowel.[18] Lynch and colleagues described a clinical condition characterized by hereditary site specific nonpolyposis colon cancer that is inherited as an autosomal dominant trait with 90 per cent penetrance.[19] Features include multiple colon cancers developing at a relatively young age. The majority of cancers are located in the proximal colon, and the development of flat adenomas in other parts of the colon indicates the need for thorough colonoscopy. A variant of the Lynch syndrome (the so-called Lynch type II) is associated with colon cancer and other adenocarcinomas, most commonly endometrial, ovarian, breast, or gastric.[19]

Predisposing Colon Disease

Previous history of colorectal cancer and neoplastic polyps confers a threefold or higher risk of subsequent development of colon cancer. Inflammatory bowel diseases, notably ulcerative colitis, confer a well-recognized increased risk (up to 20- to 30-fold) of colon cancer in patients. Extent of bowel involvement, age at onset, severity, and duration of the disease are very important with respect to ulcerative colitis. A number of retrospective studies have attempted to assess the cumulative risk of cancer in this population. However, the rates vary widely, changing from about 35 per cent at 25 years in some studies from Sweden[20] to less than 1 to 2 per cent at 20 years in other studies from Czechoslovakia, Denmark, and Israel.[21] While surveillance in this population is intellectually compelling and has been the norm in many places, there is no conclusive evidence that surveillance is beneficial. Being involved in a surveillance program does not guarantee that lethal cancers will not develop, because it is very difficult to identify the highest risk area of the target organ. Many of the cancers develop in flat mucosa. Often dysplasia is multifocal, leading to a large sampling error, and the morphologic description of increasingly severe dysplasia remains qualitative. Even if some patients benefit, it is not clear that this justifies the large cost of surveillance, which is estimated to be about $200,000 for each cancer found.[21] In people with a high risk of developing colon cancer, several markers have been postulated to predict early or future cancer occurrence. Most of these are tumor-associated antigens detected by monoclonal antibodies and some are biochemical markers such as ornithine decarboxylase deficiency[22] or increasing expression of sucrase isomaltase.[23] Such early studies warrant further large scale analyses before any conclusions can be made regarding application to conventional screening approaches.

Molecular Genetics of Colon Cancer

The most exciting research in the area of molecular biology of solid tumors is in proving the old concept of multistep colon carcinogenesis. While the identification of the putative gene responsible for familial polyposis has stimulated enthusiasm to search for more general chromosomal changes during colon cancer development, concurrent studies on the role of various dominant proto-oncogenes has led to a beginning delineation of their role in colon carcinogenesis. Bos and coworkers have identified ras mutations in over 40 per cent of colon cancers.[24] Other oncogenes, such as myc, have been implicated in colon cancer progression.[25] Vogelstein and others have extended these observations in providing their postulate of a multistep process in colorectal cancer development involving a progressive mutational activation of multiple oncogenes, as well as inactivation of what undoubtedly will become numerous tumor suppressor genes.[26] Allelic loss on chromosome 5 (FAP locus) and other events in the nucleus, such as DNA hypomethylation, may lead to a hyperproliferative state in the "initiated" colon mucosa. A second set of events, such as ras mutation, may lead to colorectal adenoma formation. Ras mutations have been identified in about half of the colorectal adenomas and colorectal cancers.[26] A large proportion are in the Ki-ras gene. Since these mutations are present in both adenomas and carcinomas, it is suggested that ras mutations precede emergence of malignant phenotype. After one or more of these dominant oncogenic mutations, inactivation of tumor suppressor genes seems to occur with the development of malignant phenotype. Vogelstein and coworkers have identified that the p-53 gene (mapped to chromosome 17) seems to be inactivated in the majority of colorectal cancers studied.[27] P-53 gene encodes a nuclear protein that may play a role in cell cycle regulation. As these mutations are identified along with chromosome 17 deletions, it is postulated that this acts as a tumor suppressor gene and the mutational deactivation of this gene by allelic loss may lead to "transformation" of the colon mucosa.

A second tumor suppressor gene, located on the long arm of chromosome 18 (18 q), has now been associated with colorectal cancer progression.[26] In more than 70 per cent of colorectal cancers studied, at least one copy of this gene, called DCC (deleted in colorectal cancer), was missing. It is largely unknown at present as to the genetic changes involved in the further evolution of the metastatic phenotype. Since DCC gene seems to be encoding for a cell adhesion molecule, it is intriguing to postulate that further changes in the genes encoding for cell migration, attachment, and enzymatic degradation of basement membrane may complete the whole spectrum of colon cancer transformation including the metastatic phenotype. Undoubtedly, our understanding of the complexity of enhancer and suppressor genes involved will increase as will the functional interaction between these genes' products and numerous colorectal mucosal- and stromal-related growth factors.

DIAGNOSIS AND SCREENING

In most patients with colon cancer initially occurring symptoms may be vague. Even rectal bleeding has a very low predictive value in the diagnosis of colon cancer. Characteristically, left colon cancers occur with obstruction and right colon tumors with low-grade, chronic bleeding. A minority present with obstruction or perforation. Duration of symptoms do not correlate directly with the prognosis, and in some situations the reverse may be true. Anemia and palpable abdominal mass are other frequent findings. While perforation and obstruction occur acutely, chronic changes can result in change of bowel habits alternating between diarrhea and constipation; chronic perforation with fistula formation to adjacent organs may be involved in the presenting symptoms. In 5 to 10 per cent of patients, distant metastases, most notably in the liver, may be the presenting manifestation.

Screening programs to detect colorectal cancer for the population at large remain of unproven value. Outside of a study setting, screening of asymptomatic patients cannot be justified in an era of cost-benefit analysis. The current empiric American Cancer Society recommendations are:

1. Yearly digital rectal examination for men and women over 40 years of age.
2. Yearly stool guaiac examination for men and women 50 years of age or above.
3. For men and women over 50 years of age, proctosigmoidoscopy every three to five years after two initial negative examinations a year apart.

The screening objectives are to identify and remove premalignant lesions, to detect early stage colorectal cancer, and to provide less extensive surgery in select groups (e.g., local excision for small rectal cancer). Another objective could be to offer reassurance to higher risk patients.

While screening for the asymptomatic population at large is not justified, does screening for high-risk patients satisfy the major rationales?

1. Better outcome in early stage disease—Yes.
2. Important and prevalent illness in society—Yes.
3. Inexpensive, safe, and acceptable—Lack of uniformity of opinion.
4. Treatment plan for screen positive patients—Yes.

Winawer has analyzed the results of stool occult blood testing worldwide.[28] The compliance rate among the total population of 309,000 studied varied widely in the studies from 50 to 90 per cent. Overall, the stool guaiac positivity rate was 1.0 to 2.5 per cent. In some of the studies, the sensitivity was as low as 50 per cent, while the specificity (if the tests were performed appropriately) could be as high as 97 per cent. However, the predictive value, which denotes the detection of adenomas and carcinomas, is only 22 to 58 per cent. Among the cases diagnosed, there was stage "downshifting" to Dukes A and B lesions in 65 to 90 per cent of patients. Diagnostic strategies for patients with positive fecal occult blood tests have also been evaluated. Double contrast barium enema was compared with colonoscopy. The sensitivity was 90 per cent and 95 per cent respectively for double contrast barium enema and colonoscopy in detecting early colon cancers. The cost was roughly similar for both categories in this report, but other studies have shown colonoscopy to be more expensive by a factor of 2 to 3.[6] When compared with colonoscopy, the barium enema was sensitive only in 35 per cent for small polyps (< 1 cm) and specific only in 83 per cent for all polyps taken together. The important caveats to bear in mind are that the fecal occult blood testing is false positive in 2 per cent and false negative in 40 per cent of the cases. The use of air contrast barium enema versus colonoscopy will depend on the risk group being screened. For the average risk population, air contrast barium enema is perhaps more acceptable, while in high-risk populations, colonoscopy will increase the detection rate for small polyps and could be therapeutic in the performance of polypectomy.

The effect of routine screening of the colonic mucosa in the context of physical examination was applied in a study of more than 21,000 patients subjected to routine yearly proctosigmoidoscopy and polypectomy, conducted over many years in Minnesota.[29] It is estimated that 85 per cent of the expected rectosigmoid carcinomas have not appeared in this cohort. No deaths from colorectal cancer were recorded over a period of seven years. Data from other programs of yearly proctosigmoidoscopy suggest a similar reduction in colon cancer incidence by up to 80 per cent. However, prospective randomized trials are not mature enough to make strong recommendations about pancolonic mucosal surveillance and subsequent reduction of the colon cancer risk versus morbidity of the screening procedure itself.

The application of screening techniques outside the setting of physical examination has been even more difficult to evaluate. One such example is the hemoccult screening program carried out by the American Cancer Society in the greater Chicago area.[30] After several days of televised public education, 106,551 people ordered hemoccult test. Of these, 45,658 properly completed and returned their kits; 591 were found to be positive and 508 of these patients saw a physician. Despite this, only 67 patients received an appropriate set of diagnostic studies once they reached a physician. Fifteen of the 22 cancers found in the study were Dukes A and B lesions. Despite the various analytic approaches the study may provide in cost-benefit estimation, the single most important consideration was the fact that most physicians apparently did not know what appropriate diagnostic studies should be performed after stool was found to contain occult blood.

Screening programs for high-risk populations have been well substantiated. For families with familial polyposis coli, colonic mucosal surveillance is recommended starting at age 12. Patients with this syndrome who undergo colon resection with retained rectum should undergo rigid proctoscopy with fulguration of polyps every six months for the rest of their lives. Patients with Lynch syndrome should probably undergo complete colonoscopy annually, starting five years before the age at which the first family member developed colon cancer. If that information is not available, colonoscopy beginning at age 20 is recommended. The caveat of colonoscopic screening for patients with ulcerative colitis has been previously outlined. Other high-risk groups to whom annual flexible sigmoidoscopy is recommended are women with gynecologic malignancies, men with prostate cancer, and any patient who has had pelvic irradiation or who is a first-degree relative of a patient with colorectal cancer.

POLYPS AND COLON CANCER

Neoplastic and non-neoplastic polyps occur in the large bowel. Neoplastic polyps, otherwise called adenomas, may be tubular or villous and are felt to be precursors of colorectal cancers. Dysplastic changes occur in these adenomas, and are forerunners to carcinoma transformation. Dysplasia can be graded from mild to severe. The incidence of carcinoma in polyps is related to size. It varies from 1 per cent in polyps about 0.5 cm in diameter to 45 per cent or more in polyps larger than 3 cm in diameter.[31] Approximately 25 per cent of patients with one polyp will have other adenomas. Villous adenomas are reported to have eight to 10 times the probability of cancer than tubular adenomas.[32] Studies have addressed the rate of recurrence of polyp formation (metachronous) after index polypectomy. Recent colonoscopic studies have demonstrated a recurrence rate of 20 to 60 per cent of new polyps after initial excision.

Cancers invasive only to the level of muscularis mucosa in the polyps do not have access to lymphatic pathways and hence are judged to be cured by endoscopic polypectomy. The factors that should be taken into consideration when considering colon resection after removal of polyps with cancer are the level of invasion, degree of differentiation, presence of lymphatic or blood vessel invasion, and the margin of endoscopic resection. For example, polypectomy can be curative in most patients with moderate or well-differentiated cancer limited to the head of a pedunculated polyp (levels I and II) with no evidence of vessel invasion and clear margins at the stalk.[33] The polypectomy site should, however, be re-examined at approximately six months to confirm lack of recurrence. On the other hand, polyps showing level III or IV invasion (stalk or the submucosa) that are poorly differentiated and show evidence of vessel invasion should be considered as high risk for local or nodal metastatic cancer and be treated with the standard surgical approach as though they have a primary colon cancer. Interestingly enough, adenomatous polyps with the worst prognostic sign cancers in them may be biologic bad actors despite adequate colonic resection subsequent to the polypectomy.

STAGING OF COLON CANCER

Dukes classification has been the practical staging system used in colorectal cancer for 50 years. Various modifications have been incorporated into the original Dukes classification. The most popular modifications are shown in Table 6–2. Despite the long utility of Dukes staging or one of its modifications, the revised and unified tumor, node, and metastasis classification system (TNM) is becoming widely used in the world.[6] The TNM classification system will mitigate some of the confusion that has existed over the years among those using the various Dukes-based classifications. The most salient features in changing to a unified TNM classification are:

1. Shifting of B_1 stage from the old system stage II to stage I in the new TNM classification (B_1 equals T_2N_0 lesions).
2. Inclusion of the Gastrointestinal Tumor Study Group's modifications (B_3 as T_4N_0 category).
3. Comparison between studies under the revised system is simpler and considers the important prognostic factors of depth of penetration of the primary tumor plus the number of positive nodes (N_1 versus N_2).

PREOPERATIVE AND INTRAOPERATIVE CONSIDERATIONS

The routine preoperative evaluation should include a careful history for familial incidence of colon cancer and other cancers, physical examination

TABLE 6–2. STAGING SYSTEMS FOR COLON CANCER**

Classification	Stage A	Stage B		Stage C	
		B_1	B_2	C_1	C_2
Dukes, 1948	Limited to wall	Spread by direct		Regional	Glands
Kirklin, 1949	Limited to mucosa	To muscularis propria	Through muscularis propria	Lymph node involvement	
Aster/Coller, 1954	Limited to mucosa	To muscularis propria	Through muscularis propria to wall; nodes positive	Tumor limited	Tumor through the wall; nodes positive
*GITSG, 1984	Limited to mucosa	To muscularis propria	Through muscularis propria	1–4 positive nodes	More than 5 lymph nodes positive
AJCC/UICC, nodes		*Stage I* T_1: To submucosa	*Stage II* T_3: Through muscularis propria into subserosa	*Stage III* N_1: 1–3 pericolic lymph	

*Later modification included B_3 and C_3 to denote spread through serosa into contiguous organs.
**Stage D or Stage IV refers to distant metastases, M_1.

to look for any abdominal masses and to rule out metastasis, and laboratory data including complete blood count, CEA, and liver chemistries. Since about 4 per cent of patients will have synchronous cancers and perhaps a higher percentage will have synchronous polyps, the remainder of the colon should be evaluated with colonoscopy or an air contrast barium enema combined with sigmoidoscopy. A preoperative computed tomography (CT) scan or ultrasound study of the liver as baseline is often performed, but the cost benefit is questionable. An x-ray of the chest is obtained for anesthetic evaluation and to rule out metastases. If preoperative evaluation of proximal colonic mucosa is obviated by an obstructing lesion, colonoscopy or double contrast enema should be performed within three months after operation.

A formal complete surgical exploration is performed during surgery. Bimanual palpation of the liver is very sensitive in detecting occult liver metastasis undetected by preoperative evaluation. The use of intraoperative ultrasound to screen apparently normal livers remains investigational. The primary treatment approach in patients with colon cancer involves en bloc surgical resection with excision of adequate colon proximally and distally, adequate lateral margins of the tumor in case it is adherent to contiguous structure, and removal of regional lymphatics. The extent of colonic resection for colon cancer is determined not only by the biology of local tumor growth intramurally, but more so by the requirement of regional lymphadenectomy requiring ligation and division of multiple vascular trunks (Fig. 6–1). Segmental or sleeve resections of colon for treatment of primary colon cancer should be condemned except in those circumstances when it is done for palliation in the presence of distant metastasis. The dogma of no-touch technique was based on the prevention of intraoperative vascular dissemination of tumor cells via the portal vein. Current concepts suggest, however, that the micrometastases are already established prior to the laparotomy in most patients with colon cancer. Hence a more extensive lymph node dissection including peri-iliac, hypogastric, and periaortic lymph nodes as part of the en bloc resection of colon cancer as proposed by Enker and coworkers and most recently by Heald is not recommended.[34] The biology of colon cancer implies that once spread to the periaortic lymph nodes has occurred, the cancer is most likely systemic and not curable by regional surgery. Increased complications entailed by routine radical lymph node dissection and no-touch ligation are therefore not justified. Even in the series of Enker et al, a clear demonstration of delay in regional and systemic recurrence has not been provided in any randomized controlled trial.

SPECIAL CIRCUMSTANCES

Familial Polyposis Coli

The traditional recommendation has been to perform a total proctocolectomy and an end ileostomy. However, during the last 15 years, the technical advance of performing a "Park's procedure" with continent anal ileostomy has improved the functional outlook of these young patients with decades of normal life ahead of them.[35] However, the Park's pouch should be done only by surgeons specially trained in performing the various procedures and familiar with the careful preoperative and postoperative

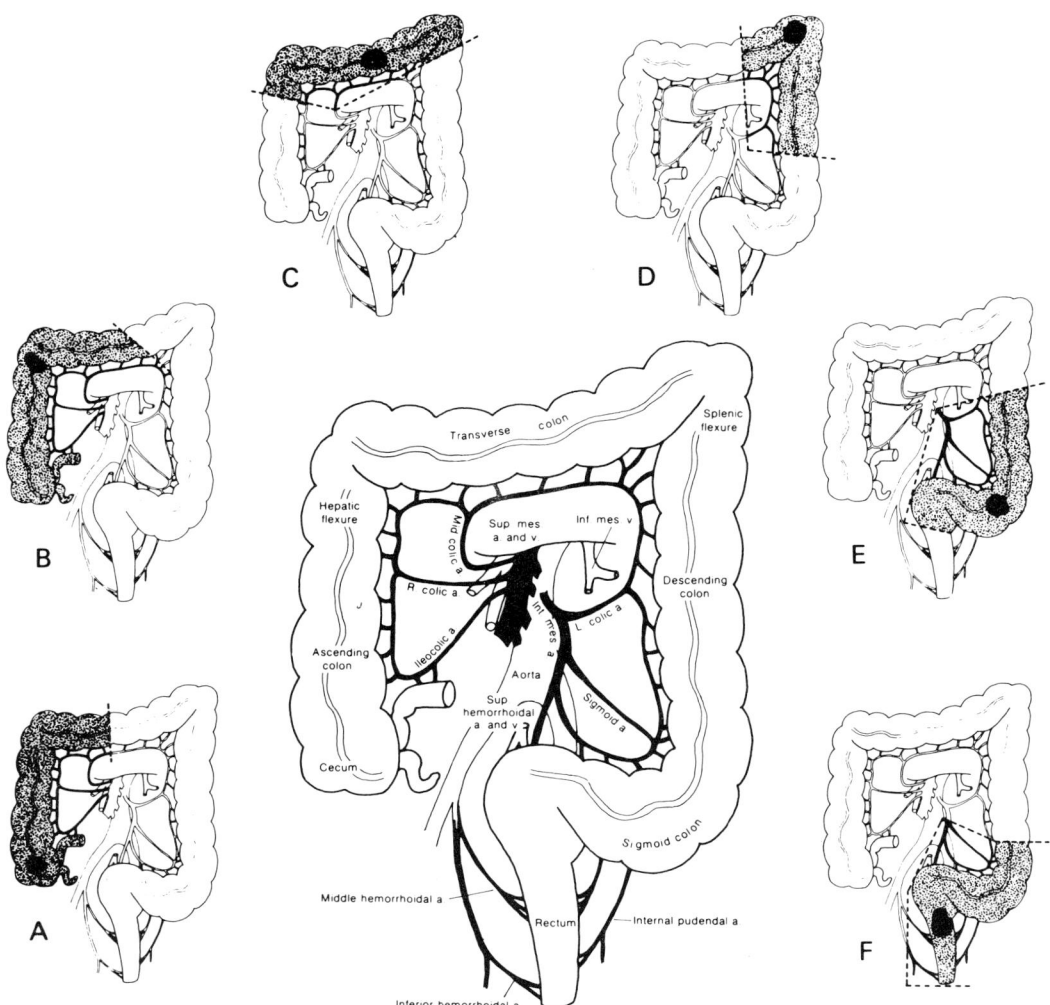

Figure 6–1. Anatomic segments, arterial and venous blood supply, and surgical resections of the colon and rectum. (Redrawn and modified from Jones T, Shepard WC: A Manual of Surgical Anatomy. Philadelphia, Saunders, 1945; and Collier, JA: Cancer of the Colon and Rectum. New York, American Cancer Society, Inc., 1956).

management entailed. In some patients, surgeons have recommended total colectomy with preservation of rectal mucosa in circumstances where the rectum is relatively spared. In such situations, three to six monthly proctoscopic surveillances are essential with removal of any developing polyps.

Prophylactic Oophorectomy

Synchronous ovarian metastases occur in 2 to 8 per cent of women with colorectal cancer; about 4 to 5 per cent of patients undergoing potentially curative resections for colon cancer subsequently develop ovarian metastasis.[36] This has been the rationale for advocating prophylactic oophorectomy along with the curative resection for colon cancer (especially of rectosigmoid or sigmoid). However, there is no evidence that prophylactic oophorectomy changes the survival of women who have undergone colon cancer surgery. O'Brien et al, in their retrospective study of 268 women, have suggested that although prophylactic oophorectomy does not enhance the cure rate of colon cancer, it may obviate the need for reoperation for palliation in a finite number of women.[37] Most studies report a greater risk of ovarian metastasis in node positive patients in premenopausal women. Another factor in recommending oophorectomy prophylactically is that it would reduce or eliminate the risk of subsequent primary ovarian cancer in approximately 1 per cent of women over the age of 40. While in the majority of perimenopausal and postmenopausal women prophylactic oophorectomy should be considered, such recommendation in a premenopausal woman who may desire childbirth is not warranted.

Contiguous Organ Involvement

Approximately 38 to 70 per cent of adhesions between primary colon tumor and an adjacent organ or structure are carcinomatous.[3] Surgeons must, therefore, assume the worst and include the contiguous organ or at least the adjacent part in the en bloc tumor resection. Such en bloc removal is relatively safe and is compatible with prolonged survival (i.e., "cure") in 24 to 64 per cent of patients.[3]

Perforation and Obstruction

Perforation or obstruction of bowel cancer worsens prognosis. Patients with free perforations of their colon cancer have almost no chance of surviving disease-free five years later. Adverse effects on prognosis in patients with obstructing cancers of the colon are likely due to the preponderance of highly invasive lesions. A three-stage procedure is rarely performed for obstructing cancers except in extenuating circumstances. Most such ascending and transverse colon cancers can be treated by a one-stage resection and ileocolon anastomosis. In left-sided obstructing colonic lesions, a two-stage procedure using the so-called Hartmann's pouch is normally used: the tumor is resected with an end colostomy and rectal turn-in. Colon continuity can be established in a second operation after the patient has proven a lack of regional recurrence.

RESULTS AND PROGNOSIS

Five-year survival rates after surgical resection of colon cancer have improved progressively in recent years. A more appropriate and careful staging based on perioperative CT scan and ultrasound, better pathologic grading of resected tumors, and perhaps more widespread application of principles of cancer surgery techniques have contributed to improved survival figures. Cure rates at five years for node negative patients range from 90 per cent for T_1 lesions to about 60 per cent for even T_4 lesions. For any given T classification, the cure rates for node positive patients drop by about 15 per cent. The number of nodes involved is a determinant. The Gastrointestinal Tumor Study Group reported that if four or fewer nodes were involved, a five-year survival of 56 per cent could be expected, while only 26 per cent of patients with more than four nodes survived five years.[38] While the depth of penetration and the number of positive nodes dictate the final outcome to a large part, several other prognostic variables influence the patient's survival.

Age at Presentation

Colon cancer in patients less than 45 years of age occurs at a more advanced stage than in older patients. Furthermore, the percentage of mucinous adenocarcinomas and undifferentiated tumors are higher in younger patients. When one controls for all these variables, there is perhaps no difference in the relative prognosis for the young age groups, simply on the basis of age alone.

Sex

While some studies find no difference in the prognosis between men and women, many studies showed an improved survival for women.

Presenting Features

Features upon presentation such as duration of symptoms, complications such as perforation and obstruction, size of the tumor, and the location of the primary tumor have been looked at as independent prognostic variables. The duration of symptoms does not confer any adverse impact on the ultimate outcome; in fact, some studies propose that symptoms lasting longer than six months may have a favorable impact on long-term survival.[39] Obstruction and/or perforation categorically reduce survival. Multi-institutional studies such as those by the National Surgical Adjuvant Breast and Bowel Project (NSABP) and the Gastrointestinal Tumor Study Group (GITSG) used multivariate analysis to examine obstruction as a prognostic variable.[40,41] Obstruction was an important predictor for prognosis independent of Dukes stage. The relative risk increases up to three-fold. Tumor size in colon cancers and its impact on long-term survival is debatable. While the majority of the retrospective studies report no adverse relationship, some prospective analyses demonstrate increasing size to have a positive effect on overall and disease-free survival.

Pathologic Features

The degree of differentiation, grade, and morphologic types of the primary tumor have been correlated with outcome. Poorly differentiated tumors are noted for local, regional and distant metastasis, and poor outcome.

Morphologic tumor grading is fraught with the problems associated with nonuniformity among pathologists and heterogeneity of pattern seen within a given primary tumor. Just as in poorly differentiated tumors, colloid carcinomas have poor prognosis with increased chance of local, regional, and distant failures. The survival in patients with colloid carcinomas is less than half of noncolloid carcinomas in a given stage. Symonds and Vickery reported that only 34 per cent of patients with colloid colorectal carcinomas were alive at five years.[42] Similarly, a high proportion of stage C or D tumors are colloid carcinomas. In multivariate analysis, blood vessel and lymphatic invasion are independent prognostic variables.

Blood Transfusion

The immunosuppressive effect of blood transfusion has been suggested to have a negative effect on survival of patients with colonic cancer.[43] This was demonstrated regardless of the stage of the primary cancer. The number of units transfused seems to have a strong prognostic value in colon cancer.[44] These reports need further confirmation.

Biomarkers

Carcinoembryonic antigen (CEA) is the best studied biomarker in colon cancer. The preoperative CEA level correlates highly with venous invasion and perhaps extent of tumor burden. The preoperative CEA level is correlated with prognosis in a negative manner in most but not all studies.[45] In addition, in prospective studies for evaluation of postoperative monitoring of patients after resection of the colon cancer, CEA has been shown consistently to be the best overall indicator of early recurrence and response to subsequent therapy.[46]

Tumor DNA Content

Abnormalities in DNA content of primary tumors have recently been associated with a poor prognosis in colorectal and other cancers. Scott et al and Kokal and associates showed an increased percentage of nondiploid tumors among more advanced lesions in colon cancers.[47, 48] A high proportion of patients with colorectal cancer had aneuploid tumors (42 per cent); patients with well-differentiated tumors but tumor aneuploidy had survival similar to poorly differentiated cancer. These data are now emerging in colorectal cancer, and we must await larger studies, as in breast cancer, before tumor DNA content can be used as a prognostic indicator for adjuvant therapy and other interventional diagnostic or treatment modalities.

Novel Gene Products

The products of mutational activations of Ras genes and other markers such as laminin-receptor expression are currently being evaluated in the prediction of aggressive behavior of colon cancer.[49, 50] Ideally, such molecular markers will be applicable at the time of tumor biopsy. This would allow establishment of high-risk subsets prior to pathologic examination of resected specimens. Only then will preoperative or neoadjuvant protocols for colon cancer become possible.

FOLLOW-UP AFTER POTENTIALLY CURATIVE SURGERY

1. Physical examination every three to four months for two to three years, then every six months for two years.
2. Fecal occult blood and sigmoidoscopy, the same frequency as physical examination.
3. Colonoscopy, if not done preoperatively, three to four months postoperatively and then every year. If colon was deemed free of any polyps for two years in a row, extend the frequency to every third year.
4. CEA and liver chemistries should be obtained every three months for two years, then every six months.
5. Chest x-ray yearly.

As we have reported extensively elsewhere and summarized previously, the appropriate follow-up plans will be determined by patient and physician "venue." Only if diagnosis of recurrence will make a difference in conventional or experimental treatment plans is follow-up directed at making such a diagnosis justifiable.

PATTERNS OF RECURRENCE

The liver is the major organ at risk for colorectal cancer failure. In about a third of the patients dying from colon cancer, the liver remains the only site of failure. About 70 per cent of patients with recurrence have hepatic metastasis at some time or other. Local/regional recurrence accounts for about 30 to 40 per cent of failures; however, isolated local recurrence (i.e., suture line recurrence) occurs in less than 5 per cent of those who have failed.[51, 52] Welch and Donaldson analyzed the incidence of recurrence at various sites in their review of 177 patients with recurrent colorectal cancer.[52] Recurrence rates that were reported as "only site" and "with other site" were, respectively: liver—13 per cent, 45 per cent; abdomen—7 per cent, 23 per cent; pelvis—30 per cent, 45 per cent; lung—4 per cent, 32 per cent; bone—0 per cent, 7 per cent; and brain—1 per cent, 6 per cent. The histologic grade of tumor appears to influence the incidence of regional recurrence. Olsen et al reported approximately a 10 per cent incidence of distant metastasis for all tumor grades but diffuse regional recurrences rose from 9 per cent with well-differentiated tumors to 15 per cent for moderately differentiated tumors to 22 per cent with poorly differentiated tumors.[53] Local/regional recurrence correlates with transmural penetration of the primary tumor and particularly with adherence to or invasion of adjacent viscera or structures. The regional failure rate also increases with increasing lymph node involvement, approaching 50 per cent with five or more positive mesenteric lymph nodes. In ascending and descending colon tumors, posterior penetration of the cancer in the area of the colon devoid of serosa may increase local recurrence rate and justify regional adjuvant therapy studies for such colon cancer subsets. The incidence of peritoneal seeding has been difficult to evaluate, but ultimate failure rates of 32 to 58 per cent with peritoneal carcinomatosis have been reported in various studies.[5, 52]

ADJUVANT THERAPY

Both radiation therapy and chemotherapy have been used in the adjuvant setting following resection of colon cancers with a high risk of recurrence. Radiation therapy has been used to minimize local/regional recurrence and to minimize peritoneal failure. While radiation therapy directed at reducing regional recurrence (cecum, ascending colon, descending colon, and sigmoid colon) has met with some success in uncontrolled, single institution, anecdotal studies, data on whole abdominal radiation for patients with high risk of developing peritoneal carcinomatosis are even more equivocal.[54, 55]

Adjuvant Systemic Therapy

Despite our intellectually satisfying advocacy of early detection and adherence to surgical principles in curative resection of colon cancer, 50 to 60 per cent of colorectal cancer patients show tumors that penetrate the serosa or involve the regional lymph nodes. Most tumors in this category will eventually recur and ultimately death will result. Adjuvant trials for colon cancer were initiated in the 1950s in order to identify effective systemic treatment for patients who were presumed to have disease spread at the time of surgery or already beyond the bounds of resection before surgery. Despite the fact that 5-fluorouracil (5-FU) achieves only a 10 to 20 per cent response rate in patients with advanced disease, this remains the most active drug in colon cancer. There have been numerous randomized and nonrandomized studies that compared surgery alone with surgery plus 5-FU or one of the combinations of 5-FU and other drugs. Buyse and coworkers have recently reviewed all randomized controlled trials of adjuvant therapy of colon cancer published up to December 1986 in the English language.[56] They have performed a meta-analysis of 17 trials comparing chemotherapy with control (surgery alone) groups in patients with high-risk colorectal cancer. A total of 6791 patients forms this analysis cohort. Regimens containing 5-FU resulted in only a small benefit in terms of overall survival. The mortality odds ratio was 0.83 in favor of therapy. All other treatment combinations failed to show statistically significant differences between treated and control arms. Only one of the five trials using combinations of 5-FU and methyl-CCNU reported a borderline survival benefit in patients who received the so-called MOF regimen (methyl CCNU, vincristine, and 5-FU). MOF resulted in 67 per cent five-year survival versus 58 per cent for controls. This survival advantage has become less obvious with additional follow-up. The combination of immunotherapy using BCG, BCG-MER, or Levamisole has also been attempted. BCG treatment alone had no discernable impact on overall survival.

Verhaegen and coworkers reported preliminary results regarding the usefulness of Levamisole as an immunomodulating agent in advanced colorectal cancer patients in the early 1980s.[57] Based on these data, the North Central Cancer Treatment Group (NCCTG) began a randomized trial testing adjuvant Levamisole alone, Levamisole with 5-FU, and surgery only in patients with Dukes B_2 or C colon cancer. In this study, comprising 408 patients and a median follow-up of 56 months, the Levamisole plus 5-FU and Levamisole regimens improved disease-free survival for patients with Dukes B and C lesions.[58] Subset analysis demonstrated that stage C patients who received Levamisole and 5-FU had prolonged survival. A larger confirmatory intergroup trial was launched in 1984, and the enrollment was completed in October, 1987. In this trial, 1296 patients with resected colon cancer (stage B_2 and C) were randomly assigned to observation or adjuvant treatment for one year with Levamisole combined with 5-FU or Levamisole alone.[59] Levamisole was administered orally 50 mg every eight hours for a period of three days, with the cycle being repeated every two weeks for one year. After the initial loading dosage, weekly 5-FU (450 mg/m^2) was continued for one year. With the median follow-up of three years, treatment of the Levamisole plus 5-FU reduced the risk of cancer recurrence by 41 per cent ($p < .0001$), overall mortality was reduced by 33 per cent ($p = .006$). Levamisole alone had no detectable effect. The results in patients with Dukes stage B_2 disease were equivocal.

An NIH Consensus Development Conference on adjuvant therapy for patients with colon and rectal cancer was held in April, 1990. The following are the consensus panel's recommendations: Patients with stage I disease are at low risk of recurrence and should not receive adjuvant treatment. Optimal adjuvant therapy for stage II and stage III colon cancer has been devised. Continued clinical trials in this disease are essential to discover more active adjuvant therapies. Based on the current clinical trial data, stage III patients unable to enter clinical trial should be offered adjuvant 5-FU and Levamisole as administered in the intergroup trial. The panel did not recommend any specific adjuvant therapy for stage II patients outside of clinical trials. Studies are currently underway to identify the characteristics of tumor in this subset that could increase the benefit of adjuvant therapy. DNA flow analysis may be one such marker. T_4 lesions and cancers with nondiploid DNA content have recently been identified as the highest risk categories in stage II patients. Perhaps the next generation of studies will address the role of 5-FU and Levamisole in this subset of patients.

Other trials will evaluate the usefulness of 5-FU modulators such as leucovorin or possibly α-interferon in the adjuvant situation and after identification of genetic and biologic markers that can more precisely define who is at highest risk for recurrence.

Adjuvant Liver Infusion Therapy

In 1975, Taylor and coworkers reported preliminary data on adjuvant liver perfusion with 5-FU for Dukes B_2 and C colorectal cancer patients.[60] Since the liver is the predominant site of distant failure in colon cancer, eradication of micrometastases in the liver in the perioperative period was a good rationale for this approach. Follow-up data by Taylor showed improved survival (death rate reduction by 55 per cent) and decreased liver recurrence (reduced by 77 per cent) following portal vein infusion using 5-FU at a dosage of 500 mg/m^2 for seven consecutive days, starting within five days of surgery.[61] Confirmatory trials were initiated soon thereafter by eight separate groups including recent trials by the NSABP and NCCTG.[6] Recent updates (median follow-up time over five years) reveal a uniform lack of benefit in reducing liver recurrence but a split in that half show some slight decrease in distant recurrence diffusely and a slight improvement in survival after portal vein infusion and half show no survival benefit whatever. Current thinking is that adjuvant portal vein infusion may be a complex way to deliver systemic therapy and cannot be recommended outside of a clinical trial setting.

CONCLUSIONS

Scientific proof of any effective colon cancer prevention techniques remains to be documented. If screening in asymptomatic patients not at high risk is to become practicable, a substantial contribution will have to be made by primary care physicians. This has not happened and probably will not happen until present rapid advances in the basic science of colon cancer lead to a rapid, predictive blood or tissue test that can be applied in the physician's office. Delineation of the "multistep" process of colon carcinogenesis provides the clinician now, nevertheless, with numerous opportunities for intervention. Markers of malignant transformation can be identified in polyps and therapeutic and diagnostic plans tailored to the patient. Once the primary cancer is detected, modern staging will eventually include not only the TNM classification, but a panel of biologic markers denoting high risk of recurrence or possibly even site-specific recurrence. The surgical oncologist must play a crucial role, not only in delivering primary tumor care, but in coordinating the multimodal care in concert with the pathologist, gastroenterologist, and other oncologists. The surgeon should also be the focal point for many of the basic science applications as they are tested to provide diagnostic or therapeutic options for the near future.

REFERENCES

1. Silverberg, E., and Lubera, J.A.: Cancer statistics 1989. CA *39*:3–20, 1989.
2. Phillips, R.K., Hittinger, R., Blesovsky, L., et al.: Local recurrence following "curative" surgery for large bowel cancer. I. The overall picture. Br. J. Surg. *71*:12–16, 1984.
3. Steele, G., Jr., and Osteen, R.T.: Surgical treatment of colon cancer. *In* Steele, G., Jr., and Osteen, R.T. (Eds.): Colorectal Cancer. New York, Marcel Dekker, Inc., 1986, pp. 127–162.
4. Cass, A.W., Milton, R.R., and Pfaff, W.W.: Patterns of recurrence following surgery alone for adenocarcinomas of the colon and rectum. Cancer *37*:2861–2865, 1976.
5. Russell, A.H., Pelton, J., Reheis, C.E., et al.: Adenocarcinoma of the colon: An autopsy study with implications for new therapeutic strategies. Cancer *56*:1446–1451, 1985.
6. Cohen, A.M., Shank, B., and Friedman, M.A.: Colorectal cancer. *In* DeVita, V.T., Jr., Hellman, S., and Rosenberg, S.A. (Eds.): Principles and Practice of Oncology, 3rd Edition. 1989, pp. 895–964.
7. Bruce, W.R.: Recent hypothesis for the origin of colon cancer. Cancer Res. *47*:4237–4242, 1987.

8. Garland, C., Shekelle, R.B., Barrett-Connor, E. et al.: Dietary vitamin D and calcium and risk of colorectal cancer: A 19-year prospective study in man. Lancet *1*:307–309, 1985.
9. Lipkin, M., and Newmark, H.: Effect of added dietary calcium on colonic epithelial-cell proliferation in subjects at high risk for familial colonic cancer. N. Engl. J. Med. *313*:1381–1384, 1985.
10. Dion, P.W., Bright-See, E.B., Smith, C.C., and Bruce, W.R.: The effect of dietary ascorbic acid and α-tocopherol on fecal mutagenicity. Mutat. Res. *102*:27–37, 1982.
11. Reddy, B.S., Sharma, C., Simi, B., et al.: Metabolic epidemiology of colon cancer: Effect of dietary fiber on fecal mutagens and bile acids in healthy subjects. Cancer Res. *47*:644–648, 1987.
12. van Dokkum, W., de Boer, B.C., van Faassen, A., et al.: Diet, faecal pH and colorectal cancer. Br. J. Cancer *48*:109–110, 1983.
13. Winawer, S.J., Flehinger, B.J., Buchalter, J., et al.: Declining serum cholesterol levels prior to diagnosis of colon cancer: A time-trend, case-control study. JAMA *263*:2083–2085, 1990.
14. Bodmer, W.F., Bailey, C.J., Bodmer, J., et al.: Localization of the gene for familial adenomatous polyposis on chromosome 5. Nature *328*:614–616, 1987.
15. Vogelstein, B., Fearon, E.R., Hamilton, S.R., et al.: Genetic alterations during colorectal tumor development. N. Engl. J. Med. *319*:525–532, 1988.
16. Gardner, E.J.: Follow-up study of a family group exhibiting dominant inheritance for a syndrome including intestinal polyps, osteomas, fibromas and epidermal cysts. Am. J. Hum. Genet. *14*:376–390, 1962.
17. Oldfield, M.C.: The association of familial polyposis of the colon with multiple sebaceous cysts. Br. J. Surg. *41*:534–541, 1954.
18. Turcot, J., Despres, J.P., and Pierre, F.: Malignant tumors of the central nervous system associated with familial polyposis of the colon. Report of two cases. Dis. Colon Rectum *2*:465–468, 1959.
19. Lynch, H.T., Albano, W.A., Lynch, J.F., et al.: Recognition of the cancer family syndrome. Gastroenterology *84*:672–673, 1983.
20. Kewenter, J., Ahlman, H., and Hulten, L.: Cancer risk in extensive ulcerative colitis. Ann. Surg. *188*:824–828, 1978.
21. Collins, R.H., Jr., Feldman, M., and Fordtran, J.S.: Colon cancer, dysplasia, and surveillance in patients with ulcerative colitis. N. Engl. J. Med. *316*:1654–1658, 1987.
22. Luk, G.D., and Baylin, S.B.: Ornithine decarboxylase as a biologic marker in familial colonic polyposis. N. Engl. J. Med. *311*:80–83, 1984.
23. Wiltz, O., O'Hara, C.J., Steele, G.D., Jr., and Mercurio, A.M.: Expression of enzymatically active sucrase-isomaltase is a ubiquitous property of primary and metastatic colon adenocarcinoma but not of normal colon mucosa. Gastroenterology *(in press)*.
24. Bos, J.L., Fearon, E.R., Hamilton, S.R., et al.: Prevalence of ras gene mutations in human colorectal cancer. Nature *327*:293–297, 1987.
25. Finley, G.G., Schulz, N.T., Hill, S.A., et al.: Expression of the myc gene family in different stages of human colorectal cancer. Oncogene *4*:963–971, 1989.
26. Fearon, E.R., and Vogelstein, B.: A genetic model for colorectal tumorigenesis. Cell *61*:759–767, 1990.
27. Vogelstein, B., Fearon, E.R., Kern, S.E., et al.: Allelotype of colorectal carcinomas. Science *244*:207–211, 1989.
28. Winawer, S.: American Cancer Society Workshop in "Imaging for Cancer." January, 1990.
29. Gilbertsen, V.A., McHugh, R., Schuman, L., et al.: The earlier detection of colorectal cancer: A preliminary report on the studies of the Occult Blood Study. Cancer *45*:2899–2901, 1980.
30. Winchester, D.P., Schull, J.H., Scanlon, E.F., et al.: A mass screening program for colorectal cancer using chemical testing for occult blood in the stool. Cancer *45*:2955–2958, 1980.
31. Shinya, H., and Wolff, W.I.: Morphology, anatomic distribution and cancer potential of colonic polyps: An analysis of 7000 polyps endoscopically removed. Ann. Surg. *190*:679–683, 1979.
32. Appel, M.F., Spjut, H.J., and Estroda, R.G.: The significance of villous component in colonic polyps. Am. J. Surg. *134*:770–771, 1977.
33. Lambert, R., Sobin, L.H., Waye, J.D., and Stalder, G.A.: The management of patients with colorectal adenomas. CA *34*:167–176, 1984.
34. Enker, W.E., Laffer, V.T., and Block, G.E.: Enhanced survival of patients with colon and rectum cancer is based upon wide anatomic resection. Ann. Surg. *190*:350–360, 1979.
35. Taylor, B.A., Wolff, B.G., Dozois, R.R., et al.: Ileal pouch–anal anastomosis for chronic ulcerative colitis and familial polyposis coli complicated by adenocarcinoma. Dis. Colon Rectum *31*:358–362, 1988.
36. Cutait, R., Lesser, M.L., and Enker, W.E.: Prophylactic oophorectomy in surgery for large bowel cancer. Dis. Colon Rectum *26*:6–11, 1983.
37. O'Brien, P.H., Newton, B.B., Metcalf, J.S., and Rittenbury, M.S.: Oophorectomy in women with carcinoma of the colon and rectum. Surg. Gynecol. Obstet. *153*:827–830, 1981.

38. Gastrointestinal Tumor Study Group: Adjuvant therapy of colon cancer: Results of a prospectively randomized trial. N. Engl. J. Med. *310:*737–743, 1984.
39. McDermott, F.T., Hughes, E.S.R., Paihl, E., et al.: Prognosis in relation to symptom duration in colon cancer. Br. J. Surg. *68:*846–849, 1981.
40. Wolmark, N., Wieand, H.S., Rockette, H.E., et al.: The prognostic significance of tumor location and bowel obstruction in Dukes B and C colorectal cancer: Findings from the NSABP clinical trials. Ann. Surg. *198:*743–752, 1983.
41. Steinberg, S.M., Barkin, J.S., Kaplan, R.S., et al.: Prognostic indicators of colon tumors: The Gastrointestinal Tumor Study Group experience. Cancer *57:*1866–1870, 1986.
42. Symonds, D.A., and Vickery, A.L., Jr.: Mucinous carcinoma of colon and rectum. Cancer *37:*1891–1900, 1976.
43. Burrows, L., and Tartter, P.: Effect of blood transfusions on colonic malignancy recurrence rate. Lancet *2:*662, 1982.
44. Corman, J., Arnoux, R., Peloquin, A., et al.: Blood transfusions and survival after colectomy for colorectal cancer. Can. J. Surg. *29:*325–329, 1986.
45. Wanebo, H.J., Rao, B., Pinsky, C., et al.: Preoperative carcinoembryonic antigen levels as a prognostic indicator in colorectal cancer. N. Engl. J. Med. *299:*466–451, 1978.
46. Steele, G., Jr., Ellenberg, S., Ramming, K., et al.: CEA monitoring among patients in multi-institutional adjuvant GI therapy protocols. Ann. Surg. *196:*162–168, 1982.
47. Scott, N.A., Rainwater, L.M., Wieand, H.S., et al.: The relative prognostic value of flow cytometric DNA analysis and conventional clinicopathologic criteria in patients with operable rectal carcinoma. Dis. Colon Rectum *30:*513–520, 1987.
48. Kokal, W.A., Gardine, R.L., Sheibani, K., et al.: Tumor DNA content in resectable, primary colorectal carcinoma. Ann. Surg. *209:*188–193, 1989.
49. Ravikumar, T.S., Wolf, B., Cocchiaro, C., et al.: Ras gene activation and EGFr expression in colon cancer. J. Surg. Res. *47:*418–422, 1989.
50. Mafune, K., Ravikumar, T.S., Wong, J.M., et al.: Expression of Mr 32,000 Laminin-binding protein messenger RNA in human colon carcinoma correlates with disease progression. Cancer Res. *50:*3888–3891, 1990.
51. Enker, W.E., and Alipshen, S.J.: Patterns of failure resulting after definitive resections for rectal or colonic cancer. Cancer Treat. Symposia *2:*173–180, 1983.
52. Welch, J.P., and Donaldson, G.A.: Detection and treatment of recurrent cancer of the colon and rectum. Am. J. Surg. *135:*505–511, 1978.
53. Olson, R.M., Perencevich, N.P., Malcolm, A.W., et al.: Patterns of recurrences following curative resection of adenocarcinoma of the colon and rectum. Cancer *45:*2969–2974, 1980.
54. Duttenhaver, J.R., Hoskins, R.B., Gunderson, L.L., and Tepper, J.E.: Adjuvant postoperative radiation therapy in the management of adenocarcinoma of the colon. Cancer *57:*955–963, 1986.
55. Wong, C.S., Harwood, A.R., Cummings, B.J., et al.: Total abdominal irradiation for cancer of the colon. Radiother. Oncol. *2:*209–214, 1984.
56. Buyse, M., Zeleniuch-Jacquotte, A., and Chalmers, T.C.: Adjuvant therapy of colorectal cancer: Why we still don't know. JAMA *259:*3571–3578, 1988.
57. Verhaegen, H., DeCree, J., DeCock, W., et al.: Levamisole therapy in patients with colorectal cancer. *In* Terry, W.B., and Rosenberg, S.A. (Eds.): Immunotherapy of Human Cancer. New York, Excerpta Medica, 1982, pp. 225–229.
58. Laurie, J.A., Moertel, C.G., Fleming, T.R., et al.: Surgical adjuvant therapy of large bowel carcinoma: An evaluation of levamisole and the combination of levamisole and fluorouracil: The North Central Cancer Treatment Group and the Mayo Clinic. J. Clin. Oncol. *7:*1447–1456, 1989.
59. Moertel, C.G., Fleming, T.R., MacDonald, J.S., et al.: Levamisole and fluorouracil for surgical therapy of colon carcinoma. N. Engl. J. Med. *322:*352–358, 1990.
60. Taylor, I., West, C.R., and Rowling, J.T.: Adjuvant cytotoxic liver perfusion for colorectal cancer. Br. J. Surg. *66:*833–837, 1979.
61. Taylor, I., Machin, D., Mullee, M., et al.: A randomized controlled trial of adjuvant portal vein cytotoxic perfusion in colorectal cancer. Br. J. Surg. *72:*359–362, 1985.

7

RECTAL AND ANAL CARCINOMA

by J. Milburn Jessup, M.D., and Glenn Steele, Jr., M.D.

Adenocarcinoma of the rectum is a common cancer while squamous carcinoma of the anus is seen infrequently in the practice of the surgical oncologist. Adenocarcinomas more than 6 cm from the anal verge are surgically treated by anterior resection, while abdominoperineal resection is the standard operation for rectal carcinomas that are closer to the anal verge. Patients whose tumors penetrate the rectal wall or involve regional lymph nodes should also receive adjuvant radiotherapy and chemotherapy. Patients with adenocarcinomas within 6 cm of the anal verge that have not penetrated the rectal wall may be candidates for sphincter-sparing procedures in which local excision of the cancer is followed by chemotherapy and radiotherapy. Conservative management of these carcinomas with low metastatic potential may achieve local control and survival similar to that achieved by radical resection alone. Squamous carcinoma of the anus should be treated with combination chemotherapy and radiotherapy unless chemoradiation fails or carcinoma occurs initially that encircles more than two-thirds of the anal circumference.

INTRODUCTION

Adenocarcinoma of the rectum will be diagnosed in about 40,000 patients in the United States during 1991 and about half of these patients will die of their cancer.[1] This cancer is the fifth most common carcinoma and constitutes a large part of the oncologic practice of many general surgeons and surgical oncologists. Since the report of Miles[2] in 1908, abdominoperineal resection, the resection of anus, rectum, and a portion of the rectosigmoid colon has been the standard treatment for carcinomas within 12 cm of the anal verge. Abdominoperineal resection has achieved local control of rectal cancer in approximately three-quarters of patients. However, it has a 10 to 50 per cent incidence of bladder dysfunction, impotence, and infection, and about a 5 per cent mortality rate.[3-13] Many patients also find it hard to accept a permanent colostomy. Since more conservative surgical procedures combined with chemotherapy and radiotherapy have achieved survival results similar to that for radical resection in breast cancer and skeletal and soft tissue sarcoma with improved quality of life, considerable enthusiasm has been generated for procedures that spare rectal sphincters, avoid a permanent colostomy, and yet achieve both local control and cure at rates similar to that of radical resection. This chapter reviews the management of adenocarcinoma of the rectum and squamous carcinoma of the anus. Our focus is on those cancers that are in the low rectum (0 to 6 cm from the anal verge), because lesions in the mid (6 to 12 cm from the anal verge) or high (12 to 15 cm from the anal verge) rectum may be treated successfully by anterior resection to achieve sphincter preservation. We will first review the anatomy that forms the basis for the surgical management of rectal and anal cancer and then describe the options available for treatment.

SURGICAL ANATOMY OF THE RECTUM AND ANUS

A carcinoma situated within 6 cm of the anal verge is in a difficult area to approach surgically because of its proximity to internal and external sphincter muscles and the narrow confines of the bony pelvis and the levator ani muscles. Huber and colleagues[14] have described this surgical anatomy in detail and have shown that the sphincter muscles extend approximately 3 cm from the anal verge to about 1 cm above the dentate line. The rectum lies within a funnel whose neck is formed by the fusion of the levator ani muscles with the muscularis propria of the rectum at the sphincter muscles and whose base is 6 cm from the anal verge and extends 3 to 6 cm around the posterior and lateral rectum to the coccyx posteriorly and the bladder or vagina anteriorly. This funnel is filled with the mesorectum, which is, in turn, covered by Waldeyer's fascia. Posterior and lateral low rectal cancers that penetrate the rectal wall directly invade the mesorectum and may produce micrometastases in the adipose tissue. Low rectal cancers that penetrate the muscularis propria of the anterior rectal wall invade Denonvilliers' fascia and then either the prostate and bladder in the male or the vagina in the female. Thus, the majority of rectal cancer recurrences arise from contiguous spread and occur either at the base of the bladder, prostate, vagina, or adjacent to the sacrum.[15]

The lymphatic drainage of a cancer determines its pattern of nodal metastases. Since lymphatics follow arteries, the distribution of the arterial supply defines the lymphatic drainage. The high and mid rectum are supplied by the superior hemorrhoidal artery that is the termination of the inferior mesenteric artery, whereas the low rectum has three sources of arterial supply. The inferior hemorrhoidal arteries supply the distal 2 cm of the rectum and anus while the middle hemorrhoidal arteries with contributions from the superior hemorrhoidal artery supply the 2 to 4 cm from the anal verge. Since the inferior and middle hemorrhoidal arteries are branches of the internal iliac arteries, lymphatics that course along these arteries drain to lateral pelvic (obturator, iliac) nodes. Thus, lymphatic metastases from low rectal or anal carcinomas may produce metastases in iliac and obturator nodes as well as metastases to the inferior mesenteric and para-aortic nodes.

Invasion of the inferior and the middle hemorrhoidal veins permits rectal carcinoma cells direct access to the systemic circulation and accounts for the higher incidence of lung metastases in rectal cancer compared with that in colon cancer.[16] Carcinoma cells that invade the superior hemorrhoidal vein from the low rectum enter the portal circulation and traverse the liver first. Thus, a rectal carcinoma may spread to either the lungs or the liver depending on whether it invades the superior or inferior-middle hemorrhoidal lymphatics or veins.

RECURRENCE PATTERNS IN RECTAL CANCER

Several areas are at high risk for local or regional recurrence of rectal carcinoma based on the anatomy previously described: the obvious regions of contiguous spread in adjacent viscera and sacrum but also the internal iliac lymph nodes in the pelvic side wall. Proximal superior hemorrhoidal, inferior mesenteric, or para-aortic nodes may be involved in advanced carcinomas. However, if superior hemorrhoidal or more proximal lymph nodes are involved with metastatic carcinoma, the prognosis is uniformly dismal. The superior hemorrhoidal and inferior mesenteric lymph nodes may be resected as part of the standard abdominoperineal resection by a high ligation of the inferior mesenteric artery, but their resection does not appear to significantly improve survival and may increase the morbidity of the abdominoperineal resection.[17] The incidence of lateral pelvic lymphatic metastasis in low rectal cancer is 9 to 23 per cent.[18-20] This has been used to justify the performance of lateral hypogastric node dissection. However, such a pelvic node dissection has a high morbidity rate with a 57 per cent incidence of urologic complications (neurogenic bladder, impotence) in patients who have either an abdominoperineal or anterior resection[20] and incontinence in those patients who have an anterior resection.[21] Enker, Block, and their colleagues have suggested that the lateral pelvic node dissection should be part of the standard treatment of rectal cancer.[22,23] However, the benefit in survival may occur only in patients with Dukes C lesions who have metastases in pararectal nodes; none of the patients in their series with lateral pelvic node metastases survived more than five years.[22] Similarly, lateral pelvic nodal metastasis, if present, carries a very poor prognosis since only one of 48 patients with lateral pelvic node metastasis survived five years in the study by Hojo et al.[18] Stearns and Deddish[20] observed that only one of 64 patients (2 per cent) with Dukes A and B lesions subsequently developed lateral pelvic nodal metastases compared with 10 of 58 patients (17 per cent) with Dukes C lesions. Thus, metastases to lateral pelvic nodes may occur as a late event after metastasis to pararectal nodes, perhaps because the flow of lymph is altered by the obstruction of lymph flow through pararectal nodal metastases. Surgical clearance of the lateral pelvic nodes would not seem to warrant the morbidity of the extended dissection, since dissemination to systemic sites has probably already occurred if these nodes contain tumor. Control of these nodal metastases by radiotherapy may be appropriate if the morbidity of radiation is low.

PROGNOSTIC FACTORS IN RECTAL CARCINOMA

Radical resection of low rectal cancers may be avoided without compromising cure if objective criteria accurately separate the cancers that are nonmetastatic from the cancers that produce metastases. Those histopathologic characteristics that are directly associated with the production of lymph node and distant metastases are: increased penetration into or through the rectal wall by the primary tumor; progressive loss of differentiation of the neoplastic cells; a high content of mucin in the primary tumor; a border of the tumor that infiltrates rather than pushes into the surrounding margin of tissue; invasion of adjacent blood vessels, lymphatics, or nerves; and ulceration of the tumor. Cohen et al[24] demonstrated that in tumors that were well or moderately differentiated, less than 3 cm in diameter, and exophytic the probability of metastasis in regional lymph nodes was only 10 per cent. Similar results were reported by Morson.[25] Furthermore, Jass et al[26] demonstrated that only a 5 mm invasion of the perirectal tissue by the primary carcinoma significantly increased the recurrence of rectal carcinoma. Twenty to 30 per cent of carcinomas that penetrate the serosa (T_3) metastasize to regional pararectal lymph nodes compared with 10 to 15 per cent of carcinomas that invade the submucosa (T_1) or the muscularis propria (T_2).[24-28] The importance of these prognostic factors to identify the risk of recurrence is demonstrated by Pilipshen et al[29] who reported that 96 per cent of patients who developed a pelvic recurrence died of their disease compared with only 23 per cent of patients who did not develop such a local or regional failure.

Performance of a radical resection does not necessarily prevent recurrence of rectal carcinoma. Abdominoperineal resection or anterior resections performed for cure provide five-year survivals of 72 to 88 per cent for Dukes A lesions ($T_{1-2}N_0$), 57 to 77 per cent for Dukes B (T_3N_0), and 33 to 55 per cent for Dukes C ($T_{1-3}N_{1-2}$) carcinomas (Table 7–1). In addition, local recurrences occur in these patients after radical resections for cure in direct proportion to their stage of disease (0 to 27 per cent for Dukes A, 12 to 83 per cent for Dukes B, and 27 to 71 per cent for Dukes C) (Table 7–2). Recurrence does not depend on the proximal and distal margins as much as it does the lateral margin in the mesorectum or pararectal tissues closest to adjacent pelvic viscera. Quirke et al[36] observed that 14 of 52 patients who underwent a potentially curative operation for low rectal carcinoma had a positive lateral margin and that 12 of these patients developed a local

TABLE 7–1. FIVE-YEAR SURVIVAL FOR RADICAL RESECTION OF RECTAL CARCINOMA: % ALIVE AT 5 YEARS WITH INITIAL DUKES STAGE

Series	A	B	C
Enker et al[22]	88	63	50
Pilipshen et al[29]	84	64	39
Whittaker and Goligher[30]	80	62	33
Williams et al[31]	81	77	55
Freedman et al[32]	72	57	35

Dukes A carcinoma is limited to bowel wall ($T_{1-2}N_0$), Dukes B carcinoma is through bowel wall but not spread to regional lymph nodes (T_3N_0), and Dukes C carcinoma is spread to regional lymph nodes but not beyond ($T_{1-3}N_{1-2}$).

TABLE 7–2. LOCAL RECURRENCE OF RECTAL CARCINOMA AFTER POTENTIALLY CURATIVE RADICAL RESECTION: % RECURRED IN PELVIS AFTER SURGERY FOR INITIAL DUKES STAGE

Series	A	B	C
Enker et al[22]	9	12	28
Pilipshen et al[29]	14	30	40
Williams et al[31]	18	21	53
Moossa et al[33]	0	17	27
McDermott et al[34]	27	35	31
Gunderson and Sosin[35]	—	83	71

Dukes stage as described above
—No patients at risk with Dukes A carcinoma

recurrence. All patients with negative lateral margins remained free of local recurrence for a median of 23 months. Chan et al[37] reported that the lateral margin was less than 6 mm for both Dukes B and C carcinomas that had been resected for cure in a series of 50 patients. Because of the narrow funnel of the pelvis, the lateral margin is often quite close in an abdominoperineal resection. Microscopic disease in this margin causes the local recurrences in pelvic viscera and around the sacrum. In fact, Heald et al[38] advocate total excision of the mesorectum because they found microscopic deposits of carcinoma several centimeters beyond the distal edge of the rectal cancer in the mesorectum that would have been left in situ if an extended dissection of the mesorectum was not performed. There were no local recurrences in 50 patients whose mesorectum did not demonstrate any micrometastases. Thus, the amount of tissue removed by an abdominoperineal resection does not guarantee an adequate lateral margin because the narrow confines of the pelvis may force the surgeon to compromise on a wide resection. As a result, local failure often results from contiguous spread of rectal carcinoma into tissues that are not removed by the surgeon, because removal of such tissues may cause high morbidity or an alteration of lifestyle that is not acceptable to the patient. Gunderson and Sosin[35] demonstrated that local recurrence in the perineum or midpelvis was a component of 92 per cent of all recurrences in rectal carcinoma and was the only site of failure in approximately 50 per cent of cases that failed. Since these sites are encompassed within a standard pelvic radiation port, the addition of other treatment modalities such as radiation therapy may sterilize micrometastases in the mesorectum and regional nodes.

The importance of contiguous spread as the source of recurrence is confirmed by a series of reports on the importance of computerized tomography (CT) or magnetic resonance imaging (MRI) in the detection of recurrences after surgery for low rectal carcinoma.[39–43] The majority of lesions in these reports were either at the base of the bladder, the vagina, or in the presacral space at the level of the rectal cancer. Thus, local recurrence is the inevitable result if negative lateral margins are not achieved.

PREOPERATIVE RADIOTHERAPY IN RECTAL CANCER

Since neither abdominoperineal nor anterior resection eliminate local recurrence in the pelvis, investigators have attempted to add other treatments to improve local control of rectal cancer. Gunderson and Sosin[35] analyzed patients at the University of Minnesota who underwent second-look surgery and observed that most local recurrences of rectal carcinoma are within the pelvic port of a radiotherapy field and that postoperative radiotherapy should decrease recurrence. Rich et al[44] later demonstrated in a nonrandomized study at the Massachusetts General Hospital that postoperative adjuvant radiotherapy significantly decreased local recurrences for each stage of rectal carcinoma. Romsdahl and Withers[45] observed a similar reduction in local recurrence with postoperative radiotherapy but did not notice any improvement in patient survival. The administration of 20 to 45 Gy prior to operation has the theoretical advantage that undisturbed, oxygenated tissues should be more susceptible to ionizing radiation than the relatively avascular planes created by surgery that are treated with postoperative radiation. Furthermore, more than two-thirds of nodal metastases are less than 4 mm in diameter[46] and, hence, may be controlled by radiotherapy. When radiotherapy was administered preoperatively in either a randomized[47] or nonrandomized[48] study, there appeared to be significant downstaging of regional disease since the frequency of lymphatic metastases was decreased in irradiated patients. However, Cedermark et al[49] did not observe any significant improvement in local control or survival in a randomized trial of preoperative radiotherapy in which patients received 25 Gy to the tumor and pelvis one week prior to surgery, nor did a subsequent trial by the Veterans Administration confirm their first study.[50]

However, the dosage of preoperative radiotherapy may need to be greater than 25 Gy to achieve a measurable biologic effect. Marks and colleagues have aggressively pursued this by irradiating patients with 40 to 55 Gy preoperatively and then performing sphincter-saving operations for low and mid rectal carcinomas with good results.[51, 52] Only seven of 43 patients (16 per cent) with carcinoma within 6 cm of the anal verge developed a local recurrence while 86 per cent of patients were continent after resection.[52] Relatively few patients underwent local excision after preoperative radiotherapy, possibly because healing in the irradiated field may be difficult. Fleshman and colleagues[53] reported similar results with anterior resection for rectal carcinomas after 20 to 45 Gy in which local recurrence was less than 2 per cent in a series of 102 patients, 23 of whom were Dukes C lesions. Fleshman et al[53] stressed that successful healing after preoperative operation required the advancement of nonradiated descending colon into the pelvis to provide sufficient blood supply to heal the anastomosis.

COMBINED CHEMOTHERAPY AND RADIOTHERAPY FOR RECTAL CARCINOMA

While preoperative radiation therapy may decrease local recurrence, it has not been widely accepted presumably because it may downstage the disease and hinder healing. However, radiotherapy should be part of the postoperative adjuvant therapy of rectal cancer that has penetrated the rectal wall or metastasized to regional nodes. The Gastrointestinal Tumor Study Group randomized patients with Dukes B_2 or C lesions to receive either surgery alone, postoperative radiotherapy (40 to 48 Gy), adjuvant 5-fluorouracil and methyl-CCNU, or combined chemotherapy and radiotherapy.

Postoperative radiotherapy combined with 5-fluorouracil and methyl-CCNU significantly decreased local recurrence with an insignificant decrease in distant metastasis.[54] Neither radiotherapy nor chemotherapy alone achieved the same effect on either local or distant recurrence in these patients. The effect of combined chemoradiotherapy has translated into a significant improvement in survival with longer follow-up.[55] A significant effect of adjuvant chemotherapy on survival was observed in the National Surgical Adjuvant Bowel and Breast Project protocol R-01.[56] Patients with Dukes B_2 or C rectal carcinoma were randomized to either surgery alone, chemotherapy with methyl-CCNU, 5-fluorouracil, and vincristine, or radiotherapy. Both chemotherapy and radiotherapy significantly decreased local recurrence, but only chemotherapy significantly improved the disease-free survival of patients. Unfortunately, this R-01 trial did not contain an arm that combined radiotherapy with chemotherapy. However, a third study from the North Central Cancer Treatment Group supports the Gastrointestinal Tumor Study Group (GITSG) study and demonstrates a decrease in local recurrence and improved disease-free survival in patients with rectal cancer who receive both chemotherapy and radiotherapy.[57] Thus, the standard of practice for adenocarcinomas of the rectum that penetrate the rectal wall (Dukes B_2) or involve regional lymph nodes (Dukes C) is a radical resection followed by chemotherapy and radiotherapy.

THE ROLE OF LOCAL EXCISION IN THE TREATMENT OF RECTAL CANCER

In the narrow confines of the pelvis a local excision of a primary cancer with en bloc removal of mesorectal fat may have a lateral margin that is comparable to that of a standard radical resection. If patients are carefully selected so as to decrease the chance of lymph node metastasis, it may be possible to locally excise rectal carcinomas and achieve cure rates similar to that of radical resection. Morson et al[58] articulated a "policy" for the total excision of rectal cancer in which local excision was the definitive therapy for lesions that were confined to the submucosa, well or moderately differentiated, without vascular invasion or mucin production, and completely excised with negative margins. When this policy is followed in T_1 and T_2 low rectal cancers, local control ranges between 79 and 100 per cent in patients followed for at least two years (Table 7–3). This rate of local control is similar to that achieved with radical resection for Dukes A lesions (see Table 7–2).

Excision is usually performed by the transanal approach, although several series used a posterior parasacral or trans-sphincteric technique. While the transanal approach is easier and may be accomplished with a low complication rate, the posterior sacral approaches have the advantage that the surgeon may evaluate the mesorectum where small deposits of metastatic carcinoma may be found that would otherwise have escaped detection. The trans-sphincteric technique was popularized by York Mason[68,69] although the trans-sacral method of Kraske[70] provides similar exposure by removing the coccyx. Posterior and lateral rectal cancers within 6 cm of the anal verge are easily excised by either posterior sacral approach and anterior rectal cancers can be removed through the posterior wall of the rectum.

TABLE 7–3. LOCAL CONTROL AND SURVIVAL FOR T_{1-2} RECTAL CARCINOMA WITHIN 6 CM OF THE DENTATE LINE TREATED BY LOCAL EXCISION ALONE

Series	Number of Patients	% Local Control	% 5-Year Survival
Deddish[59]	85	92	84
Stearns et al[60]	29	90	90
Grigg et al[61]	16	94	100
Whiteway et al[62]	19	100	84
Biggers et al[63]	234	79	96
Killingback[64]	28	82	82
Cuthbertson and Simpson[65]	25	75	—
Hager et al[66]	59	90	90 (T_1) / 78 (T_2)
Willett et al[67]	36	92	89

Our current policy at the New England Deaconess Hospital is to attempt local excision of those adenocarcinomas of the distal rectum that clinically are less than 4 cm in diameter or 30 per cent of rectal circumference, mobile, nonulcerated, well or moderately differentiated without mucin production. A pelvic CT scan is obtained to exclude patients with detectable pararectal or pelvic lymph node metastases. A posterior or parasacral approach is our method of choice so that the mesorectum may be removed intact with the primary carcinoma and may be palpated for small metastases. Since adjuvant chemoradiotherapy has decreased local recurrence in more advanced rectal carcinoma, patients are then given 5-fluorouracil and 45 Gy to the pelvis and tumor bed after recovery from operation. While the initial incidence of wound infection and fistula may be as high as 29 per cent,[72] the long-term functional results of local excision by the posterior sacral approach with postoperative radiotherapy are good with 91 to 95 per cent of patients fully continent six to eight weeks after surgery and another 5 per cent only having slight soiling at night.[72, 73] Experience with local excision combined with postoperative radiotherapy is limited, although local control ranges from 86 to 100 per cent with a five-year survival of 71 to 100 per cent (Table 7–4). In a prospective trial at the M.D. Anderson Hospital, Rich et al[72] treated 36 patients with T_{1-2} lesions with a 92 per cent local control after a median follow-up of 18 months. While these results need to be followed further, they suggest that favorable adenocarcinomas may be treated by local excision and chemoradiotherapy with sphincter preservation and outcome similar to

TABLE 7–4. LOCAL CONTROL AND SURVIVAL FOR T_{1-2} RECTAL CARCINOMA WITHIN 6 CM OF THE DENTATE LINE TREATED BY LOCAL EXCISION AND RADIOTHERAPY

Series	Number of Patients	% Local Control	% 5-Year Survival
Ellis et al[74]	9	100	100
Willett et al[67]	22	86	96
Ramming et al[75]	8	100	100
Rich et al[76]	17	95	—
Rich et al[77]	36	92	71

that achieved by radical resection for Dukes A to B_1 lesions. Since endorectal ultrasonography assesses the depth of rectal wall invasion by tumor with 85 to 95 per cent sensitivity and specificity,[78–82] patients with T_1 or T_2 carcinomas may now be objectively identified. Two similar prospective trials of local excision and chemoradiotherapy for $T_{1-2}N_0$ rectal carcinomas are currently under way in the Radiation Therapy Oncology Group and the Cancer and Leukemia Group B cooperative groups. During the next few years it may be possible to preserve sphincter function in a greater proportion of low rectal carcinomas and to determine the relative importance of chemotherapy and radiotherapy.[83]

CARCINOMA OF THE ANUS

Carcinoma of the anus constitutes 2 per cent of the cancers of the rectum[84] and includes squamous, basosquamous, basaloid, and cloacogenic carcinomas. Epidermoid carcinoma often arises in association with other anorectal pathology, e.g., condylomata, fistulae, fissura, abscesses, and hemorrhoids.[85] Prognosis is determined by the degree of keratinization of the tumor.[86] These cancers arise in the anal skin and the anal canal with size being an important prognostic factor. Like the adenocarcinomas that arise at or above the dentate line, these carcinomas may metastasize to inguinal or pelvic (obturator) lymph nodes through lymphatics that follow the inferior and middle hemorrhoidal arteries. The cancers that arise in the anal canal appear to be more aggressive,[87] although Paradis et al[88] did not observe any difference in survival between anal margin or canal lesions. Anal canal lesions tend to be less differentiated and invade the submucosa and sphincter ani muscles and their lymphatics earlier than anal margin cancers penetrate the dermis.

Surgical management of carcinoma of the anus is largely reserved to two situations. The first relates to the size of the lesion and the second relates to treatment of the failures of chemoradiotherapy. In the first situation, anal margin carcinomas may attain large size, especially in patients who have poor hygiene. Women with squamous carcinoma of the anus may have associated squamous carcinoma of the vulva with a number of lesions that range from in situ to frankly invasive carcinomas. For these patients surgery represents the best treatment because the carcinomas behave as though they arise in a field of dysplastic perineal epithelium. Radiation will not change this biology and a radical vulvectomy with abdominoperineal resection is sometimes required to clear all neoplastic disease. Skin grafts and myocutaneous flaps may be necessary to cover the perineum. These patients may do quite well even though they have primary and margin cancers that are greater than 10 cm in diameter, so long as their carcinoma does not involve the anal canal.

Surgery, usually an abdominoperineal resection, is required for those patients whose cancers do not respond to chemoradiation. Since the advent of the Nigro regimen of 5-fluorouracil and mitomycin-C administered with 30 Gy of external beam radiation, the five-year survival of carcinoma of the anus has improved to 79 per cent with more than 90 per cent of patients having complete resolution of their carcinoma without excision.[89] However, primary anal canal carcinomas that encircle more than two-thirds the circumference of the anus, that are greater than 5 cm in diameter, that present with incontinence, or that are poorly differentiated, are less likely to disappear after chemoradiotherapy. Evaluation of these patients may be difficult because as the carcinomas shrink they may be replaced by fibrosis. Biopsy is difficult because full thickness incisional biopsies may not heal after the chemoradiation. Evaluation under anesthesia is recommended with biopsy performed by fine-needle aspiration if an experienced cytologist is available. The chemoradiation may take four to six months to achieve its effect, further complicating the evaluation of possible residual disease. Thus, patients should be examined for up to six months after chemoradiation, possibly with the aid of endorectal ultrasound, before therapy is considered to have failed. If biopsy reveals residual or recurrent disease, an abdominoperineal resection is often required because the chemoradiation makes healing problematic. Recurrences of squamous carcinoma of the anal canal are often poorly differentiated adenocarcinomas that are located deep in the sphincter muscles. Fortunately, abdominoperineal resections are required now in less than 5 per cent of patients.

REFERENCES

1. Silverberg, E., and Lubera, J.A.: Cancer statistics, 1989. CA 39:3–20, 1989.
2. Miles, W.E.: A method of performing abdominoperineal excision for carcinoma of the rectum and of the terminal portion of the pelvic colon. Lancet 2:1812–1813, 1908.
3. Weinstein, M., and Roberts, M.: Sexual potency following surgery for rectal carcinoma. Ann. Surg. 185:295–300, 1977.
4. Danzi, M., Ferulano, G.P., Abate, S., and Califano, G.: Male sexual function after abdominoperineal resection for rectal cancer. Dis. Colon Rectum 26:665–668, 1983.
5. Balslev, I., and Harling, H.: Sexual dysfunction following operation for carcinoma of the rectum. Dis. Colon Rectum 26:785–788, 1983.
6. Williams, J.T., and Slack, W.W.: A prospective study of sexual function after colorectal surgery. Br. J. Surg. 67:722–774, 1980.
7. Yeager, E.S., and van Heerden, J.A.: Sexual dysfunction following proctocolectomy and abdominoperineal resection. Ann. Surg. 191:169–170, 1980.
8. Kinn, A-C., and Ohman, U.: Bladder and sexual function after surgery for rectal cancer. Dis. Colon Rectum 29:43–48, 1986.
9. Fowler, J.W., Bremner, D.N., and Moffat, L.E.F.: The incidence and consequences of damage to the parasympathetic nerve supply to the bladder after abdominoperineal resection of the rectum for carcinoma. Br. J. Urol. 50:95–98, 1978.
10. Gerstenberg, T.C., Nielsen, M.L., Clausen, S., et al.: Bladder function after abdominoperineal resection of the rectum for anorectal cancer: Urodynamic investigation before and after operation in a consecutive series. Ann. Surg. 191:81–86, 1980.
11. Lea, J.W., Covington, K., McSwain, B., and Scott, H.W.: Surgical experience with carcinoma of the colon and rectum. Ann. Surg. 195:600–607, 1982.
12. Hughes, E.S.R., McDermott, F.T., Masterton, J.P., et al.: Operative mortality following excision of the rectum. Br. J. Surg. 67:49–51, 1980.
13. Payne, J.E., Chapuis, P.H., and Pheils, M.T.: Surgery for large bowel cancer in people aged 75 years and older. Dis. Colon Rectum 29:733–737, 1986.
14. Huber, A., von Hochstetter, A.H.C., and Allgower, M.: Transsphincteric surgery of the rectum: Topographical anatomy and operation technique. Berlin, Springer-Verlag, 1984, pp. 1–83.
15. Cass, A.W., Million, R.R., and Pfaff, W.W.: Patterns of recurrence following surgery alone for adenocarcinoma of the colon and rectum. Cancer 37:2861–2865, 1976.
16. Brown, C.E., and Warren, S.: Visceral metastasis from rectal carcinoma. Surg. Gynecol. Obstet. 66:611–621, 1938.
17. Sugarbaker, P.H., and Corlew, S.: Influence of surgical techniques on survival in patients with colorectal cancer: A review. Dis. Colon Rectum 25:545–557, 1982.
18. Hojo, K., Kyama, Y., and Moriya, Y.: Lymphatic spread and its prognostic value in patients with rectal cancer. Am. J. Surg. 144:350–354, 1982.
19. Sauer, I., and Bacon, H.E.: A new approach for excision of carcinoma of the lower portion of the rectum and   al canal. Surg. Gynecol. Obstet. 95:229–242, 1952.

20. Stearns, M.W., Jr., Deddish, M.R.: Five-year results of abdominopelvic lymph node dissection for carcinoma of the rectum. Dis. Colon Rectum 2:169–172, 1959.
21. Glass, R.E., Ritchie, J.K., Thompson, H.R., and Mann, C.V.: The results of surgical treatment of cancer of the rectum by radical resection and extended abdominoiliac lymphadenectomy. Br. J. Surg. 72:599–601, 1985.
22. Enker, W.E., Laffer, U.T., and Block, G.E.: Enhanced survival of patients with colon and rectal cancer is based upon wide anatomic resection. Ann. Surg. 190:350–360, 1979.
23. Enker, W.E., Heilweil, M.L., Hertz, R.E., et al.: En bloc pelvic lymphadenectomy and sphincter preservation in the surgical management of rectal cancer. Ann. Surg. 203:426–433, 1986.
24. Cohen, A.M., Wood, W.C., Gunderson, L.L., and Shinnar, M.: Pathological studies in rectal cancer. Cancer 45:2965–2968, 1980.
25. Morson, B.C.: Factors influencing the prognosis of early cancer of the rectum. Proc. R. Soc. Med. 59:607–608, 1966.
26. Jass, J.R., Atkin, W.S., Cuzick, J., et al.: The grading of rectal cancer: Historical perspectives and a multivariate analysis of 447 cases. Histopathology 10:437–459, 1986.
27. Schmitz-Mormann, P., Himmelmann, G.W., Baum, U., and Nilles, M.: Morphological predictors of survival in colorectal carcinoma: Univariate and multivariate analysis. J. Cancer Res. Clin. Oncol. 113:586–592, 1987.
28. Spratt, J.S., Jr., and Spjut, H.J.: Prevalence and prognosis of individual clinical and pathologic variables associated with colorectal carcinoma. Cancer 20:1976–1985, 1967.
29. Pilipshen, S.J., Heilweil, M., Quan, S.H., et al.: Patterns of pelvic recurrence following definitive resections of rectal cancer. Cancer 53:1354–1362, 1984.
30. Whittaker, M., and Goligher, J.C.: The prognosis after surgical treatment for carcinoma of the rectum. Br. J. Surg. 63:384–388, 1976.
31. Williams, N.S., Dixon, M.F., and Johnston, D.: Reappraisal of the 5 centimetre rule of distal excision for carcinoma of the rectum: A study of distal intramural spread and of patients' survival. Br. J. Surg. 70:150–155, 1983.
32. Freedman, L.S., Macaskill, P., and Smith, A.N.: Multivariate analysis of prognostic factors for operable rectal cancer. Lancet 2:733–736, 1984.
33. Moossa, A.R., Ree, P.C., Marks, J.E., et al.: Factors influencing the local recurrence after abdominoperineal resection for cancer of the rectum and rectosigmoid. Br. J. Surg. 62:727–730, 1975.
34. McDermott, F.T., Hughes, E.S., Pihl, E., et al.: Local recurrence after potentially curative resection for rectal cancer in a series of 1008 patients. Br. J. Surg. 72:34–37, 1985.
35. Gunderson, L.L., and Sosin, H.: Areas of failure found at reoperation (second or symptomatic look) following "curative surgery" for adenocarcinoma of the rectum. Cancer 34:1278–1292, 1974.
36. Quirke, P., Durdey, P., Dixon, M.F., and Williams, N.S.: Local recurrence of rectal adenocarcinoma due to inadequate surgical resection. Lancet 2:1, 1986.
37. Chan, K.W., Bey, J., Wong, S.K.: A method of reporting radial invasion and surgical clearance of rectal carcinoma. Histopathology 9:1319–1327, 1985.
38. Heald, R.J., Husband, E.M., and Ryall, R.D.: The mesorectum in rectal cancer surgery: The clue to pelvis recurrence? Br. J. Surg. 69:613–616, 1982.
39. Wilking, N., Herrera, L., Petrelli, N.J., and Mittelman, A.: Pelvic and perineal recurrences after abdominoperineal resection for adenocarcinoma of the rectum. Am. J. Surg. 150:561–563, 1985.
40. Thompson, W.M., Halvorsen, R.A., Foster, W.L., Jr., et al.: Preoperative and postoperative CT staging of rectosigmoid carcinoma. AJR 146:703–710, 1986.
41. Roman, G., de Rosa, P., Vallne, G., et al.: Intrarectal ultrasound and computed tomography in the pre- and postoperative assessment of patients with rectal cancer. Br. J. Surg. S117–S119, 1985.
42. Freeny, P.C., Marks, W.M., Ryan, J.A., and Blen, J.W.: Colorectal carcinoma evaluation with CT: Preoperative staging and detection of postoperative recurrence. Radiology 158:347–353, 1986.
43. Schiessel, R., Wunderlich, M., and Herbst, F.: Local recurrence of colorectal cancer: Effect of early detection and aggressive surgery. Br. J. Surg. 73:342–344, 1986.
44. Rich, T., Gunderson, L.L., Lew, R., et al.: Patterns of recurrence of rectal cancer after potentially curative surgery. Cancer 52:1317–1329, 1983.
45. Romsdahl, M.M., and Withers, H.R.: Radiotherapy combined with curative surgery. Arch. Surg. 113:446–453, 1978.
46. Herrera-Ornelas, L., Justiniano, J., Castillo, N., et al.: Metastases in small lymph nodes from colon cancer. Arch. Surg. 122:1253–1256, 1987.
47. Roswit, B., Higgins, G.A., Jr., and Keehn, R.J.: Preoperative irradiation for carcinoma of rectum and rectosigmoid colon: Report of a National Veterans Administration randomized study. Cancer 35:1597–1602, 1975.
48. Mendenhall, W.M., Bland, K.I., Rout, W.R., et al.: Clinically resectable adenocarcinoma of

the rectum treated with preoperative irradiation and surgery. Dis. Colon Rectum *31*:287–290, 1988.
49. Cedermark, B., Theve, N.O., Rieger, A., et al.: Preoperative short-term radiotherapy in rectal carcinoma: A preliminary report of a prospective randomized study. Cancer *55*:1182–1185, 1985.
50. Higgins, G.A., Humphrey, E.W., Dwight, R.W., et al.: Preoperative radiation and surgery for cancer of the rectum: Veterans Administration Surgical Oncology Group Trial II. Cancer *58*:352–359, 1986.
51. Mohiuddin, M., and Marks, G.J.: High dose preoperative radiation and sphincter preservation in the treatment of rectal cancer. Int. J. Radiat. Oncol. Biol. Phys. *13*:839–842, 1987.
52. Marks, G., Mohiuddin, M., and Goldstein, S.D.: Sphincter preservation for cancer of the distal rectum using high dose preoperative radiation. Int. J. Radiat. Oncol. Biol. Phys. *15*:1065–1068, 1988.
53. Fleshman, J.W., Kodner, I.J., Fry, R.D., et al.: Adenocarcinoma of the rectum: Results of radiotherapy and resection, endocavitary irradiation, local excision, and preoperative clinical staging. Dis. Colon Rectum *28*:810–815, 1985.
54. Gastrointestinal Tumor Study Group: Prolongation of the disease-free interval in surgically treated rectal carcinoma. N. Engl. J. Med. *312*:1465–1472, 1985.
55. Thomas, P.R., and Lindblad, A.S.: Adjuvant postoperative radiotherapy and chemotherapy in rectal carcinoma: A review of the Gastrointestinal Tumor Study Group experience. Radiother. Oncol. *13*:245–252, 1988.
56. Fisher, B., Wolmark, N., Rockette, H., et al.: Postoperative adjuvant chemotherapy or radiation therapy for rectal cancer: Results from NSABP protocol R 01. J. Natl. Cancer Inst. *80*:21–29, 1988.
57. Moertel, C.G.: Surgical adjuvant treatment of large bowel cancer. J. Clin. Oncol. *6*:934–936, 1988.
58. Morson, B.C., Bussey, H.J.R., and Samoorian, S.: Policy of local excision for early cancer of the colorectum. Gut *18*:1045–1050, 1977.
59. Deddish, M.R.: Local excision. Surg. Clin. N. Am. *54*:877–880, 1974.
60. Stearns, M.W., Jr., Sternberg, S.S., and DeCosse, J.J.: Treatment alternatives: Localized rectal cancer. Cancer *54*:2691–2694, 1984.
61. Grigg, M., McDermott, F.T., Pihl, E.A., and Hughes, E.S.R.: Curative local excision in the treatment of carcinoma of the rectum. Dis. Colon Rectum *27*:81–83, 1984.
62. Whiteway, J., Nicholls, R.J., and Morson, B.C.: The role of surgical excision in the treatment of rectal cancer. Br. J. Surg. *72*:694–697, 1985.
63. Biggers, O.R., Beart, R.W., and Ilstrup, D.M.: Local excision of rectal cancer. Dis. Colon Rectum *29*:374–377, 1986.
64. Killingback, M.J.: Indications for local excision of rectal cancer. Br. J. Surg. *72*:s54–s56, 1985.
65. Cuthbertson, A.M., and Simpson, R.L.: Curative local excision of rectal adenocarcinoma. Aust. N. Z. J. Surg. *56*:229–231, 1986.
66. Hager, T., Gall, F.P, and Hermanek, P.: Local excision of cancer of the rectum. Dis. Colon Rectum *26*:149–151, 1983.
67. Willett, C.G., Tepper, J.E., Donnelly, S., et al.: Patterns of failure following local excision and local excision and postoperative radiation therapy for invasive rectal adenocarcinoma. J. Clin. Oncol. *7*:1003–1008, 1989.
68. York Mason, A.: The place of local resection in the treatment of rectal carcinoma. Proc. R. Soc. Med. *63*:1259–1262, 1970.
69. York Mason, A.: Surgical access to the rectum—a transsphincteric exposure. Proc. R. Soc. Med. *63*(Suppl):91–94, 1970.
70. Kraske, P.: Zur extirpation hochsitzenden mastdarmkrebs verhandle deutsch gesellsch. Verh. Otsch. Gs. Chir. *14*:464–474, 1885.
71. Steele, G.D., Jr., Busse, P., Huberman, M.S., et al.: A pilot study of sphincter sparing management of adenocarcinoma of the rectum. Arch. Surg. *126*:696–702, 1991.
72. McCready, D.R., Ota, D.M., Rich, T.A., et al.: Prospective phase I trial of conservative management of low rectal lesions. Arch. Surg. *124*:67–70, 1989.
73. Westbrook, K.C., Lang, N.P., Broadwater, J.R., and Thompson, B.W.: Posterior surgical approaches to the rectum. Ann. Surg. *195*:677–685, 1982.
74. Ellis, L.M., Mendenhall, W.M., Bland, K.I., and Copeland, E.M., III: Local excision and radiation therapy for early rectal cancer. Am. Surg. *54*:217–220, 1988.
75. Ramming, K.P., Juillard, G., Parker, R., and Eilber, F.: Management of carcinoma of the rectum and anus without abdominoperineal resection. Am. J. Surg. *152*:16–47, 1986.
76. Rich, T., Weiss, D.R., Mies, C., et al.: Sphincter preservation in patients with low rectal cancer treated with radiation therapy with local excision or fulguration. Radiology *156*:527–531, 1985.
77. Rich, T.A., Ota, D.M., Ames, F.C., et al.: Local excision and external beam irradiation for rectal cancer. Submitted for publication.

78. Holdswoth, P.J., Johnston, D., Chalmers, A.G., et al.: Endoluminal ultrasound and computed tomography in the staging of rectal cancer. Br. J. Surg. 75:1019–1022, 1988.
79. Hildebrandt, U., and Feifel, G.: Preoperative staging of rectal cancer by intrarectal ultrasound. Dis. Colon Rectum 28:42–46, 1985.
80. Mosnier, H., Guivarc'H, M., and Barbagelata, M.: Endorectal ultrasonography of the rectum. A method of evaluation of locoregional extension of rectal carcinoma. Gastroenterol. Clin. Biol. 11:307–311, 1987.
81. Accarpio, G., Scopinaro, G., Claudiani, F., et al.: Experience with local rectal cancer excision in light of two recent preoperative diagnostic methods. Dis. Colon Rectum 30:296–298, 1987.
82. Rifkin, M.D., McGlynn, E.T., and Marks, G.: Endorectal sonographic prospective staging of rectal cancer. Scand. J. Gastroenterol. 21(suppl. 123):99–103, 1986.
83. Steele, G.D., Jr., Hamilton, J.M., and Karr, J.P.: A rational next step in the treatment of some rectal adenocarcinomas. J. Clin. Oncol. 7(8):988–990, 1989.
84. Stearns, M.W., and Quan, S.H.: Epidermoid carcinoma of the anorectum. Surg. Gynecol. Obstet. 131:953–957, 1970.
85. Brennan, J.T., and Stewart, C.F.: Epidermoid carcinoma of the anus. Ann. Surg. 176:787–790, 1972.
86. Morson, B.C.: The pathology and results of treatment of squamous cell carcinoma of the anal canal and margin. Proc. R. Soc. Med. 53:414–420, 1960.
87. Wolfe, H.R.I., and Bussey, H.J.R.: Squamous cell carcinoma of the anus. Br. J. Surg. 55:295–301, 1968.
88. Paradis, P., Douglas, H.O., and Holyole, E.D.: The clinical implications of a staging system for carcinoma of the anus. Surg. Gynecol. Obstet. 141:411–416, 1975.
89. Nigro, N.D., Vaitkevicius, V.K., and Considine, B., Jr.: Dynamic management of squamous cell cancer of the anal canal. Invest. New Drugs 7:83–89, 1989.

8

PRIMARY AND METASTATIC CANCER OF THE LIVER

by William V. McDermott, Jr., M.D.,
Roger L. Jenkins, M.D., Blake Cady, M.D.,
and Glenn Steele, Jr., M.D.

EPIDEMIOLOGY

It is impossible to establish any universal data on cancer of the liver because of the tremendous variation that occurs with geography. Even within the two major categories of primary and metastatic liver cancer, there is also a wide range of biologic behavior and prognosis in relation to age and cell type in the primary tumors and, in the case of metastatic cancer, to the location and staging of the primary lesion, to the number and distribution of the metastases within the liver, to the interval between resection of the primary, and to the appearance of metachronous disease and the presence or absence of spread to other organs.

Throughout Africa and Asia, *primary hepatocellular cancer* is one of the most common malignant tumors encountered; the epidemiology has been related both to the widespread occurrence of the hepatitis B virus often with accompanying micronodular cirrhosis and also to contamination of stored grain with aflatoxins produced by *Aspergillus flavus*. For obvious reasons, accurate data as to absolute occurrence, survival, and pathology are not easily available. One must rely on selected series in the most sophisticated population centers.[1]

On the other hand, in North America and Western Europe, primary hepatocellular cancer, in the absence of parenchymatous liver disease, is relatively rare. With established cirrhosis, however, single or multiple primary cancers are common in the United States. Reported incidence rates range from approximately 2 per cent in alcoholic cirrhosis to as high as 20 per cent occurring over a 10-year period of recognized disease in the macronodular cirrhotic process seen with hemochromatosis. When one looks at secondary liver cancer, again one sees a totally different picture of the disease in Asia and Africa from that encountered in western civilization. This reverse geographic discrepancy occurs because cancer of the colon (the usual primary source of metastatic liver cancer) is the most frequent nonepidermal malignancy of both sexes in the United States, whereas it is quite rare in Africa and Asia presumably because of the high fiber content of the diet in these countries.[1]

In this particular discussion, the data presented reflect our own personal departmental experience in a western medical center. Thus, the information and conclusions from it may not be applicable throughout the world.

Evaluation and Diagnosis

When a suspected liver tumor presents for study, a reasonably accurate preoperative assessment can be made by modern technology with a fairly high degree of accuracy and without needle biopsy. We have not personally recommended this approach to establish an accurate histologic diagnosis except in instances of clearly incurable disease in which the theoretical and occasionally demonstrable risk of spread of the tumor would not destroy any theoretical chance of cure. In addition, the risk of hemorrhage from primary hepatocellular cancer following needle biopsy is significant.

Some biologic markers may be useful, such as a rise in carcinoembryonic antigen (CEA) levels, which may have been the factor that led to the initial suspicion of metastatic cancer, usually from colon or rectum. Levels of α-fetoprotein may provide a lead in differential diagnosis. However, because of the inconsistent elevations found in this particular marker, it is not as useful as might have been the case if a more consistent pattern was evident.

Radiologic techniques are particularly vital in terms of recognition, definition, evaluation, and assessment of the tumor, and the subsequent development of an appropriate plan of therapy. The liver/spleen scan is simple, noninvasive, and sufficiently accurate, making it useful as a quick and relatively inexpensive screening test in suspicious cases. However, ultrasonic scanning has generally replaced radionucleotide scanning because it is simple, safe, economical, and particularly useful in defining consistency, thus permitting the elimination of simple asymptomatic cysts from further consideration of any interventional surgery.

The CT scan is an almost essential tool in evaluating the nature, location, and extent of primary or secondary liver disease. It is also useful in expanding the information developed from a preliminary screening by isotopic or ultrasonic scanning.

Magnetic resonance imaging (MRI) is a recently introduced technique that, at the moment, can be considered only as supplementary to the other more standardized techniques with which more experience has been gathered. In our institution, we believe that MRI with or without dynamic scanning can make a major contribution in differentiating hemangiomas from other space-occupying liver lesions. Whether it has any better resolution capacity for primary hepatocellular carcinomas or a variety of metastatic lesions to the liver when compared with external ultrasound or the most recent generation of CT scan is uncertain. We are currently very enthusiastic about MRI angiography, which noninvasively provides an internal road map of the intrahepatic vascular anatomy in a three-dimensional manner and which allows more precise operative planning in situations in which resection is possible.

Celiac and superior mesenteric angiography has been an almost essential tool in determining the ultimate therapy to be utilized in any given instance. Not only can the procedure aid in accuracy of location and define the vascularity of a lesion, but it may help clarify the nature of the tumor. Abnormalities of the arterial inflow are frequent; if surgeons have foreknowledge of these, they can handle the technical problems much more easily. These invasive studies are accompanied by a not insignificant series of complications in which even deaths have been reported. In experienced hands and with appropriate patient selection and preparation, however, the morbidity and mortality can be minimized and the information obtained is invaluable. The precise anatomic images generated today by CT and MRI scans now often avoid the need for angiography in the hands of a surgeon experienced with variations in extrahepatic arterial anatomy.

Intraoperative ultrasonic scanning of the liver should be mentioned at this point, although basically our utilization of this has been as much as an adjunct to certain types of therapy as it is a part of a preresection assessment. This extension of a radiologic technique has proved to be extraordinarily useful in identifying otherwise occult lesions and, not infrequently, avoiding a planned resection that, under the circumstances, would have been unnecessarily life threatening. In addition to its usefulness in assessment, we have also employed this technique in conjunction with a radiologic procedure in directing the introduction of probes utilized for cryosurgical therapy. We will do no more than include a brief reference to this technology under sections on therapy because our experience is too limited to present any more than this somewhat premature comment.

PRIMARY CANCER

Pathology and Classification

The two common varieties of primary cancer of the liver should be divided into *primary hepatocellular carcinoma* (PHC) and *primary cholangiocarcinoma* (PCC). However, there have been many classifications and subdivisions of these tumors that, if scrutinized critically, have shown mixed histologic patterns. The most important subdivisions in our experience have been the fibrolamellar and the clear cell varieties of PHC. In addition to these major divisions, there are isolated primary tumors of the liver that will be mentioned only in passing because of the rarity and the impossibility of developing any extensive experience or solid data.

Hepatoblastoma is, of course, a common malignant tumor of the liver that occurs in childhood. This carries with it a much better prognosis, if resectable, than any of the malignant primary tumors seen in the adult.

Hemangiosarcoma, although rare, is of some interest because of the subsequent development of an appropriate plan of therapy.

Cystadenocarcinoma is rare compared with its benign version, the *cystadenoma;* however, when malignant degeneration has occurred, the prognosis is still surprisingly good when the lesion is technically resectable.

One also may encounter such tumors as teratomas, carcinosarcomas, mucoepidermoid squamous cell tumors, malignant mesenchymoma, and embryonal rhabdomyosarcoma, all of which are too rare to warrant further analysis.

Lymphoma has been described as a primary tumor of the liver, but this is always suspect and, in our own experience of one case in which resection was undertaken, multiple other lesions developed elsewhere over the ensuing years. Of course one could not state categorically that these represented other manifestations of a diffuse malignancy or might by chance represent metastatic growths. The former seems much more likely. It is still open to question as to whether there is such an entity as primary lymphoma of the liver.

TREATMENT AND RESULTS

Primary malignant tumors of the liver at the New England Deaconess Hospital were reviewed over a 15-year period from 1970 to 1985[2] (Table 8–1).

Over that period of time, a total of 98 PHCs were identified, of which 61 occurred in cirrhotic livers (Fig. 8–1). In this area of the world, most of these occurred in alcoholic cirrhotics, although there were scattered instances of tumors arising in other nonalcoholic cirrhotics, including various types of macronodular cirrhosis and hemochromatosis. Of this subgroup (cirrhotics), only six tumors were resectable. There was one perioperative death from uncontrollable coagulopathy. Four others died with a median survival of only 6.9 months, but one patient, who actually had an almost pedunculated tumor hanging from the edge of the liver, is still alive after an interval of seven years. Obviously, however, the overall prognosis of PHC arising in cirrhosis is poor at best and this reflects the experience of other hospitals throughout the world. The reasons for the low resectability rate of PHC occurring in cirrhotics are probably self-evident. Under these circumstances, the cancer is often multifocal, rapidly growing, and almost terminal when discovered. The nature of the cirrhotic process tends to obscure the existence of the tumor until it has spread widely, because venous invasion is a common characteristic. Even if the tumor is localized, the derangement of liver

TABLE 8–1. RESECTIONS FOR PRIMARY HEPATOCELLULAR CANCER

	Number	Range	Survival Median	Mean
Total Resections	22			
Peri-op Death	1			
Survivors	21	2 mos–15 yrs	22 mos	48 mos
Cirrhotics	5	5 mos–6 yrs	19 mos	33 mos
Normal	16	2 mos–15 yrs	32 mos	53 mos

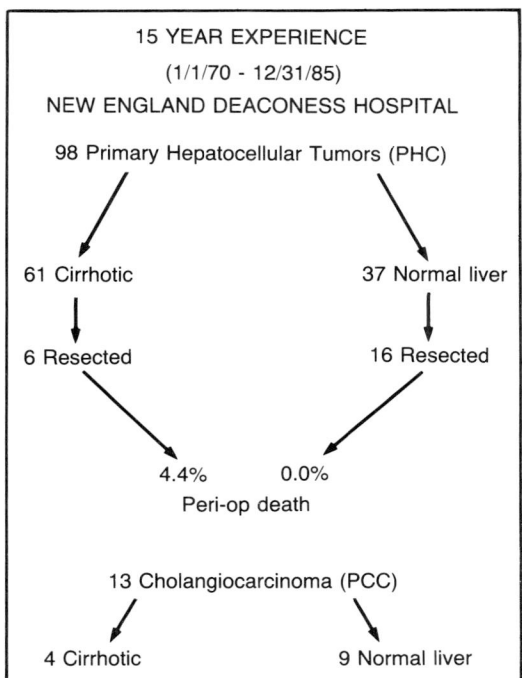

Figure 8–1. 15-year experience with primary hepatocellular carcinoma—98 cases at New England Deaconess Hospital, 1/1/70–12/31/85.

function is frequently severe and precludes any consideration of liver surgery. It is these clinical situations, however, that theoretically may respond best to total hepatectomy and orthotopic liver transplant.

There was a group of 37 PHCs that arose in an otherwise normal liver. Of these, 16 were resectable and were equally divided between men and women. The median age was 48 years. The pathology of the resectable group was PHC,[10] fibrolamellar variant,[3] clear cell variant,[2] and mixed elements,[1] which should probably, for simplicity, be kept under the major category of PHC. All resections were carried out with the intention of cure, and the survival curves of the whole group were 78 per cent (one year) to 55 per cent (four years). There is an interesting, albeit anecdotal, aspect to the group of primary carcinomas characterized as the fibrolamellar variant, inasmuch as the three patients were under 40 years of age and are still living and well, two, four, and seven years after resection. One patient (a nurse) with clear cell carcinoma was 19 years old at the time of resection and had multiple small metastatic nodules in the remaining right lobe, several of which were biopsied and shown to be similar to the primary tumor; despite this, this young woman remains alive and well without demonstrable evidence of disease 15 years after the primary resection.

Thirteen cases were ultimately categorized under the heading of primary cholangiocarcinoma (PCC). This group of liver tumors does not lend itself easily to categorization and analysis. First, there are three cases that involve bile duct carcinomas that histologically resemble the others in this group. Interestingly enough, not one of these patients in whom left hepatic lobectomy was carried out survived five years but none died of the PCC.[3] One further patient whose lesion fits more exactly into the category of cholangiocarcinoma is living and free of disease seven years after major resection; the remaining cases of PCC behaved more like PHC biologically rather than bile duct cancer. The interface of these tumors needs further histologic, biologic, and clinical study and definition.

METASTATIC CANCER

Hepatic resection for metastatic malignancy has been, in most series, primarily related to synchronous or metachronous disease from primary lesions in the colon and rectum. In the extensive watershed monograph by Foster and Berman[4] in which liver resection was analyzed in 164 cases, and in similar experiences from single institutional series, including our own multiple series,[5-8] certain conclusions may be drawn relative to results of surgical resection. We will review these conclusions as follows:

In our early institutional experience at the New England Deaconess Hospital,[5] if we eliminate scattered cases of metastases from stomach, cervix, kidney, and from primary melanomas and leiomyosarcomas elsewhere, there were 76 consecutive patients analyzed who underwent hepatic resection for colorectal cancer. Twenty-three patients were reported initially following major resection from metachronous metastases from colorectal cancer and have been followed up for a considerable period of time. In addition, there have been three cases of synchronous metastatic tumors not included in order to maintain as much homogeneity as possible in the initial series.

In analyzing factors that appeared to affect long-term survival, in this first series with longest follow-up it has become obvious that the fewer the metastases, the more sanguine one could be about long-term survival. In fact, when more than three metastases were found in the resected specimen, we have had no long-term survivors, whereas only three patients (17 per cent) with fewer than four metastatic lesions died of recurrent disease of the liver. Analysis of this subgroup showed a median survival of 38 months. This single-institution experience is quite similar to that reported by Steele et al at the Brigham and Women's Hospital,[6] in which overall survival following successful hepatic resection in a selected group of liver-only colorectal cancer recurrence patients was shown to be 50 per cent at five years following surgery. All of these patients had fewer than three metastases. Adson et al[9] in summarizing the entire experience of the Mayo Clinic, including patients with synchronous liver metastases, did not show this striking dependence on number of liver nodules.

Other reports[10-14] are difficult to compare directly, but the composite review of Hughes et al[14] showed a similar profile, in which the presence of three or more metastases carried a poorer prognosis. One might expect that a long interval between the resection of the primary and appearance of the metastases in the liver might presage a good result. However, in our experience, this is valid only when combined with evaluation of the multiplicity of the lesions.[8]

The other clear-cut indicator was the resection margin. If more than 1.0 cm of normal liver intervened between the tumor and the surgical margin, the survival was much better than otherwise.

No other patient characteristics, such as age, sex, stage of primary cancer, or size of metastases, were found to correlate consistently with survival.

In subsequent analyses of single-institutional experience at the New England Deaconess Hospital, it has become obvious that the more liberal the criteria for inclusion into hepatic resection treatment for metastatic colon and rectum cancer, the less favorable the outcome. In a recent analysis of approximately 100 consecutive patients who underwent hepatic resection for liver-only colorectal cancer, we have shown a median disease-free survival of 23 months.[8] As in most major liver resection series, operative mortality was only 3 per cent. Age, sex, location and stage of primary colon cancer, extent of hepatic resection done to encompass the tumor, flow cytometry and ploidy results, and presence or absence of satellite lesions in the pathologically examined specimen did not affect survival. Extended interval between primary and hepatic metastasis resection seemed to be associated with an increased disease-free survival. Patients with carcinoembryonic antigen values of less than 200 ng/ml prior to hepatic resection survived longer compared with patients with prehepatic metastasis resection values that were over 200. Most important and consistent with our smaller series with longer follow-up, patients with negative resection margins were found to have disease-free survival that was twice as long as in patients with positive margins. Overall five-year survival was three times higher when patients who underwent resection had free margins (33 per cent versus 10 per cent overall survival, respectively). The "ideal" candidates for hepatic resection of metastases from colorectal carcinoma have a disease-free interval between primary and hepatic metastasis of over two years, a low CEA prior to their hepatic metastasis resection, fewer than three liver nodules that are surgically encompassable, and pathologically defined negative resection margins. Such "ideal" patients in our series have a five-year disease-free survival of 54 per cent in contrast to patients who have all of the worst features with a five-year disease-free survival of only 4 per cent.

As recently reviewed by Steele and Ravikumar,[7] approximately 1000 resections of liver metastases have been performed during the past decade and have been repeatedly retrospectively analyzed. Despite the fact that between 20 and 30 per cent of such operated patients are probably cured, the following caveats are obvious. First, most patients are not cured by surgery. Second, although predictors have been proposed to select appropriate patients most likely to benefit from surgery, no predictor is discriminating in and of itself. Third, most therapy questions in this group of patients have not been and probably cannot be addressed in any formal way. Fourth, surgery for isolated regionally recurrent colon and rectum cancer remains an important stopgap only until effective systemic therapy is discovered.

Because no surgeon would ever flip a coin to determine whether or not a surgically staged potentially resectable hepatic metastasis should or should not be resected in an otherwise healthy anesthetized patient, the true benefit of surgery in such patients will remain impossible to differentiate from the selection bias of those very few patients who come to surgeons with isolated potentially resectable metastases in the first place. In attempting to define in a more rigorous way the accuracy of preoperative versus operative staging, morbidity and mortality of major liver resection in a multi-institutional setting, and survival in patients who have adequate versus inadequate margins after hepatic metastases resection, the Gastrointestinal Tumor Study Group has recently completed a formal registry of patients who have undergone resection of resectable metastases. These data were presented at the American

Society of Clinical Oncology meeting and will soon appear in the Journal of Clinical Oncology. Conclusions show that the median survival of patients who have resected tumors with pathologically proven margins free of tumor is approximately 35 months. Patients who have undergone resection but are found at pathologic examination to have inadequate margins have exactly the same median survival (19 to 20 months) as those patients operated on and not having resection because of anatomically unresectable liver metastases or previously unsuspected extrahepatic disease.

Thus, the best candidate for hepatic resection of metastatic cancer would be an individual in good general health with an otherwise normal liver, a solitary lesion anatomically satisfactory for resection, an interval of two or more years from the resection of the primary tumor, and the absence of extrahepatic disease. Nonetheless, these relatively strict criteria are only guidelines, and there are many excellent results in patients whose clinical evaluation has deviated from these ideal indicators.

OTHER TREATMENT OF HEPATIC CANCERS

CHEMOTHERAPY

Chemotherapy has not proved very effective in either primary or secondary liver cancer, although hepatic arterial infusion or bolus therapy has achieved what appears to be palliation and increased survival in some instances.

DEARTERIALIZATION

Dearterialization of the liver has been shown to be feasible with a low mortality and morbidity. This approach has been possible because of the dual blood supply of the parenchyma and the fact that malignancies may depend, initially, entirely on hepatic arterial inflow. This has been accomplished both surgically[15] and by thromboembolism via a radiologically introduced catheter.[16] These approaches have proved most effective in highly vascular tumors that induce morbidity primarily through secretory release (carcinoids, insulinomas, gastrinomas, and the like). While the approach is temporarily and often dramatically effective, the duration of response is limited by the fact that tumor clusters under 200 microns in size do not depend on arterial flow and survive via angiogenesis.[17, 18] These clusters develop a blood supply as arterial collateralization develops and ultimately the secretory syndrome returns.

CRYOSURGERY AND ULTRASONIC DELINEATION

As mentioned briefly, our experience with the intraoperative use of the ultrasonic probe has proved extremely useful in detecting and delineating otherwise unrecognizable tumor nodules. In addition, this instrument has been essential in the guidance of cryoprobes introduced into nonresectable tumor nodules as a method of ablation by freezing.[19]

It is appropriate to conclude this review of the treatment of liver tumors with a reference to the role of *orthotopic transplantation* in the management of malignant disease of the liver. Presently, this area is still in a stage of evolution and evaluation.[20] Given the disappointing outlook for survival following liver transplantation for both primary and metastatic lesions, we have approached this subject cautiously, with only 18 of almost 200 consecutive transplants being carried out for neoplasm to date. Thirteen recipients harbored hepatomas, and of those, nine presented with coexisting cirrhosis from viral hepatitis (HBsAG(+)-3-,HBsAg(-1-5) or hemochromatosis,[1] while one patient suffered from sclerosing cholangitis and three had no other associated liver disorder. There were three early deaths from graft failure or rejection. Median survival of the remaining 10 is 584 days (range 70 to 1392). One patient who presented with a well-differentiated multifocal hepatoma with cirrhosis developed a solitary recurrence at two years that was resected from the graft.

Of the three recipients harboring Klatskin-type cholangiocarcinomas, two died with recurrence within six months, while one patient remains free of disease four years after initial extended left hepatectomy and two years following transplant. One patient with a massive peripheral cholangiocarcinoma remains alive at 16 months without signs of recurrence. One additional patient with glycogen storage disease and a rising α-fetoprotein was found to have diffuse hepatic adenomata rather than hepatoma.

With the limited experience gathered to date, patient survival following transplantation for primary liver cancer appears to be best in candidates with small hepatomas arising in a background of chronic cirrhosis or in those rare individuals with the fibrolamellar variant.[21] Patients with cholangiocarcinomas generally fare very poorly despite aggressive use of preoperative chemotherapy and/or radiation. Experience with metastatic disease has been similarly disappointing and, given the scarcity of donor organs, is unlikely to represent an important disease category for transplant intervention.

With reports of continued experience, particularly by Starzl, Calne, and Pichlmayer, we should be able to evaluate the role of liver transplant in the treatment of primary cancers of that organ in the near future.

CONCLUSION

A review of the distinguishing characteristics and the effectiveness of treatment in the management of either primary or metastatic cancer in and to the liver has been presented. It has been recognized that the relative rarity of surgical application limits any conclusive evaluation of results, particularly in attempting to differentiate therapy success from biologic selection.

REFERENCES

1. McDermott, W.V., Jr.: Surgical disease in East Africa. Arch. Surg. *122*:397–402, 1987.
2. McDermott, W.V., Jr., Cady, B., Georgi, B., et al.: Primary cancer of the liver, evaluation, treatment and prognosis. Arch. Surg. *124*:552–555, 1989.
3. McDermott, W.V., Jr., and Peinert, R.A.: Carcinoma in the supra-ampullary portion of the bile ducts. Surg. Gynecol. Obstet. *149*:681–686, 1979.
4. Foster, J.H., and Berman, M.M.: Solid liver tumors. Vol 23. *In* Major Problems in Clinical Surgery. Philadelphia, W.B. Saunders, 1977.
5. Cady, B., and McDermott, W.V., Jr.: Major hepatic resection for metachronous metastases from colon cancer. Ann. Surg. *291*:204–209, 1985.
6. Steele, G., Jr., Osteen, R.T., Wilson, R.E., et al.: Patterns of failure after surgical "cure" of large liver tumors—a change in the proximate cause of death and a need for effective systemic adjuvant therapy. Am. J. Surg. *147*:544–549, 1984.

7. Steele, G., Jr., and Ravikumar, T.S.: Resection of hepatic metastases from colorectal cancer: Biologic perspectives. Ann. Surg. *210:*126–138, 1989.
8. Cady, B., McDermott, W.V., Jr., Jenkins, R.L., et al.: Hepatic resection for colorectal metastases: Prognostic features governing outcome. In preparation.
9. Adson, M.A., Van Heerden, J.A., Adson, M.H., et al.: Resection of hepatic metastases from colorectal cancer. Arch. Surg. *119:*647–651, 1984.
10. Foster, J.H.: Survival after liver resection for secondary tumors. Am. J. Med. *135:*389–394, 1978.
11. Logan, S.E., Meter, S.J., Ramming, K.P., et al.: Hepatic resection of metastatic colorectal carcinoma. Arch. Surg. *117:*25–28, 1982.
12. Fortner, J.G., Silva, J.S., Golbev, R.B., et al.: Multivariate analysis of a personal series of 247 consecutive patients with liver metastases from colorectal cancer. Ann. Surg. *199:*182–186, 1984.
13. Rajpal, S., Sasmahapatra, K.S., Ledesma, E.J., et al.: Extensive resections of isolated metastasis from carcinoma of the colon and rectum. Surg. Gynecol. Obstet. *155:*813–816, 1982.
14. Hughes, K.S., Simon, R., Songhorabodi, S., et al.: Resection of the liver for colorectal carcinoma metastases: A multi-institutional study of patterns of recurrence. Surgery *100:*278–284, 1986.
15. McDermott, W.V., Jr., Paris, A.L., Clouse, M.E., and Meissner, W.A.: Dearterialization of the liver for metastatic cancer. Clinical, angiographic and pathologic observations. Ann. Surg. *187:*38–46, 1978.
16. Clouse, M.E., Lee, R.G.L., Duszlak, E., et al.: Hepatic artery embolization for primary and secondary liver neoplasms. Radiology *147:*407–411, 1983.
17. Folkman, J.: Anti-angiogenesis. New concept for therapy of solid tumors. Ann. Surg. *175:*409, 1972.
18. Folkman, J.: Tumor angiogenesis factor. Cancer Res. *34:*2109, 1974.
19. Ravikumar, T.S., Kane, R., Cady, B., et al.: Hepatic cryosurgery with intraoperative ultrasound monitoring for metastatic colon carcinoma. Arch. Surg. *122:*402–409, 1987.
20. Ringe, B., Wittekind, C., Bechstein, W.O., et al.: The role of liver transplantation in hepatobiliary malignancy. Ann. Surg. *209:*88–98, 1989.
21. Jenkins, R.L., Pinson, C.V., and Stone, M.D.: Experience with transplantation in the treatment of liver cancer. Cancer Chemother. Pharmacol. *23:*104–109s, 1989.

9

BREAST CANCER

by Blake Cady, M.D.

The standard treatment of breast cancer in the future, even five years in the future, is difficult to predict at the present time. Significant improvements in the disease appearance, rapid accumulation of knowledge about newer therapies, and major changes in public and professional attitudes about breast cancer itself are accelerating such that what is considered standard therapy today may well become outmoded. This chapter will give a personal interpretation of the changes that have occurred and their implication for a program of management. It must be stressed that this is the author's personal viewpoint of the information available as well as a personal approach to the patient with therapeutic recommendations.

BIOLOGY OF THE DISEASE

It is apparent from studies[1-6] done in the recent years that a new comprehension of the biology of the disease has become firmly established. First, the details of local therapy do not govern survival. While local recurrence in the breast or chest wall may well depend on details of the operative management, recurrence in the breast alone if it is preserved after lumpectomy, with or without radiation therapy, does not by itself bias against survival.[7-9] All randomized trials comparing local excision versus mastectomy indicate that at long-term follow-up of 10 or more years, the same number of patients will be alive in the comparative groups.[1-4, 10, 11] These data reinforce the assumption that breast cancer cells spread from the original local site in the breast simultaneously by lymphatic and hematogenous routes and that this metastatic spread of cells may occur extremely early in the course of the disease. A local recurrence within an intact breast after lumpectomy will not add further to this risk of metastatic spread of cells and thus will not increase clinical metastatic disease as demonstrated by the identical long-term survival outcome in these controlled trials.

Second, it is apparent that lymph node metastases are "indicators but not governors"[12] of survival and that axillary lymph node dissections are prognostic and staging procedures and not therapeutic procedures in terms of impact on survival. This has been made clear in the studies of the National Surgical Adjuvant Breast Project (NSABP) B-04 in which patient outcome in various trials was compared in terms of treatment of an axilla and no treatment of the axilla and surgical dissection and radiotherapeutic treatment of the axilla.[3] The results of this trial and many earlier trials[9, 12, 13] evaluating the outcome of postmastectomy radiation therapy to regional lymph nodes have indicated that the treatment of regional lymph node basins associated with breast cancer does not alter survival outcome. Indeed, these studies[3] indicate that only half of pathologically defined lymph node metastases ever become clinically apparent in follow-up despite the absence of any treatment to the axilla. Thus, lymph node metastases, while having a marker or descriptive function, have no controlling function in the clinical course of breast cancer patients.[12]

Third, the biology of duct carcinoma in situ is becoming more apparent with the elegant studies of Lagios et al in San Francisco,[14] who treated a large number of patients with duct carcinoma in situ (DCIS) less than 2.5 cm in diameter by local excision only (without radiation therapy). These patients have demonstrated a low recurrence rate and an absence of other ipsilateral foci of DCIS in follow-up. This information and the exhaustive analysis of DCIS by whole organ sections of mastectomy specimens by Lagios et al[14] indicate that multifocal disease and occult microscopic invasion are both associated with large and extensive duct carcinoma in situ (over 4 cm in diameter), which were usually clinically apparent masses. Thus, the small DCIS, the usual form of the disease encountered with mammographic screening, when excised locally is usually cured. This would indicate that the multifocal disease of more extensive DCIS may well be the result of intraductal spread from one area of the breast to another without invasion of the basement membrane in a manner that would resemble, within the more peripheral ducts, the process seen in Paget's disease of the terminal lactiferous ducts and the nipple. Absence of the microinvasive component of DCIS in lesions less than 4 cm in diameter would indicate that extensive intraductal spread of DCIS occurs before the basement membrane is breached and the tumor becomes fully invasive in at least a significant proportion of DCIS. The studies of Holland et al[15] demonstrating the surrounding foci of DCIS associated with invasive breast cancer that extends in significant peripheral directions from the predominant invasive component illustrate the pattern usually assumed to occur in the presence of an initial focus of DCIS in many breast cancers. Thus, early invasion may well indicate a distinctive cancer cell behavior in contradistinction to purely intraductal spread.

Next, the recent data[16] on monoclonal antibody staining of bone marrow biopsy specimens in primary breast cancer patients illustrate that the mere presence of a bone marrow breast cancer cell does not necessarily indicate that such cells will become foci of clinical metastatic disease. Patients with a minimal tumor burden in their bone marrow biopsies, at least in initial short-term studies,[16] seem to have a good prognosis that is not accompanied by metastatic growth. This is in keeping with the assumption that micrometastatic disease or cell dissemination, while perhaps occurring in large numbers of patients, may be clinically significant in a much smaller proportion. This conforms to the experimental animal models that distinguish between tumor cell dissemination, lodgment, and progressive growth, which are three separate processes.

Finally, adjuvant treatment of poor-risk breast cancer patients, as determined by positive lymph nodes or prognostic marker studies, produces only a proportional reduction in recurrence or mortality and not an absolute reduction.[17] The fact that recurrence and mortality are proportionally reduced in far less than 50 per cent of the patients despite apparently effective chemotherapy at a micrometastatic stage indicates that the assumption that treatment of micrometastatic disease is the key to the success of systemic chemotherapy is not necessarily the only or best model of chemotherapeutic action in the majority of cases. Such limited success of adjuvant chemotherapy programs reemphasizes the aspects of cellular heterogeneity in metastatic disease in breast cancer and offers further challenges in the development of more successful systemic adjuvant treatments. Adjuvant chemotherapy, when utilized with radiation therapy, also reduces local recurrence rate in primary breast cancer treated by local excision.[2] The exact quantitation of this effect is to be determined. A variety of animal and human studies in the use of tamoxifen as an adjunct to treatment of primary breast cancer all emphasize the fact that tamoxifen is a suppressive agent for the growth of breast cancer cells and not a cancerocidal agent that kills breast cancer cells as is assumed in chemotherapy.[18] Long-term tamoxifen therapy may reduce the rate of recurrence after local surgery in the ipsilateral breast and seems to reduce the incidence of new contralateral primary breast cancers.[2, 18]

These various biologic aspects of the disease provide comfort in the more widespread adaptation of conservative surgery in treatment of the primary breast cancer. However, they also pose challenges in developing more effective systemic agents for the treatment of micrometastatic disease to achieve the successes that are seen with, for instance, testicular carcinoma, in which even gross metastatic disease can be treated for cure by effective chemotherapy. This testicular cancer model of human solid tumors is strikingly different from that of breast cancer because the effectiveness of later chemotherapy in metastatic testicular cancer is such that adjuvant chemotherapy after orchiectomy may not be necessary since later curative chemotherapy is so reliable. Only those patients who actually develop clinical metastatic disease require chemotherapeutic treatments. Here again is an illustration of the fact that treatment in the setting of micrometastatic disease may be less important in terms of drug effectiveness than in specificity of chemotherapeutic agents. The mediocre results of adjuvant 5-fluorouracil (5-FU) alone in colon cancer reemphasizes this point, although the addition of other agents (levamisole, leucovorin) makes 5-FU more effective.

DISEASE PRESENTATION

One of the most striking aspects of breast cancer in recent years has been the marked reduction in mean size and nodal metastatic involvement with the widespread use of screening mammography. A large number of well-controlled randomized trials comparing the offering of mammography with either physical examination alone or nothing specifically directed at breast cancer detection have indicated the effectiveness of mammography as a screening procedure to detect early disease and reduce death rate from breast cancer.[19] Large numbers of nonpalpable breast cancers are now being detected, and the data from screening trials indicate that if the entire female population over the age of 40 or 50 could be screened with mammography (with physical examination by the physician and self-examination by the patient), major reductions in breast cancer mortality could be achieved. The reduction in mortality at 5 to 7 years after mammography trials have been started is in the range of one-third.[19] This reduction is minimized or underestimated by the fact that, in every trial conducted, large numbers of patients in experimental groups failed to actually receive mammography and significant numbers of patients in control groups receive mammography anyway. Such dilution of the two assigned groups may minimize the actual achievements of mammography screening. It is apparent that we are at the threshold of a new era in primary breast cancer in which early detection may be so successful that the majority of tumors will be detected at a nonpalpable and, in many cases, noninvasive stage of disease. The overall impact of these many trials of mammography screening strongly substantiates the need to conduct true population screening with mammography in the United States. Public education, subsidy of mammography cost, and simplification of the process may lead to more universal application in women over the age of 40 or 50. When such routine screening mammography should cease is not clear, but age 70 or 75 seems appropriate.[19]

EPIDEMIOLOGY

Study of the epidemiology of breast cancer continues because the exact epidemiologic features of the vast majority of cases continue to be elusive. It seems clear that a western diet with high consumption of animal fats and high caloric intake is associated with a high incidence of postmenopausal breast cancer. In societies that are "westernizing" their traditional diet, sharp increases in breast cancer incidence develop. The exact components of the diet and the detailed nature of the causative linkage remain to be elucidated. It is also apparent that the incidence of premenopausal breast cancer is not greatly dissimilar throughout the world comparing both high-incidence and low-incidence areas. Thus, it seems that premenopausal and postmenopausal breast cancer, appearing the same under the microscope and in the clinical course of the disease, are in fact quite different in their epidemiologic and etiologic aspects. This can be surmised also by the more frequent genetic aspects of premenopausal breast cancer, which include a higher incidence of familial disease and a higher incidence of bilaterality. Risk of breast cancer in first-degree members of breast cancer patients is linked, for the most part, with premenopausal status. Risk ratios in the order of 3 to 8 based on the number of first-degree relatives and the unilateral or bilateral nature of the disease are in contrast to the risk ratios of only 1.3 to 2 when the breast cancer patient is postmenopausal. Studies of sex hormone interrelationships remain important to explain the increasing risk of breast cancer with progressive delays in first full-term pregnancy, particularly into the mid and late 30s. Thus, events in the hormonal life of women are reflected in breast cancer rates 30 to 40 years later, and these variations in parturition history affect postmenopausal, not premenopausal, breast cancer risk. Further evidence of biologic differences between premenopausal and postmenopausal breast cancer can be seen in their different responses to adjuvant chemotherapy or tamoxifen.[17]

LOBULAR CARCINOMA IN SITU

Lobular carcinoma in situ has been studied intensively over the past decades, and a common understanding of its implication is now accepted by most surgeons.[20, 21] Lobular carcinoma in situ (LCIS) is a risk indicator and not a preinvasive breast cancer. Most subsequent breast cancers in patients with LCIS are ductal carcinomas not lobular carcinomas, and later invasive breast cancer is as liable to appear in the opposite breast as the ipsilateral breast and as liable to appear in other quadrants of the ipsilateral breast as the original biopsy site. These features all substantiate the conclusion that after local excision LCIS does not lead to invasive cancer at the local site of the biopsy due to inadequate local therapy.

Thus, treatment of lobular carcinoma in situ should generally be conservative and probably by biopsy only. However, LCIS may be an additional significant risk indicator in an otherwise defined high-risk case such that prophylactic bilateral mastectomy to reduce a very high risk of invasive cancer may be selected. For instance, in a high-risk family with premenopausal first-degree relatives with invasive breast cancer, a patient who has LCIS has a risk of eventual development of invasive cancer that approaches 50 per cent. In this case, the diagnosis of LCIS might well lead to selection of prophylactic bilateral mastectomy, with or without reconstruction, in an attempt to prevent later invasive breast cancer. Unilateral mastectomy is inappropriate treatment for any lobular carcinoma in situ.

An unanswered question in LCIS is the fate of patients who have repeated biopsies of LCIS from different areas of breast tissue. Do such patients have such an increased risk of later invasive carcinoma which would make candidates for prophylactic mastectomy? No answer is apparent at the present time and such patients are few in number. I personally believe that repeated episodes of LCIS by biopsy may indicate a higher than usual background risk, even in the absence of other historic risk factors, and should at least lead to discussions about the usefulness of prophylactic bilateral mastectomy.

The cumulative risk of invasive carcinoma developing in a patient with lobular carcinoma in situ without a family history approaches 1 per cent per year. With a family history of a premenopausal first-degree relative with invasive cancer, a diagnosis of LCIS indicates a cumulative life-time risk of about 2 per cent per year, or 40 per cent in 20 years of follow-up.[22] Issues of reliability of detection by screening mammography and prognosis of cancers detected by careful follow-up then become paramount in discussion with patients about treatment options.

The fact that LCIS is more common on biopsy material and mastectomy specimens in premenopausal women than in postmenopausal women indicates that it is probably estrogen dependent. This reemphasizes the assumption that it is a risk factor since patients develop invasive breast cancer at a continuing cumulative rate despite the apparent disappearance of the marker lesion itself over time after menopause.

TABLE 9–1. INCIDENCE OF INVASIVE CANCER WHEN ORIGINAL LCIS TREATED BY BIOPSY

Years After LCIS Diagnosis	# at Risk	Cumulative Probability Ipsilateral Breast Cancer	Cumulative Probability Contralateral Breast Cancer
5	236	4%	5%
10	224	7%	8%
15	135	11%	9%
20	94	18%	12%
25	42	21%	15%

From Haagensen, C. D., Bodian, C., and Haagensen, D. (Eds.): Lobular neoplasia (lobular carcinoma in situ). *In* Breast Carcinoma Risk and Detection. Philadelphia, W. B. Saunders, 1981, p. 267.

DUCT CARCINOMA IN SITU

The large increase of duct carcinoma in situ (DCIS) being uncovered by mammography screening programs has created the opportunity to understand its biology and thus eventually to understand which DCIS lesions pose a threat to the patient and which are pathologic curiosities without apparent progressive growth.[14] The studies of Lagios et al[14] have been pioneering efforts to evaluate this disease at an early stage. When the group of DCIS lesions measuring less than 2.5 cm in diameter (which have a median diameter of less than 1 cm) are treated by local excision, only a small fraction of patients (10 to 20 per cent) develop recurrent DCIS or invasive breast cancer in the same quadrant as the biopsy. The exact risk of such local recurrence is no more than 2 per cent per year cumulatively[22] in these small DCIS lesions detected by mammography, and it may be even less. It is clear that recurrences following local excision for small DCIS appear adjacent to the previous local excision. This indicates that DCIS is indeed a preinvasive cancer in many cases and requires completely different strategies than LCIS. In Lagios' studies,[14] it is apparent that microinvasion, multifocality, and lymph node metastases occur only in DCIS larger than 4 or 5 cm in greatest diameter. In lesions less than 2.5 cm in diameter, there is no microinvasion, no multifocality, and no lymph node metastases when such patients are subsequently treated by mastectomy.

Patients early in Lagios' series[14] followed for more than eight years had approximately a 20 per cent rate of local recurrence, while later patients followed for a median of four years but up to eight years had a risk of local recurrence of only 10 per cent. Half of recurrences are again DCIS, while the others are small invasive cancers usually only a few millimeters in diameter and probably totally curable because of their very small size. No deaths from cancer have occurred in the initial reports of the series.

Thus, the typical small DCIS lesions are usually detected by mammography, as clustered calcifications that measure in total less than 2.5 cm with a median diameter of less than 1 cm. They can safely be treated by local excision if the surgical margins are clear and no other suspicious calcifications are present in the mammogram and the patient is followed carefully by repeated mammography and physical examination (Table 9–2).[23]

Few of the earlier reports of DCIS are pertinent today because they

TABLE 9–2. GUIDELINES FOR THE EVALUATION OF PATIENTS WITH MAMMOGRAPHICALLY DETECTED, NONPALPABLE LESIONS WITH MICROCALCIFICATIONS BEING CONSIDERED FOR BREAST-CONSERVING TREATMENT

1. Careful mammographic evaluation of the breast before biopsy, including magnification views, to delineate the extent of the microcalcifications.
2. Needle localization for the biopsy.
3. Specimen radiography, preferably with magnification views as well as contact views, to confirm that the lesion has been excised and to direct pathologic sampling.
4. Careful gross description of the excised specimen by the pathologist.
5. Inking of the specimen margins by the pathologist before sectioning to facilitate evaluation of margins on permanent sections.
6. On microscopic examination, description of the relation of the calcifications to the lesion and the distance of the tumor from the inked margins of resection.
7. Post-biopsy mammography with magnification views to confirm that all suspicious microcalcifications have been removed.
8. Repeat excision of the primary site if residual microcalcifications are seen on postbiopsy mammography, or if tumor involves margins of resection microscopically.

From Schnitt, S. J., Silen, W., Sadowsky, N. L., et al.: Ductal carcinoma in situ (intraductal carcinoma) of the breast. N. Engl. J. Med. *318*:898–902, 1988.

largely represented palpable lesions with diameters greater than 2.5 cm. When DCIS lesions larger than 5 cm in diameter are discovered, either by mammography or physical examination, mastectomy should be advised even today since such patients display extensive disease, frequent multifocality, a high incidence of microinvasion, and occasional axillary lymph node metastases.[14] Such patients correspond to the DCIS lesions reported in the premammographic era with a more progressive behavior pattern.

For DCIS lesions between 2.5 and 4 or 5 cm in diameter, attempts at local excision should be considered if the woman has a large enough breast to achieve a satisfactory cosmetic result, the surgical margins are clear, the postoperative mammogram is free of calcifications, and the patient understands and accepts the risks of recurrence. It is unclear at present whether the addition of radiation therapy in such patients has any role in reducing local recurrence. Separate pathologic categories of DCIS are associated with distinctive risks of recurrences, even if the lesions are less than 2.5 cm in diameter. Thus, the comedo type may have a recurrence risk of 30 per cent while papillary varieties have little or no risk of recurrence.[14]

High-Risk Noninvasive Primary Breast Pathology

Table 9–3 represents the author's estimate of the risk of eventual invasive breast cancer incidence and risk of death by treatment of these lesions by local excision and breast preservation. These are estimates of the possible price a woman might pay for the benefit of breast retention, an important component of discussion with women about therapeutic alternatives.

TABLE 9–3. ESTIMATED OUTCOME IN PATIENTS WITH HIGH-RISK, NONINVASIVE BREAST PATHOLOGY TREATED BY LOCAL EXCISION

Histology	Family History	Incidence of Invasive Cancer		Maximum Estimated 20-Year Mortality if Breast Preserved
		Annually	*At 20 Years*	
ADH	No	0.5%	10%	1%
ALH	Yes	1%	20%	2%
LCIS	No	1%	20%	2%
	Yes	2%	40%	4%
DCIS	No	2%	40%	4%
	Yes	(4%)	(60% at 15 years)	(6%)

ALH Atypical Lobular Hyperplasia
ADH Atypical Ductal Hyperplasia
LCIS Lobular Carcinoma in situ
DCIS Duct Carcinoma in situ
( ) No data available—author's estimate

NONPALPABLE INVASIVE BREAST CANCER

Nonpalpable invasive breast cancer, by definition, is detected by mammography. These lesions are now being seen in an increasing proportion in primary breast cancer patients and are in direct relationship to the mammographic application in the population. Recent estimates[24] indicate that two-thirds of women over the age of 45 or 50 have had a mammogram, but only one-third have had more than one mammogram over time. As the proportion of women who have mammography at yearly intervals increases, the proportion of breast cancers that are nonpalpable will certainly exceed 50 or 60 per cent.

At our own hospital in the past five years, the mean diameter of invasive breast cancer has dropped to 2.31 cm and the median diameter is only 2 cm.[25] Many nonpalpable breast cancers are even too small to measure and are seen only as an area of 1 or 2 mm associated with calcification or a small mass by mammography. Nonpalpable primary breast cancers of 1 cm or less have an incidence of lymph node metastases of 10 per cent or less in our hospital.[25] Thus, in such early cases, the usefulness of axillary dissection has to be questioned, as the proportion of positive dissections is so low.[26] In addition, among these patients with cancers 1 cm or smaller, almost 50 per cent have only one positive lymph node and another 30 per cent have only two positive nodes.[25] Many of these positive nodes are, in fact, micrometastases with apparently little impact on prognosis.[27] The overall prognosis of patients with nonpalpable invasive breast cancers of 1 cm or less in diameter should be at least 95 per cent at five years and probably close to that at ten years according to the long-term follow-up of the Breast Cancer Detection Demonstration Project (BCDDP) reports.[29]

These nonpalpable, small breast cancers will all be diagnosed by localization mammography and excision with mammographic control of the specimen. Principles of incision placement are discussed further on.[30] Management of these patients depends on accurate handling of the specimen removed at localization mammographic lumpectomy. The specimen removed at local excision should be carefully marked for borders, radiographed to ensure that calcification or mass is removed, and subjected to detailed pathologic analysis. Frozen section analysis of these specimens should not be undertaken since precise diagnosis and the extent of disease are so crucial. Both of these features may be significantly impaired by the frozen section analysis of the tissue block. Estrogen and progesterone receptor analysis need not be obtained in tiny cancers for the same reason; frozen section and partitioning of the tumor may destroy the chance for later sophisticated and complete analysis of microinvasion or DCIS. The margins of local excisions should be pathologically negative; occasionally such patients will require a return to the operating room for a re-excision at a later time to remove a margin found to be positive on careful pathologic examination.

Several techniques of margin analysis have been proposed. The most sophisticated technique currently involves multicolored inks applied to various surfaces of the excised specimen for both orientation and accurate analysis under the microscope of the location of the primary cancer and its proximity to resection margins. What the minimum margin should be is not at all clear but probably a 1 cm margin should be achieved.[31]

Whether radiation therapy in addition to local excision in patients with very small invasive cancers is useful or necessary remains an unanswered question at present.[2, 6, 32] Early data (unpublished) from the NSABP would indicate that the reduction in local recurrence in invasive cancers less than 1 cm in diameter amounts to no more than 15 per cent when comparing patients radiated versus patients not irradiated after lumpectomy with margins that were pathologically negative.[33] If less than a 15 per cent reduction can be achieved by the use of radiation therapy in such small invasive cancers, it probably should be avoided. Patients can be followed more accurately with a nonradiated breast because both physical examination and mammography are easier, and if recurrence appears, radiation therapy after a re-excision can be given. The expected rate of re-excision in such small cancers should be less than 20 per cent and is probably less than 15 per cent.[6, 32] If, in addition, extensive intraductal component (EIC) is diagnosed, a direct relationship to local recurrence is recognized; such patients at greatest risk of local recurrence can be selected out for management by either wider local primary excision or a high-dosage of local radiation therapy.[34, 35]

Because of the success in the treatment of such patients with conservative local excision with or without radiation therapy, excellent cosmetic appearance can be achieved.[31, 36] The details of the local surgical procedure therefore need to be re-emphasized. Indeed, it should be understood that the treatment of such small cancers is primarily surgical and therefore surgeons should assume the prime responsibility of careful management. This management includes appropriate incisions on the breast with consideration of the cosmetic results, suitable placement of incisions for the conduct of later mastectomy if that is required by patient request or disease features, and detailed follow-up to observe for local recurrence and the appearance of new primary cancers.[30] There are certain programmatic requirements for the treatment of such lesions by conservative surgery, which will be discussed further on.[37]

Other advantages to the treatment of such small nonpalpable invasive breast cancers include markedly reduced costs as these patients can be treated entirely on an out-patient basis. By avoidance of both axillary dissection and radiation therapy in the majority of such tiny invasive nonpalpable breast cancers, the psychic and physical trauma of the diagnosis of breast cancer and the surgical management can be reduced to a minimum. The marked savings and costs can easily justify the more widespread application of mammographic screening to the general population.

PALPABLE PRIMARY BREAST CANCER

Even before the widespread use of mammography there had been a progressive and steady decline of significant proportions in the mean and median diameter of invasive breast cancers seen in the United States.[38] This decline in size began after 1948 and continued through 1973 before the major impact of breast cancer screening. This decline was entirely due to public and professional education about the seriousness of breast masses. Currently, only a small minority of patients with invasive breast cancer arrives at treatment facilities in the United States with cancers larger than 5 cm in diameter.[25] Thus, even palpable primary breast cancers are decreasing in size and becoming ever more suitable for conservative surgical management with breast preservation. The incidence of lymph node metastases in palpable breast cancers greater than 1 cm in diameter still exceeds 20 per cent. Thus, these patients need to be considered for axillary node dissection for staging until prognostic features of the primary cancer can be found to be equivalent to lymph node status as indicators of long-term outcome. Rapid development of a variety of prognostic indicators in primary cancer features may well supplant the use of axillary dissection in the future, but continued studies need to be performed to substantiate this assumption.[39, 40]

Patients with a palpable mass in the breast should have a needle aspiration cytology performed on the first visit to the physician's office. In over 75 per cent of cancers the needle aspiration cytology can establish the diagnosis. A negative aspiration cytology of such lesions, however, is in no way a secure diagnosis. Patients with negative aspiration cytology need to undergo other diagnostic studies, usually including excisional biopsy before a final diagnosis is made if the surgeon is suspicious of cancer. Following the initial office visit of patients with a palpable mass in the breast, bilateral mammography should be performed if it has not been done in the immediate past. Since the purpose of mammography is not to look at palpable lesions but only to inspect the breast for nonpalpable early cancers, such mammography should in no way bear on the diagnosis and management of the palpable mass. The mammography is performed only to screen the rest of the breast tissue to look for multifocal disease and occult breast cancers in other portions of the ipsilateral or contralateral breast. A negative mammography in the presence of a palpable mass means nothing, and the normal diagnostic sequence of a palpable breast mass should continue regardless of the mammographic findings.

One of the advantages of an initial needle aspiration of a palpable breast mass is that breast cysts, with few exceptions, can be diagnosed and treated by the aspiration in the office. Such cysts need no further excision if they disappear completely, if the fluid obtained is nonbloody, and if the cyst does not repeatedly recur. However, in these patients, mammography should be obtained to rule out occult carcinoma. Most breast cysts appear in women in their 40s, when they are beginning to enter the high-risk age category for breast cancer. Thus, the opportunity for a screening mammography at this crucial stage should not be missed. Few, if any, cysts of the breasts need operation. They can either be evacuated by needle aspiration if palpable or, if seen by mammography, they can be diagnosed by ultrasound. Ultrasound is diagnostically accurate enough in nonpalpable, cystic lesions so that no further studies need be performed. An ultrasonically or mammographically guided needle biopsy can be performed to either evacuate a cyst or obtain a needle cytology aspiration if a lesion proves to be solid. Stereotactic-guided needle biopsy is now being evaluated and may be a useful technique in the future.

At the present time, breast biopsy to remove solid masses should always be performed as a lumpectomy. Thus, the mass should be excised in toto with an estimated 1 cm margin of normal breast tissue surrounding it. With adherence to this format the need for re-excision after breast biopsy can be reduced to a minimum.[31] The only breast lesions that should be subjected to an incisional biopsy are those that are large and those for which needle aspiration or core needle biopsy attempts have been unsuccessful. Such cases should be uncommon. In palpable breast cancers large enough to be difficult for total excisional biopsy, core cutting biopsy can be performed under local anaesthesia in an office setting if aspiration cytology is not diagnostic for accurate diagnosis. Indeed, enough material from repeated passes with a core cutting biopsy can be obtained so that accurate estrogen receptor and progesterone receptor determinations can be performed. Such tissue could also be analyzed for specific prognostic features since quite adequate tissue volume can be obtained by repeated core cutting samples. Table 9–4 is the author's estimate of 10-year disease-free survival of breast cancer as of 1990 by the American Joint Committee on staging.[41]

INCISIONS

The conduct of an excisional biopsy of a palpable breast cancer should recognize the cosmetic imperative of contemporary breast cancer management. Thus, skin incisions should be curvilinear to follow Langer's lines and centrally placed in the breast; some peripheral tunnelling to achieve total excision of a peripheral palpable mass is perfectly acceptable (Fig. 9–1). The incisions must be placed in such a way that later mastectomy can be

TABLE 9–4. AUTHOR'S ESTIMATION OF SURVIVAL DISEASE FREE AT 10 YEARS

T Category	N Category	Disease Free Survival 10 Years
T_{is}	N_0	100%
T_{1a} 0 to .5 cm	N_0	99%
	pN_{1ai} + micrometastasis	95%
	pN_{1bi} + macrometastasis	80%
T_{1b} .6 to 1.0 cm	N_0	95%
	pN_{1ai} + micrometastasis	90%
	pN_{1bi} + macrometastasis	75%
T_{1c} 1.1 to 2 cm	N_0	90%
	pN_{1bii} + 1–3 macrometastases	70%
	pN_{1biii} + >3 macrometastases	<50%
T_2 2.1 to 3 cm	N_0	80%
	N_1	<50%

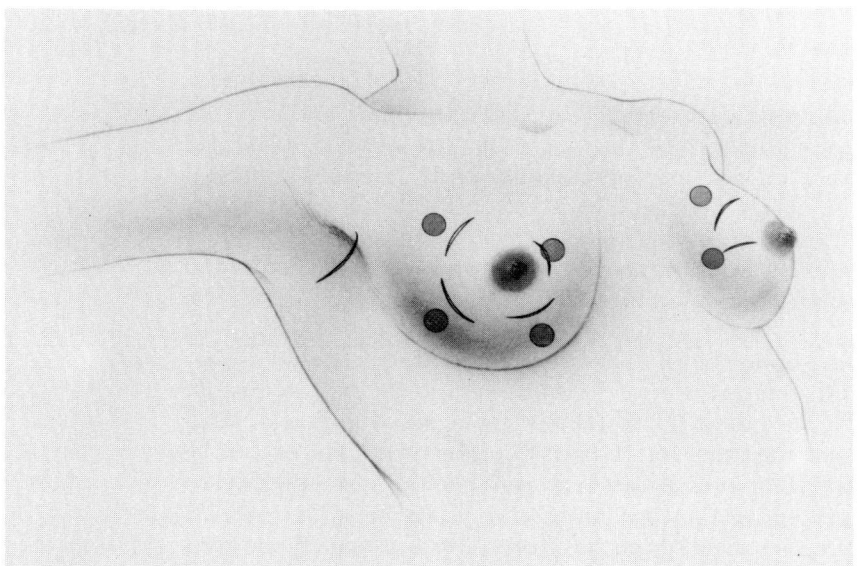

Figure 9–1. Examples of appropriate Langer's line circular incisions relatively central in the breast. The only appropriate radial incision is in the extreme medial aspect of the breast as depicted on the patient's left. Also note the small axillary dissection incision that runs below the axillary hair line and does not extend forward of the anterior axillary fold. (From Cady, B.: Choice of operations for breast cancer: Conservative surgery versus radical procedures. *In* Bland, K. I. and Copeland, E. M. III (Eds.): The Breast: Comprehensive Management of Benign and Malignant Diseases. Philadelphia, W. B. Saunders Co., 1991, p. 762.)

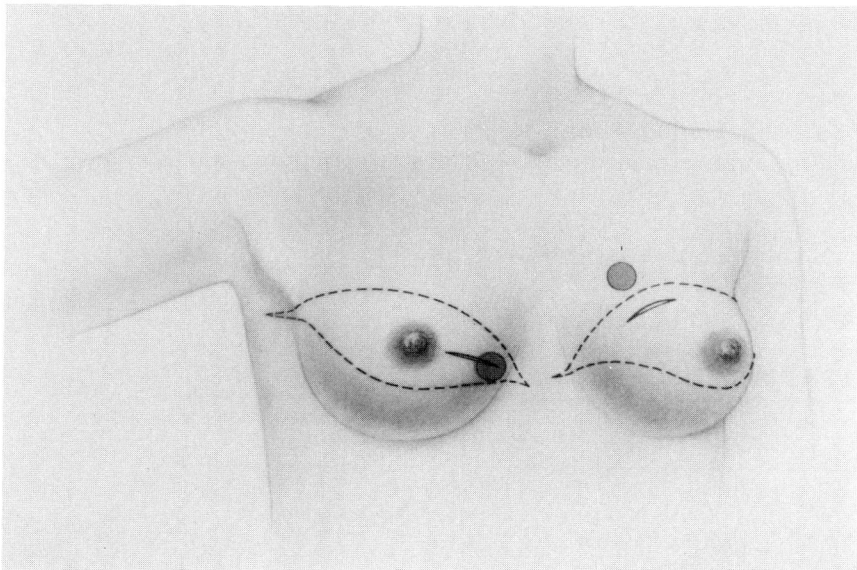

Figure 9–2. Illustration of the type of modest elliptical mastectomy incisions that can be achieved as a result of the appropriate incisions depicted in Figure 9–1. Notice that the skin sacrifice can be minimized and thus patients are suitable for immediate reconstruction with a more cosmetically satisfactory result. (From Cady, B.: Choice of operations for breast cancer: Conservative surgery versus radical procedures. *In* Bland, K. I. and Copeland, E. M. III (Eds.): The Breast: Comprehensive Management of Benign and Malignant Diseases. Philadelphia, W. B. Saunders Co., 1991, p. 763.)

performed through a horizontal elliptical incision without marked distortion and convolutions of the mastectomy flaps (Fig. 9–2). This requirement necessitates the more central placement of curvilinear incisions. The only exception to this use of circular incisions is in the extreme medial portion of the breast where a radial incision should be performed so that if a later mastectomy is required the usual horizontal elliptical incisions can be utilized with the medial corner of the elliptical incision not distorted if there is need for excision of the entire biopsy scar (Figs. 9–1 and 9–2). Since the decision regarding lumpectomy or mastectomy must await the final pathology report and subsequent discussion with the patient, it is imperative to use incisions that will lend themselves to either a cosmetically appropriate lumpectomy or mastectomy with the least sacrifice of skin to permit satisfactory reconstruction. Figures 9–3 and 9–4 represent inappropriate incision placement and the resulting problems with mastectomy incisions. Figures 9–5 and 9–6 illustrate the incision placement in mammogram-localized nonpalpable lesions. Excision of a palpable lesion with a 1 cm margin of normal tissue should be performed under local anaesthesia in an out-patient setting.

These lumpectomies should be performed without drains and preferably without external sutures after careful control of bleeding by electrocoagulation of small bleeders in the biopsy cavity wall. The actual excision of the breast mass should be done with a knife and not with cautery since generally

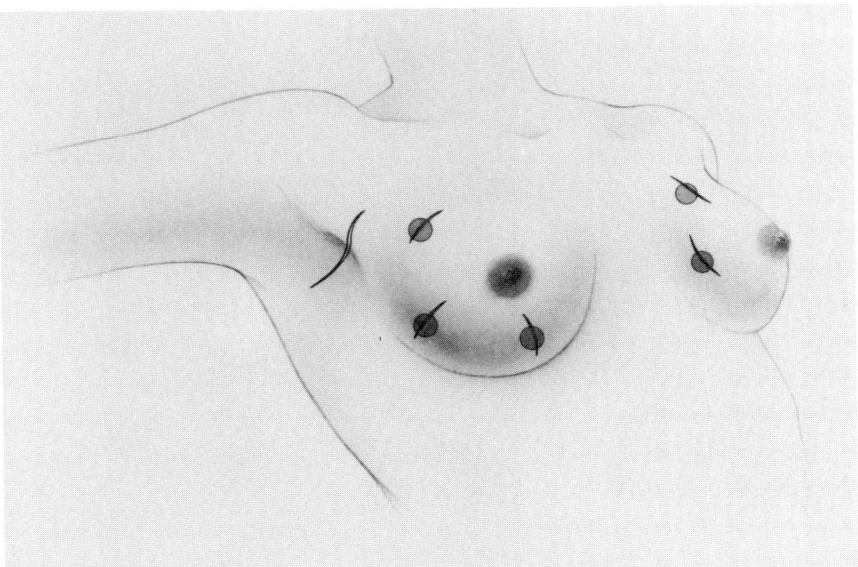

Figure 9–3. Inappropriate incisions utilized in the performance of lumpectomy. Langer's line incisions in the extreme medial part of the breast compromise later mastectomy incisions as do radial incisions at the extreme periphery of the breast. The performance of mastectomy, which sometimes is necessary or desired, may result in exaggerated incisions for the skin ellipse required after such inappropriate biopsy and lumpectomy incisions. In addition, an axillary dissection incision that runs anterior to the axillary fold imposes an unnecessary cosmetic penalty. Radial incisions almost always heal less well and are more unsightly than Langer's line circular incisions that are more centrally placed. (From Cady, B.: Choice of operations for breast cancer: Conservative surgery versus radical procedures. *In* Bland, K. I. and Copeland, E. M. III (Eds.): The Breast: Comprehensive Management of Benign and Malignant Diseases. Philadelphia, W. B. Saunders Co., 1991, p. 762.)

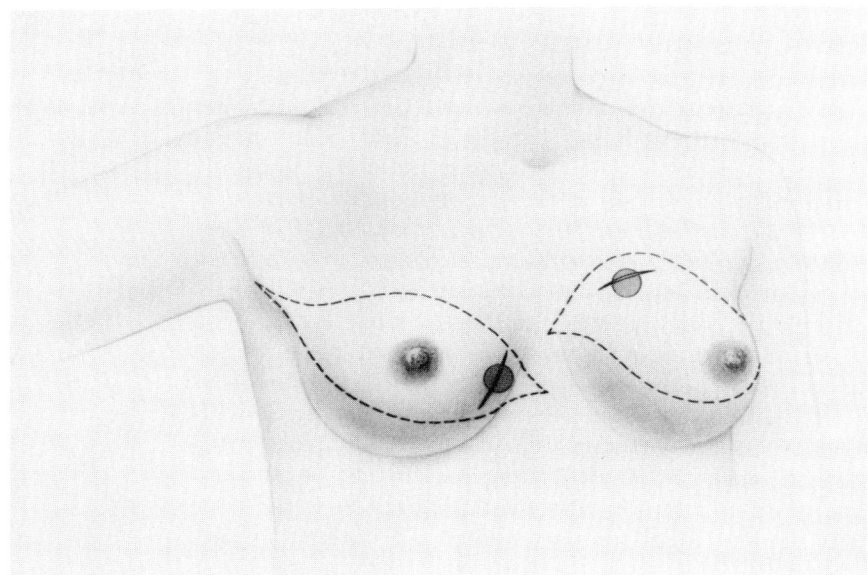

Figure 9–4. An example of the more exaggerated or distorted elliptical incisions that are required by inappropriate lumpectomy incisions as displayed previously in Figure 9–3. (From Cady, B.: Choice of operations for breast cancer: Conservative surgery versus radical procedures. *In* Bland, K. I. and Copeland, E. M. III (Eds.): The Breast: Comprehensive Management of Benign and Malignant Diseases. Philadelphia, W. B. Saunders Co., 1991, p. 763.)

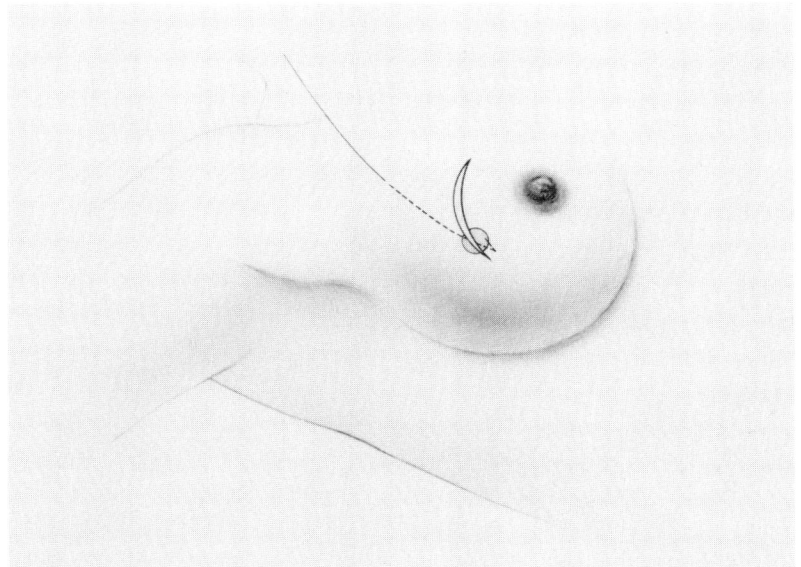

Figure 9–5. The more central curvilinear incisions previously illustrated are also utilized for mammographically detected breast lesions. Shown here is the Langer's line incision placed over the presumed location of the lesion in question. This may be at some distance from the skin entrance point of the localization wire mandated by the awkward positioning of the breast in the mammographic localizating machine. (From Cady, B.: Choice of operations for breast cancer: Conservative surgery versus radical procedures. *In* Bland, K. I. and Copeland, E. M. III (Eds.): The Breast: Comprehensive Management of Benign and Malignant Diseases. Philadelphia, W. B. Saunders Co., 1991, p. 764.)

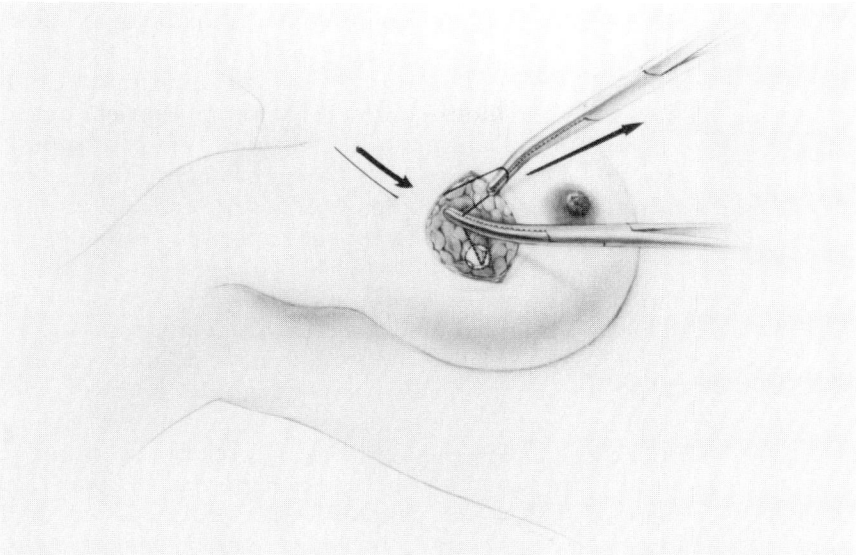

Figure 9–6. This illustrates that after the skin incision, the mammographic wire can be located either in the subcutaneous plane by elevating skin flaps if the incision is fairly close to the skin entrance site of the wire or deep in the breast on its path to the lesion for lesions at a distance from the skin entrance site of the localization wire. In either case the wire is brought into the wound at some distance from the presumed breast lesion. The wire can then be gently manipulated to help display its anchoring hook and thus guide the wide excision necessary for lumpectomy. (From Cady, B.: Choice of operations for breast cancer: Conservative surgery versus radical procedures. *In* Bland, K. I. and Copeland, E. M. III (Eds.): The Breast: Comprehensive Management of Benign and Malignant Diseases. Philadelphia, W. B. Saunders Co., 1991, p. 764.)

the estimation of estrogen receptor and progesterone receptor proteins may be altered by the use of electrocautery near a small invasive breast cancer. In all such palpable invasive breast cancers, frozen section should be obtained so that estrogen-receptor (ER) and progesterone-receptor (PR) tissue samples can be obtained promptly under pathologic control. Since these cancers are larger than the nonpalpable cancers discovered by mammography, it is important to obtain ER and PR for later aid in decisions about possible adjuvant therapy in contrast to the small, nonpalpable lesions.

Before the frozen section is obtained from the pathologist, the excised, palpable breast cancer should be carefully oriented and the margins inked for later accurate pathologic determination of margin adequacy. The most satisfactory current method of doing this is by using a variety of colored inks on the specimen, which not only mark the margin but orient the specimen for later interpretation by the pathologist under the microscope. Merely orienting the specimen by a stitch does not always translate to an accurate interpretation of which margin is positive later on after step sectioning of the tissue block and the subsequent loss of orientation.

A one-step biopsy frozen section and mastectomy should be avoided unless the patient is committed to a mastectomy beforehand after careful discussion with the surgeon. The appropriate sequence is to perform the breast biopsy and lumpectomy under local anaesthesia in an out-patient facility and then wait for a few days to a week for the final pathology report.

This report and discussion with the pathologist must be available before discussing the details of the pathology and the risk of local recurrence. Furthermore, estimations of cosmetic appearance can best be made several days after the lumpectomy. It is as inappropriate to subject all patients with invasive breast cancer to lumpectomy as it is to subject all such patients to mastectomy. Many patients have a preference for mastectomy and avoidance of radiation therapy because of lack of concern of the cosmetic appearance or difficulty in traveling for the radiation treatments.

Specific contraindications to lumpectomy as the surgical treatment of the primary breast cancer include a large cancer in a small breast whose removal would totally distort the residual breast, and patient preference for mastectomy. Relative contraindications to lumpectomy include the presence of extensive intraductal component (EIC positive), which indicates that the local recurrence rate might exceed 25 or 30 per cent. In addition, extremely young age (below the age of 35) is a relative contraindication to lumpectomy since such patients also have a high rate of local recurrence even if EIC negative.[35] In young patients who are EIC positive, the local recurrence rate exceeds 50 per cent.[35] In young patients who are EIC negative, the local recurrence rate is in the order of 20 to 25 per cent (Fig. 9–7). Other relative contraindications for conservative surgical management by lumpectomy of breast cancer would be the unavailability of radiation therapy facilities, the patient's lack of financial resources (since such treatments cost at least $6000 more than mastectomy), geographic distance from radiotherapy treatment facilities, and older age. The patient might be a poor candidate for the high-dosage radiation therapy, requiring daily transportation, or indeed may have little interest in preservation of the breast.

Since retention of the breast and feminine appearance and the acceptance of risk of local recurrence are all value judgments that are individual and personal, there are few absolutes in the decisions between lumpectomy and mastectomy. Patients should be counseled extensively and repeatedly if necessary to help them arrive at a personal decision about what to do. It is inappropriate for the surgeon to indicate which treatment is required in an authoritarian way since so many of the decisions involve value judgments

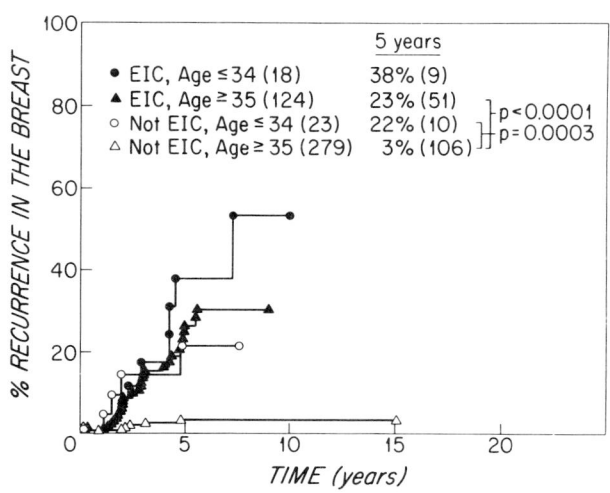

Figure 9–7. These data from the Harvard Joint Center for Radiation Therapy illustrate the principal factors in local recurrence after lumpectomy and radiation therapy. Notice that for patients older than 35 who do not have an Extensive Intraductal Component (EIC) to their tumor, the five-year actuarial recurrence rate is but 3 per cent. Notice also that for young patients with an extensive intraductal component, the recurrence rate at five years is 38 per cent and may increase still further. This information is crucial for discussing the various options with patients so that they can make a value judgment on breast retention.

that are specific to the patient. Patients, family members, and friends need to be guided and helped along the decision process; inappropriate decisions should be prevented by careful discussion and direction but a doctrinaire insistence on certain types of treatment is to be condemned.[42]

The crucial element in this decision process is the time, interest, and empathy of the surgeon, who must devote at least 30 to 60 minutes to discussion and explanation in the office. Occasionally, some patients will be unable to make a decision in such a personally important matter and may require more specific guidance or repeated instruction sessions. Since the primary breast cancer will have been removed totally by the lumpectomy, further decisions about conservative surgery versus mastectomy may occur when time is not of the essence. Patients should not feel pressured to make a decision within a restricted period of time once the invasive cancer is removed and periods of up to a month can easily be utilized by some patients to seek second opinions or consultations and to make a secure decision about which surgery to accept. While most patients make such decisions with anguish but in a reasonable time frame, others require considerable coaching and time. Thousands of women have lived satisfactorily after mastectomy and carried on with normal personal lives, so that the decision for mastectomy should in no way be considered an inferior approach to treatment of breast cancer.

If mastectomy is necessitated or selected by the patient, another discussion should be carried out and decision must be made about reconstruction. Most postmastectomy reconstruction can be performed while the patient is under anaesthesia for breast removal if the patient desires and appropriate plastic surgical talents are available.[43] Some general surgeons feel comfortable with insertion of a breast prosthesis, but by and large such reconstruction is performed by a plastic surgeon who can enter the operation at the conclusion of the mastectomy. The array of plastic surgical implants available for reconstruction of breast mound shape is large. Permanent implants and inflatable distendable implants of a variety of materials, either temporary or permanent, are all available. Immediate reconstruction at the same time as mastectomy in no way impairs healing, wound complication rates, or later survival or cancer detection. When the implants are performed in a subpectoral manner, local recurrences will be thrust forward above the surface of the implants and will not be buried. In this way, they are accessible for detection and diagnosis. Some patients may prefer or require pedicle flap reconstruction from the rectus abdominis or latissimus dorsi muscles, and these procedures can also be performed simultaneously with a mastectomy or at a later time.[44] The decision on whether to undergo reconstruction is a personal one based on value judgments by the patient; the surgeon should stand prepared to advise and guide but not command the decision process. If major doubts remain in the patient's mind about the value of reconstruction, it should be postponed and performed at a later time if she then desires it.

In our institution today, over one-half the patients who undergo mastectomy have immediate reconstruction; however, only a small fraction of those not having immediate reconstruction later elect to have a reconstruction. Most women who do not have reconstruction immediately after mastectomy find that they can live with the mastectomy perfectly satisfactorily and later do not want to be bothered with a further surgical procedure.

The resumption of breast configuration by contemporary implants and plastic surgical procedures is really quite satisfactory. While reconstructed breasts never achieve the appearance, "feel," and sensation of the normal breast, or even the breast after radiation therapy, they can be quite satisfactory and relieve the woman of the necessity of wearing an external implant and adjusting clothing styles.

Axillary lymph node metastases occur in at least 20 per cent of patients with palpable breast lesions larger than 1 cm in diameter and therefore axillary dissection should probably be a standard part of the surgical treatment of invasive palpable breast cancer. If a mastectomy is performed, of course, it will be part of that operation; however, if lumpectomy is chosen, the axillary dissection should be performed as a separate procedure through a horizontal low axillary incision that remains behind the anterior axillary border of the pectoralis major muscle for best cosmetic appearances (Figs. 9–1 and 9–3). Axillary "sampling" should generally be avoided as an axillary procedure since it is poorly defined and the number of lymph nodes obtained is not reliably sufficient to accurately separate node negative from node positive or extensive nodal involvement from minimal nodal involvement.[45] Adequate nodal dissection should preserve the long thoracic and thoracodorsal nerves, avoid skeletonizing the axillary vein, preserve the lateral pectoral nerve to the pectoral muscles, and utilize the anterior border of the latissimus dorsi muscle as the posterior extent. With these anatomic guidelines in mind, an average of 13 or more lymph nodes are obtained.[38] The resultant risk of arm edema, the major cosmetic penalty of such a procedure, is minimized but still occurs at a rate of approximately 15 per cent.[46] Despite this conservative axillary dissection, a few patients will have severe disabling arm edema and experience poor functional and cosmetic outcome as a result.[46]

Analysis of the lymph node specimen is important for understanding the patient's disease. While most pathology reports merely address the result in terms of positive or negative nodes, it is important for accurate understanding of prognosis, as well as contemporary staging, to understand whether axillary metastases are micrometastasis (less than 2 mm in diameter) or macrometastases, and exactly how many nodes are involved.[45] If such parameters are not described on the pathology report of the axillary dissection, the surgeon should insist that the pathologist accurately analyze the tissues and should go over the actual slides with the pathologist.

Because of the significant risk and expense of axillary dissection, if patients will not change the decisions regarding the administration of adjuvant therapy regardless of the lymph node pathology, axillary dissection should be avoided. Thus, if because of size, extensive lymphatic vessel involvement, or poor nuclear grade, patients will receive adjuvant therapy, which a negative axillary dissection will not alter, the dissection should be avoided. Furthermore, if the patient categorically refuses all types of adjuvant therapy because of the small size of the primary tumor or personal objections to the adjuvant treatment, there is little reason to do an axillary dissection other than to satisfy the requirements of contemporary staging. Since the axillary lymph node metastases are purely of prognostic and staging importance, and their removal is not a therapeutic procedure, the surgery needs to be carefully explained so that the patient can make a decision about the need for axillary dissection.

A small number of palpable but noninvasive breast cancers are still being discovered if the duct carcinoma in situ (DCIS) is large in extent. In Lagios' study,[14] the incidence of microinvasion in large DCIS is high and even node metastases may occur. Thus, mastectomy probably should be selected in larger (>5 cm) or multifocal or extensive DCIS. For a palpable DCIS between 2.5 and 5 cm in diameter excised in toto with negative surgical margins, lumpectomy with or without radiation therapy may be selected as appropriate treatment. In such patients, axillary dissection need not be done since there is no risk of axillary metastases. Even when such patients are found on complete analysis to have a focus of microinvasion, the risk of axillary metastasis is extremely low. Such patients need careful analysis of the pathology to look for microinvasion and complete classification. Such patients also have a higher than normal risk of a local recurrence because of the extensive nature of the DCIS; these patients are by definition EIC positive. If such patients have calcifications by mammography beyond the area of the primary DCIS, this should be assumed to be evidence of multifocal disease and mastectomy is recommended. Mammography performed after the apparent complete local excision of such larger DCIS lesions should indicate no further calcifications.

It is apparent from the previous discussions of both palpable and nonpalable invasive and noninvasive breast cancer that a myriad of treatment options exist at the present time. As a result, breast cancer management today is extraordinarily complex and requires thoughtful analysis of each case, careful discussion with the patient and the family about the various treatment options, the risks, and benefits of each course of action, and sensitivity and empathy with the patient's situation and the difficulty in selecting from the options available.

Variations in follow-up also exist that result from the treatment selections for the primary disease. If mastectomy is chosen, postoperative radiation therapy is seldom indicated. Evaluation of the mastectomy site and the dissected axilla need be undertaken no more than every six months for the first two years or so and then less frequently since further local curative therapy is not available. Adjuvant therapy may well be utilized in such patients based on primary cancer features and axillary node status. An important component of the follow-up of such patients is opposite breast mammography once a year until at least the age of 75.

Follow-up procedures for patients with lumpectomy with or without axillary dissection or radiation therapy need to be much more detailed. Since the risk of local recurrence in the breast is both real and highly curable, careful inspection of the breast should be made at three-month intervals for at least the first two years with inspection perhaps every six months thereafter until five years. Mammography of the affected breast should be performed every six months during the first two years and then at least yearly thereafter. Mammography of the opposite breast should be conducted once a year.

Physical examination of the treated breast is easier if radiation therapy has not been utilized because of the absence of skin thickening, edema, or shrinkage. Evidence of local recurrence needs to be determined. In any suspicious lesion in the area of the primary breast cancer, needle aspiration cytology should be obtained or, if necessary, a core cutting needle biopsy should be done. Open biopsy should be done whenever the situation is indeterminate and the needle biopsy is negative; however, it should not be utilized indiscriminately since repeated local open biopsies worsen the scarring, retraction, and disfigurement that may occur after radiation therapy. If suspicious calcifications reappear on follow-up mammography, localization mammogram and biopsy is performed in the usual manner.[47]

If local recurrence in the retained breast appears after lumpectomy, most patients will require mastectomy.[5, 9] However, if the recurrence is small, if it is in situ disease, or if it can be excised with clear margins, the breast can be retained in a significant proportion of cases. If the original excision was not accompanied by adjuvant breast radiation therapy, the re-excision of an invasive cancer recurrence should be accompanied by radiation therapy after obtaining negative surgical margins.

If mastectomy is required because of patient demand or the features of the local recurrent breast cancer in the retained breast, plastic surgical reconstruction should be considered. If the skin is badly damaged by the radiation therapy and elasticity is minimal, such reconstruction may be better with a flap reconstruction from the latissimus dorsi or rectus abdominis muscle. Subpectoral implant sometimes can be performed despite the thickened skin and radiation effect from the primary breast cancer treatment. Even if the latter is possible the eventual cosmetic appearance is less satisfactory because of the extra fibrosis and scarring that occurs after radiation therapy of the entire effected area.

ADVANCED LOCAL INVASIVE BREAST CANCER

Even today, a small proportion of patients enter treatment facilities because of advanced localized primary disease. This may occur in the form of a primary cancer larger than 5 cm in diameter or because of a diffuse involvement of the breast by extensive cancer with marked lymphatic invasion or inflammatory breast cancer. If a large primary breast cancer is unaccompanied by palpable axillary lymph nodes, it still may be suitable for treatment as described above in palpable breast cancer. However, in the majority of cases with advanced local disease, multidisciplinary management of the primary cancer is probably more appropriate.[48] Biopsy can be performed by core cutting needle or incisional biopsy. Primary chemotherapy and radiation therapy can frequently control local disease. Mastectomy in such patients can be reserved for those who develop progressive local disease as evidenced by increasing mass, skin involvement, ulceration, or other advanced local features that are progressive. The majority of such patients with advanced local disease will ultimately die of the breast cancer, and over half need no mastectomy because the local cancer is controlled by the combination of chemotherapy and radiation therapy. However, at any time in the disease course, if the primary breast cancer escapes control, with or without metastatic disease, mastectomy may be an appropriate procedure. This may require flap reconstruction with latissimus dorsi or rectus abdominis muscle because of extensive skin sacrifice from the advanced local disease. Axillary dissections are not required in such cases of advanced local disease since the clinical parameters of the primary cancer by themselves indicate the need for adjuvant chemotherapy and radiotherapy. The addition of axillary nodal tissue for further prognostication is usually not required and the simplicity of management can be improved by avoiding axillary dissection whenever suitable.

In recent years, the long-term outcome of patients with inflammatory breast cancer, diagnosed either clinically or because of dermal lymphatic tumor cells, has improved significantly. A large proportion of such patients will have a prolonged disease course, frequently with retention of the breast, after combined radiotherapy and chemotherapy. Long-term follow-up with careful analysis of the local breast control is required of such patients and repeated surgical input into their management is essential. Such patients seem to be decreasing in number and improving in initial presentation so that outcomes are more satisfactory. A small proportion even survive disease-free for periods beyond five years and the disease may be permanently controlled.

RADIATION THERAPY OF A RETAINED BREAST

Radiation therapy of a preserved breast should be regarded as an adjuvant to conservative surgical therapy. This statement is made to emphasize the surgeon's crucial role in the satisfactory cosmetic outcome of breast preservation and to emphasize that in the future many small breast cancers detected by mammography will be treated by local surgery only, without radiation therapy in any form. Patients who are being considered for breast preservation conservative surgery and adjuvant radiation therapy should be seen by the radiation therapist early during the decision process if possible. Frequent communication between radiotherapist and surgeon is helpful for the conduct of the initial treatment and is reassuring for the patient as well as the radiotherapist and surgeon.[49] A close working relationship with a radiotherapist is essential to achieve maximum cosmetic effect and local control.

There are two basic approaches to radiotherapy of the retained breast today. The NSABP program is whole breast radiation therapy to 5000 cGy without a boost.[2] The other program is whole breast radiation therapy of about 4500 cGy and then a boost to the local area to achieve over 6000 cGy in the local breast cancer site.[49] This latter approach is advocated by the Joint Center of Radiation Therapy at Harvard Medical School. While survival results are unchanged by variations in radiotherapy technique, it seems from the Joint Center studies that a local radiation dosage of over 6000 cGy is desirable to minimize a local recurrence.[49] Certainly, radiation therapy of the entire breast to 5500 or 6000 cGy produces poor cosmetic results. Therefore, the total breast dosage should be kept to a minimum and the local tissue dosage at the site of the primary breast cancer should probably be carried to the level of 6000 cGy.

It may well be in the future that radiation of the tumor bed in the local area of the cancer itself will be the preferred method. Total breast radiation to 4500 cGy or even 5000 cGy has little effect on the development of new primary breast cancers in other areas of the ipsilateral breast. Since radiation therapy is utilized to reduce local recurrence rate, it most logically should be directed to the primary site only. Such a program has been attempted and early results indicate little if any penalty in terms of local recurrence. It can be assumed, however, that the cosmetic result may be significantly improved.

Radiation therapy to the draining lymph nodes has been repeatedly demonstrated not to alter prognosis while adversely effecting the rate of edema of the arm. Therefore, all regional lymph node radiation should be avoided entirely in breast preservation conservative cancer management.

TAMOXIFEN

The anti-estrogen drug tamoxifen is utilized currently in high-risk node-positive postmenopausal women with estrogen-receptor or progesterone-receptor–positive tumors.[17, 18] It has been demonstrated to be a tumor suppressive agent that reduces recurrence and perhaps mortality by roughly 20 per cent. It is orally administered, easily tolerated, and virtually without major toxicities. Its use not only reduces the appearance of metastatic disease by 20 per cent or so but may also reduce local recurrence in the breast and the appearance of new opposite contralateral breast cancers. This latter feature, while not conclusively demonstrated, is highly suggested by control trials.

Whether anti-estrogen medication is useful as an adjuvant in premenopausal women with estrogen-receptor–positive tumors in addition to adjuvant chemotherapy is a matter of some controversy at the present time. Further clinical trials will be required to completely define that aspect of its use.

ADJUVANT CHEMOTHERAPY

Adjuvant chemotherapy should be used for premenopausal breast cancer patients with a poor prognosis.[17] Poor prognosis defined by positive axillary lymph nodes or prognostic features of the primary breast cancer itself should be utilized in decision-making for adjuvant chemotherapy since the toxicity and cost of adjuvant chemotherapy is significant. The standard chemotherapy at the present time is CMF (Cytoxin-methotrexate-5-fluorouracil) given in cycles for six months. A variety of other chemotherapeutic agents frequently including Adriamycin have been studied and evaluated, but the exact details of such other chemotherapeutic program benefits are not widely accepted or firmly established. Whether systemic chemotherapy in postmenopausal women has a role to play in addition to or instead of the tamoxifen is a matter of some controversy. Most studies show no benefit. In women who are postmenopausal under the age of 65 who have either estrogen-receptor–negative tumors that are node negative or have node metastases chemotherapy might be utilized on an individual basis.

REFERENCES

1. Veronesi, U.: Rationale and indications for limited surgery in breast cancer: Current data. World J. Surg. *11:*493–498, 1987.
2. Fisher, B., Redmond, C., Poisson, R., et al.: Eight-year results of a randomized clinical trial comparing total mastectomy and lumpectomy with or without irradiation in the treatment of breast cancer. N. Engl. J. Med. *320:*822–828, 1989.
3. Fisher, B., Redmond, C., Fisher, E.R., et al.: Ten-year results of a randomized clinical trial comparing radical mastectomy and total mastectomy with or without radiation. N. Engl. J. Med. *312:*674–681, 1985.
4. Lacour, J., Bucalossi, P., Cacares, E., et al.: Radical mastectomy versus radical mastectomy

plus internal mammary dissection: Five-year results of an international cooperative study. Cancer 37:206–214, 1976.
5. Spitalier, J.M., Gambarelli, J., Brandone, H., and Ayme, Y.: Breast-conserving surgery with radiation therapy for operable mammary carcinoma: A 25-year experience. World J. Surg. 10:1014–1020, 1986.
6. Greening, W.P., Montgomery, A.D.V., Gordon, A.B., and Gowing, N.C.F.: Quadrantic excision and axillary node dissection without radiation therapy: The long-term results of a selective policy in the treatment of stage I breast cancer. Eur. J. Surg. Oncol. 14:221–225, 1988.
7. Kurtz, J.M., Amalric, R., Brandone, H., et al.: Results of salvage surgery for mammary recurrence following breast-conserving therapy. Ann. Surg. 207:347–351, 1988.
8. Recht, A., Schnitt, S.J., Connolly, J.L., et al.: Prognosis following local or regional recurrence after conservative surgery and radiotherapy for early stage breast carcinoma. Int. J. Radiat. Oncol. Biol. Phys. 16:3–9, 1989.
9. Kurtz, J.M., Amalric, R., Brandone, H., et al.: Local recurrence after breast-conserving surgery and radiotherapy, frequency, time course, and prognosis. Cancer 63:1912–1917, 1989.
10. Findlay, P., Lippman, M., Danforth, D., et al.: A randomized trial comparing mastectomy to radiotherapy in the treatment of stage I–II breast cancer: A preliminary report. Proc. Am. Soc. Clin. Oncol. 5:246–263, 1986.
11. Sarrazin, D., Le, M., Rousees, J., et al.: Conservative treatment versus mastectomy in breast cancer tumors with macroscopic diameter of 20 millimeters or less. Cancer 53:1209–1213, 1984.
12. Cady, B.: Lymph node metastases: Indicators, but not governors, of survival. Arch. Surg. 119:1067–1072, 1984.
13. Ferguson, D.J., Sutton, H.G., and Dawson, P.J.: Late effects of adjuvant radiotherapy for breast cancer. Cancer 54:2319–2323, 1984.
14. Lagios, M.D., Margolin, F.R., Westdahl, P.R., and Rose, M.R.: Mammographically detected duct carcinoma in situ: Frequency of local recurrence following tylectomy and prognostic effect of nuclear grade on local recurrence. Cancer 63:618–624, 1989.
15. Holland, R., Veling, S.H.J., Mravunac, M., and Hendriks, J.H.C.L.: Histologic multifocality of T_{is}, T_{1-2} breast carcinomas. Implications for clinical trials of breast-conserving surgery. Cancer 56:979–990, 1985.
16. Mansi, J.L., Berger, U., McDonnell, T., et al.: The fate of bone marrow micrometastases in patients with primary breast cancer. J. Clin. Oncol. 7:445–449, 1989.
17. Henderson, I.C., and Mouridsen, H.: Effects of adjuvant tamoxifen and of cytotoxic therapy on mortality in early breast cancer, an overview of 61 randomized trials among 28,896 women. N. Engl. J. Med. 319:1681–1692, 1988.
18. Jordan, V.C. (Ed.): Estrogen/Antiestrogen Action and Breast Cancer Therapy. Madison, WI, University of Wisconsin Press, 1986.
19. Tabar, L., and Dean, P.B.: The control of breast cancer through mammography screening. What is the evidence? Radiol. Clin. North Am. 25:993–1004, 1987.
20. Haagensen, C.D., Lane, N., Lattes, R., and Bodian, C.: Lobular neoplasia (so-called lobular carcinoma in situ) of the breast. Cancer 42:737–769, 1978.
21. Haagenson, C.D., Bodian, C., and Haagenson, D. (Eds.): Lobular neoplasia (lobular carcinoma in situ). In Breast Carcinoma Risk and Detection. Philadelphia, W.B. Saunders, 1981, pp. 238–291.
22. Cady, B.: New diagnostic, staging, and therapeutic aspects of early breast cancer. Cancer 65:634–647, 1990.
23. Schnitt, S.J., Silen, W., Sadowsky, N.L., et al.: Current concepts, ductal carcinoma in situ (intraductal carcinoma) of the breast. N. Engl. J. Med. 318:898–902, 1988.
24. Shapiro, S.: Determining the efficacy of breast cancer screening. Cancer 63:1873–1880, 1989.
25. Cady, B.: Unpublished data, 1991.
26. Reger, V., Beito, G., and Jolly, P.C.: Factors affecting the incidence of lymph node metastases in small cancers of the breast. Am. J. Surg. 157:501–502, 1989.
27. Attiyeh, F.F., Jensen, M., Huvos, A.G., and Fracchia, A.: Axillary micrometastasis and macrometastasis in carcinoma of the breast. Surg. Gynecol. Obstet. 144:839–842, 1977.
28. Fisher, E.R., Swamidoss, S., Lee, C.H., et al.: Detection and significance of occult axillary node metastases in patients with invasive breast cancer. Cancer 42:2025–2031, 1978.
29. Baker, E.: Breast cancer detection demonstration project: Five-year summary report. Cancer 32:194–225, 1982.
30. Cady, B.: Choice of operations for breast cancer: Conservative surgery versus radical procedures. In Bland, K., and Copeland, E. (Eds.): The Breast: Comprehensive Management of Benign and Malignant Diseases. Philadelphia, W.B. Saunders, 1991, pp. 753–769.
31. Rose, M.A., Olivotto, I., Cady, B., and Koufman, C.: Conservative surgery and radiation

therapy for early breast cancer, long-term cosmetic results. Arch. Surg. *124:*153–156, 1989.
32. Lagios, M.D., Richards, V.E., Rose, M.R., and Yee, E.: Segmental mastectomy without radiotherapy, short-term follow-up. Cancer *52:*2173–2179, 1983.
33. Fisher, B.: Presentation. International Breast Cancer Symposium, Venice, Italy, June 1989.
34. Schnitt, S., Connolly, J., Recht, A., and Silver, B.: Breast relapses following primary radiation therapy for early breast cancer. II. Detection, pathologic features, and prognostic significance. Int. J. Radiat. Oncol. Biol. Phys. *11:*1277–1284, 1985.
35. Recht, A., Connolly, J.L., Schnitt, S.J., et al.: The effect of young age on tumor recurrence in the treated breast after conservative surgery and radiotherapy. Int. J. Radiat. Oncol. Biol. Phys. *14:*3–10, 1988.
36. Olivotto, I.A., Rose, M.A., Silver, B., et al.: Late cosmetic outcome after conservative surgery and radiotherapy for early I–II carcinoma of the breast treated with primary radiotherapy. Int. J. Radiat. Oncol. Biol. Phys. *12:*1575–1582, 1986.
37. Cady, B., and Stone, M.D.: Selection of breast-preservation therapy for primary invasive breast carcinoma. Surg. Clin. North Am. *70:*1047–1059, 1990.
38. Cady, B.: Changing clinical, pathologic, therapeutic, and survival patterns in differentiated thyroid carcinoma. Ann. Surg. *184:*541–553, 1976.
39. Van de Vijver, M.J., Peterse, J.L., Moot, W.J.H., et al.: Neu-protein overexpression in breast cancer, association with comedo-type ductal carcinoma in situ and limited prognostic value in stage II breast cancer. N. Engl. J. Med. *319:*1239–1282, 1988.
40. Clark, G.M., Dressler, L.G., Owens, M.A., et al.: Prediction of relapse or survival in patients with node-negative breast cancer by DNA flow cytometry. N. Engl. J. Med. *320:*627–632, 1989.
41. Beahrs, O.H., Henson, D.E., Hutter, R.V.P., and Myers, M.H. (Eds.): Manual for Staging of Cancer, 3rd ed. American Joint Committee on Cancer. Philadelphia, J.B. Lippincott, 1988, p. 147.
42. Wilson, R.G., Hart, A., and Dawes, P.J.D.K.: Mastectomy or conservation: The patient's choice. Br. Med. J. *297:*1167–1169, 1988.
43. Johnson, C.H., van Heerden, J.A., Donohue, J.H., et al.: Oncological aspects of immediate breast reconstruction following mastectomy for malignancy. Arch. Surg. *124:*819–824, 1989.
44. Bostwick, J., Paletta, C., and Hartrampf, C.R.: Conservative treatment of breast cancer, complications requiring reconstructive surgery. Ann. Surg. *203:*481–490, 1986.
45. Fisher, B., Bauer, M., Wickerham, L., et al.: Relation of number of positive axillary nodes to the prognosis of patients with primary breast cancer, an NSABP update. Cancer *52:*1551, 1983.
46. Miller, T.A.: Surgical approach to lymphedema of the arm after mastectomy. Am. J. Surg. *148:*150–156, 1984.
47. Solin, L.J., Fowble, B.L., Troupin, R.H., and Goodman, R.L.: Biopsy results of new calcifications in the postirradiated breast. Cancer *10:*1956–1961, 1989.
48. Sheldon, T., Hayes, D.R., Cady, B., and Parker, L.: Primary radiation therapy for locally advanced breast cancer. Cancer *60:*1291, 1987.
49. Recht, A., Connolly, J.L., Schnitt, S.J., et al.: Conservative surgery and radiation therapy for early breast cancer: Results, controversies, and unsolved problems. Semin. Oncol. *13:*434–449, 1986.

10

ENDOCRINE GLAND CANCERS

by Blake Cady, M.D.

ETIOLOGY, INCIDENCE, AND RISK GROUP DEFINITION

Thyroid cancer is divided into three major categories: differentiated, undifferentiated, and medullary. Medullary carcinoma actually occurs in the parafollicular C cells and therefore technically is not a cancer of thyroid follicular cells but arises in the thyroid anatomically. Medullary carcinoma makes up about 4 per cent of cases. Differentiated thyroid carcinoma in the United States today constitutes about 95 per cent of thyroid gland cancers. The undifferentiated giant cell and spindle cell or rare small cell forms have gradually decreased in incidence over the past 30 years so that they are no longer common and compose no more than 2 per cent of cases. Other malignancies such as thyroid lymphoma (uncommon) and squamous cell carcinoma (rare) also occur in the thyroid gland. The thyroid gland may also harbor metastatic disease particularly from renal cell carcinoma, melanoma, and lung cancer.

Thyroid carcinoma is an uncommon disease. There are approximately 1025 deaths per year from all forms of thyroid cancer in the United States and there are roughly 12,100 cases of thyroid cancer recorded statistically each year according to the American Cancer Society. In addition to the recorded cases, however, it is known that microscopic foci of papillary carcinoma of the thyroid are extremely common in routine autopsy studies and routine histologic inspection of thyroid glands removed for a variety of benign conditions. The incidence rates of these occult, clinically insignificant, microscopic papillary carcinoma foci in the thyroid gland range from 6 to 15 per cent in glands removed in the United States to over 30 per cent in glands seen in routine autopsy studies in some other parts of the world (Colombia and Japan).

The incidence of microscopic foci of papillary and other forms of thyroid cancer is somewhat a function of the number and spacing of pathologic sections taken through the thyroid gland at autopsy or surgical pathology gland inspection.[1] Indeed, many of the cases reported in tumor registries in the United States are actually incidentally discovered microscopic foci of papillary carcinoma of the thyroid in glands that are removed for other reasons but recorded as thyroid carcinoma. Thus, they are not truly clinical cancers at all. Even taking the lowest reported incidence of 6 per cent, there would be 15,000,000 such cases in the United States. This enormous incidence of occult microscopic disease, with relatively few registered cancers reported (12,100) and even fewer deaths (1025), has produced enormous controversy and confusion about the biology of thyroid cancer and the appropriate surgery for differentiated thyroid carcinoma.

Another aspect of differentiated thyroid carcinoma that has caused great misunderstanding and difficulty in interpreting data is the striking difference in outcome between clinical cancers in older patients and those in younger patients.[2-4] On the basis of age only, in no other human cancer is there such a marked difference in outcome with similar histologic appearance of lesions of the same organ. Thus, it is extremely uncommon (<2 per cent of cases) for men under the age of 40 and women under the age of 50 to die of this disease, whereas the death rate in selected older patients at high risk may be as high as 40 or 50 per cent. Recent reports by both the Mayo Clinic and the Lahey Clinic indicate that risk group separations can be made so efficiently that the death rate ratio between low-risk patients and high-risk patients is in the order of 1:23 to 1:26.[5,6] Since almost 90 per cent of patients fit into the low-risk category, it is apparent that the basic risk group definition of the individual patient is the crucial clinical and biologic feature that must be appreciated before embarking on therapeutic and surgical decisions in thyroid cancer. The most basic risk group consists of those separated by age, which distinguishes the two-thirds of patients who are women under 50 and men under 40 from older patients. This low-risk age separation may be expanded to include almost 90 per cent of patients by excluding younger patients with distant metastatic disease (chest x-ray) and including older patients with small (less than 5 cm) intrathyroid cancers that do not extend through the thyroid gland capsule to involve surrounding tissue.

CLINICAL PRESENTATION

The low-risk younger patients generally have a mass in the thyroid or a lymph node metastasis in the neck that may accompany either a palpable mass in the thyroid or a small or even microscopic primary site that is not palpable clinically. The later presentation occurs in about 25 per cent of children and young adults. With increasing public awareness and more detailed physical examination and diagnostic work-ups, the great majority of thyroid cancer patients today in both young and old age groups have primary cancers less than 2 cm in diameter. In older patients the clinical occurrence is almost always that of a mass in the thyroid itself, although in 10 per cent the lymph node metastasis may also be palpable and cause the clinical mass. Patients may occasionally speak with a hoarse voice resulting from involvement of the recurrent laryngeal nerve. Strident respiration may result from direct invasion of the tracheal wall, particularly in advanced undifferentiated cancers and lymphomas. Because of the small size of the cancers currently seen, symptoms generally are not part of the malignancy. When symptoms occur, they generally are of a mild discomfort or fullness in the neck area with mild dysphasia and the physical appearance of a mass in the lower neck. It is currently rare for patients with differentiated cancer of the thyroid to present with distant metastatic disease. When this does occur it is usually as a result of bone metastases from follicular carcinomas or lung metastases from papillary carcinomas. The histologic appearance of metastatic thyroid carcinoma is usually distinctive. Occult primary thyroid carcinoma does not need to be considered as a primary site of metastatic disease of unknown primary site unless the biopsy of the metastatic lesion is histologically typically that of thyroid.

EPIDEMIOLOGY

The epidemiology of thyroid carcinoma is not completely elucidated.[7-9] Follicular and undifferentiated cancers are proportionately more common in iodine-deficient geographic areas, whereas papillary carcinomas are more common in areas where there is ample dietary iodine. The overall incidence of thyroid cancer is also apparently increased in iodine-deficient areas. Until the 1950s, children were sometimes given radiation therapy because of enlarged thymus, adenoid, or tonsillar tissue or for acne treatment. In long-term follow-up a significant proportion of these patients develop thyroid nodules. Approximately 20 per cent of such thyroid nodules occur with an associated differentiated thyroid carcinoma (either the nodule itself or tissue adjacent to the nodule). There was an average delay of over 20 years between the childhood radiation therapy and the appearance of the clinical nodule. With the cessation of such radiation therapy in children, however, this association has ceased as a component of thyroid carcinoma etiology. It is important to recognize that in no study ever recorded has the clinical behavior of radiation-associated thyroid carcinoma been different from that of carcinomas not associated with radiation therapy.[10-13]

DIAGNOSTIC WORK-UP AND NEEDLE BIOPSY

The selection of patients for surgery of thyroid carcinoma is considerably more accurate now because of the widespread application of thyroid needle aspiration cytology.[14-16] Although thyroid function tests, radioactive iodine scans, and thyroid ultrasounds have traditionally been done for thyroid nodules, such expensive tests are not helpful in selecting patients at risk for cancer. The advent of needle aspiration cytology now provides fairly precise selection for surgery by displaying the cytology of the nodule. Needle aspiration of thyroid nodules is so safe, non-traumatic, non-painful, and inexpensive in making a specific recommendation for surgery, that a strong argument can be made for needle aspiration cytology as the first diagnostic study to be performed on thyroid nodules. Only in cases that reveal benign aspiration cytology should functional studies (TSH, T_3, T_4) or anatomic studies (scans, ultrasound) be done to provide more diagnostic information for nonoperative management.

Thyroid function tests have no role in surgical decisions because thyroid cancers are essentially never functional. Furthermore, patients with thyroid cancer have been shown to have a "cold" thyroid scan in no greater frequency than patients with benign adenomas or adenomatous nodules.

The largest pool of patients subjected to aspiration cytology and later operation for suspicion of thyroid carcinoma consists of patients with clinically solitary palpable nodules. However, multinodular glands in which one particular nodule or area may be harder, firmer, or less mobile may indicate carcinoma arising on the background of a multinodular gland. In previous decades almost as many thyroid carcinomas were found on the background of multinodular glands as solitary nodules. However, in more recent times, because of the gradual disappearance and control of multinodular goiters as a result of iodine replacement and thyroid suppression, the majority of thyroid cancers today are found in patients who initially have a solitary thyroid nodule.[17]

Needle aspiration biopsy technique can be performed either with a needle for aspirate cytology or with a large-gore–cutting needle biopsy. The latter, however, has a higher incidence of complications (bleeding), is a little more difficult to perform, and less tolerated by patients because of the size of the needle, the incision needed in the skin, and the occurrence of more frequent bleeding. The literature indicates that the accuracy, sensitivity, and specificity are as good with fine-needle cytology as they are with large-needle–cutting biopsies. Aspiration cytology with either a fine (#22) or a larger (#19 or #18) needle is thus the current standard for thyroid biopsy. Obviously a mass large enough to produce symptoms or cosmetic abnormalities has indication enough to warrant surgery, and needle aspiration is not necessarily useful for surgical selection but may provide useful preoperative diagnostic information when performed.

Most patients referred to surgeons for consideration of therapy have been referred by endocrinologists and internists who have performed a full thyroid work-up that includes function tests, thyroid scans, and thyroid ultrasounds despite their lack of help in surgical selection. If the patient first consults the surgeon, however, the most efficient way of handling the clinical problem is to initially do the thyroid needle biopsy. In time, the endocrinologist and internist will also appreciate the advantage of initial thyroid needle aspiration in evaluation of thyroid nodules for risk of cancer.

Thyroid needle aspiration usually (90 to 95 per cent) produces enough cellular material so that an experienced cytologist can make discriminations among colloid goiter, thyroiditis, a follicular lesion, and papillary carcinoma. Thyroid cytology should be reported in four categories: (1) malignant, essentially 100 per cent accurate; (2) suspicious, usually indicating a follicular lesion because microfollicular patterns cannot distinguish between follicular carcinoma, follicular adenoma, and adenomatous follicular nodule; (3) benign, which has less than a 1 per cent rate of a false-negative reading; and (4) insufficient material for diagnosis, which implies that a repeat needle biopsy should be done.

All suspicious microfollicular lesions or papillary lesions need to be operated on, since it is impossible to tell the difference between adenomatous nodules in a goiter, benign follicular adenoma, and follicular adenocarcinoma by cellular examination. As in other endocrine glands, the diagnosis of cancer is made on the abnormal location of cells rather than on their histologic appearance. In the thyroid gland, abnormally located follicular cells appear in the pseudocapsule of the thyroid tumor, in blood vessels, or in lymph nodes. Since accurate discrimination between the three types of follicular lesions cannot be made on cytology or histology, and follicular adenomas apparently are the antecedent to follicular adenocarcinomas, all such follicular lesions should be excised. Papillary carcinoma of the thyroid is usually diagnosed definitively by needle aspiration cytology. Less than 1 per cent of aspirate cytology read as benign will later be found to harbor carcinoma. In case of doubt, or if insufficient material is reported on the cytologic analysis, repeated aspirations of the thyroid gland can be easily performed.

The largest group of cases that can be spared surgical exploration of the thyroid gland are those with distinctive colloid and a macrofollicular pattern on the aspirate and those in which the clinical situation is such that the lesions are small enough as not to require surgery for cosmetic or symptomatic purposes. Approximately 30 to 50 per cent of patients who would have previously been subjected to exploration to rule out carcinoma currently can be spared the need for thyroid exploration by needle aspirate cytology. The thought that the majority of thyroid operations could be eliminated completely by thyroid cytology has not proved to be true, but nevertheless substantial reductions in numbers of thyroid operations for benign diseases can be achieved. For instance, less than 50 per cent of thyroid cysts can be eventually controlled by aspiration and thus not require operation. If a cyst recurs more than three times it should be removed. Furthermore, since papillary carcinomas can appear as cystic or mixed cystic solid lesions, aspirated material from thyroid cysts should be sent for cytologic analysis.

Thyroid needle aspiration cytology, like all other thyroid studies, is merely one test that helps the surgeon make a decision about the need for operation. Thyroid aspirate cytology can be most useful when it is utilized for separation of patients to be operated on from patients that do not require surgery. Any attempt to get precise diagnoses by aspirate cytology is misdirected because of the features about endocrine tumors described previously and is unrewarding and potentially harmful since 30 or 40 per cent of patients with suspicious but nondiagnostic cytology will have carcinoma.

PATHOLOGY

Differentiated thyroid carcinomas can be divided into pure follicular carcinomas and carcinomas that have papillary features of any extent.[18] Mixed papillary and follicular carcinomas may have greater or lesser proportions of follicular features. However, as long as papillary features are observed, they all behave in a similar biologic manner and have a similar prognosis. While there are differences in the clinical pattern of metastases and spread of follicular carcinomas in contrast to papillary and mixed papillary and follicular carcinomas, the most important prognostic feature for all differentiated cancers is the age of the patient and the extent of the primary cancer. Follicular carcinomas, when metastatic, tend to spread to the lung, liver, and bone, and uncommonly go to lymph nodes. Papillary carcinomas, in contrast, commonly metastasize to regional lymph nodes and occasionally metastasize to the lungs.[19, 20] Papillary carcinoma may be multifocal throughout the thyroid gland in a significant percentage of cases (±20 per cent), whereas follicular carcinoma is almost entirely unifocal. The multifocality of papillary carcinoma is usually microscopic but may occasionally be clinically palpable. When the thyroid gland is exposed at surgery, careful palpation of the opposite lobe may reveal separate nodules that warrant surgical removal. A palpably normal contralateral thyroid lobe at surgery is consistent with clinically insignificant changes, although the final pathology report may indicate areas of multiple microscopic papillary carcinoma outside the primary lesion in the ipsilateral gland. Such cases do not require further surgery.

The incidence of regional lymph node metastases from papillary carcinoma of the thyroid is very high (±75 per cent) when routine neck dissections are performed. In childhood papillary carcinoma of the thyroid, upward of 80 per cent of patients will have clinical lymph node metastases and these are usually multiple. In young adults, the incidence of lymph node metastases, when routine node dissections are performed, will be in the range of 40 to 60 per cent. In older patients with follicular carcinoma, the incidence of lymph node metastases is very low, and even papillary carcinoma has an incidence of lymph node metastases of less than 20 per cent in older patients.

Follicular adenocarcinoma is diagnosed by tumor cell invasion of the pseudocapsule or blood vessels by follicular cells. The most reliable separation between follicular cancers of very low risk and follicular cancers of high risk consists of an estimate of the extent of the tumor pseudocapsular involvement by follicular cells. With "minor" capsular involvement there is no alteration of the age-adjusted–survival curve from the normal population. However, in "major" capsular invasion or extrathyroidal involvement by follicular carcinoma, the mortality rate may be as high as 50 per cent or more. Almost 10 per cent of older patients have follicular carcinoma with major capsular involvement. In young patients, however, follicular carcinomas with major capsular involvement constitute less than 5 per cent of cases but contribute heavily to the number of deaths in young patients with differentiated thyroid carcinoma. The differential between "minor" and "major" pseudocapsular involvement by follicular cells is readily achieved by the experienced pathologist. Minor involvement includes scattered cells in a portion of the tumor pseudocapsule with occasional blood vessel invasion, while major involvement implies extensive breaching of the tumor pseudocapsule, extensive blood vessel involvement, or thyroid follicular cells outside the tumor pseudocapsule. Cases fall readily into these two categories.

OPERATIVE APPROACH

Patients should be selected to undergo surgery who show large, cosmetically unacceptable, symptomatic, or suspicious nodules on physical examination or who have nodules with suspicious or definitive histology indicated by thyroid needle aspiration cytology. Nodules that have any clinical suspicion by physical examination because of hardness, firmness, or fixation, or calcification by x-ray or other features should be resected regardless of the needle aspiration cytology report. Masses developing within glands diagnosed as Hashimoto's thyroiditis should be considered suspicious, since thyroid lymphoma and differentiated thyroid carcinoma seem to arise with a higher frequency in such a background. Patients with a background of childhood radiation who have a clinically palpable nodule should undergo operation, but whether such patients with only an abnormal scan should undergo operation is problematic.

The determined presence of lymph node metastases of papillary carcinoma, by clinical examination or proved by needle biopsy, obviously warrants surgery to resect the ipsilateral thyroid and the metastatic cervical lymph nodes. Open biopsy of any suspicious nodes is not necessary and should be avoided as a first step in obtaining histologic material.

Patients selected for thyroid surgery can be handled in an expeditious manner, since the operation is physiologically and anatomically not disturbing and the operative mortality is essentially zero. Operative morbidity is very low, particularly when conservative procedures are utilized for thyroid removal.[21-23] Because of the low risk of complications, patients with thyroid nodules can be selected for surgery in equivocal situations. Postoperatively, some patients can be discharged the following day, although most patients require a brief hospitalization. Narcotics for pain are necessary in only about 50 per cent of patients. Careful preoperative reassurance of patients about the low risk of the surgery and the rapidity of recovery helps greatly in their acceptance. Admission to the hospital the morning of surgery is a common practice today, since preoperative preparation is minimal in the usual case.

Position on the operative table is crucial for successful conduct of thyroid surgery. A blanket roll placed beneath the shoulders with the neck extended and the head thrust back and the patient in a semi-sitting position are most useful for wide exposure. The essentials of thyroid surgery involve adequate exposure, hemostasis, and protection of adjacent motor nerves and the parathyroid glands. Controversy arises about the need for dividing the strap muscles for exposure; however, high division of the strap muscles helps greatly in exposure and organization of the operative field. Retraction of the captured ends of the strap muscles, lateral retraction of the carotid artery, jugular vein, and sternocleidomastoid muscle, and medial retraction of the thyroid lobe with a triple hook clamp provide wide exposure and ease in dissecting crucial structures near the posterior surface of the thyroid gland capsule.

The basic operation should include a total lobectomy on the side of the primary nodular lesions, but less than total lobectomy is justified with removal of small lesions of the anterior thyroid or the isthmus. Careful palpation of the contralateral lobe during the conduct of the procedure is essential, and multifocal cancers require bilateral operations. When total thyroid lobectomy is performed, the entire course of the recurrent laryngeal nerve needs to be demonstrated up to the point at which it enters the cricothyroid membrane. While the dissection of the recurrent laryngeal nerve has traditionally been emphasized and still is crucial, the superior laryngeal nerve also needs to be identified and preserved for normal postoperative laryngeal function. The fibers of the superior laryngeal nerve intertwine the branches of the superior thyroid artery and occasionally loop laterally over the medial portion of the upper thyroid lobe. Therefore, extreme care must be taken in dissection of this area. In order to achieve this, the superior thyroid vessels should be identified and ligated separately directly on the surface of the upper thyroid.

The steps in dissecting a thyroid lobe are as follows: (1) Divide the strap muscles and expose the anterior surface of the thyroid gland. (2) Dissect free the middle thyroid vein laterally and, after its division, pull the sternocleidomastoid muscle, carotid artery, and jugular vein laterally with a retractor. Retract the thyroid lobe anteriorly and medially with the use of a triple hook placed into a portion of the normal thyroid lobe. (3) Identify and dissect free the recurrent laryngeal nerve, observing its course through the branches of the inferior thyroid artery and to its entrance into the larynx. (4) Divide the inferior attachments to the thyroid lobe, which include the inferior thyroid veins. (5) Divide the isthmus by dissection through the avascular plane between the isthmus and the trachea. (6) Separate the upper pole of the thyroid from the lateral larynx with careful observation of the superior laryngeal nerve and the branches of the superior thyroid artery and vein. (7) Identify the parathyroid glands on the posterior thyroid gland capsule and preserve them by dissecting them off the thyroid with the blood supply to the inferior thyroid artery remaining intact. (8) Finally, remove the thyroid lobe by careful dissection from the lateral portion of the trachea and the suspensory ligament of the thyroid with careful visualization and preservation of the parathyroid glands, recurrent laryngeal nerve, and superior laryngeal nerve. These various steps are more explicitly described and illustrated in other texts.

Lymph node dissections can be performed with an extension of the thyroid collar incision upward into the neck as far as the mastoid process if necessary. Lymph node metastases from thyroid adenocarcinoma should be resected with a functional neck dissection if they can be palpated prior to surgery. They should be dissected from the immediate thyroid bed only if they are not palpable preoperatively but are palpable within the thyroid operative field (limited dissection). Finally, if no lymph node metastases are clearly palpated either prior to surgery or intraoperatively, no formal node dissections need to be performed. When neck dissections are performed cosmetic and functional result should always be considered. Thyroid carcinoma, particularly papillary carcinoma, does not implant in operative wounds. Therefore, formal en bloc node dissections do not need to be performed. A modified dissection may or may not preserve the sternocleidomastoid muscle or jugular vein but should always preserve the spinal accessory nerve. Even "berry-picking" lymph node dissections are an acceptable procedure as long as adequate lymphatic tissue and the bulk of the palpable and obvious lymph node metastases can be removed.

It has been amply demonstrated that lymph node metastases in differentiated lymph node metastases have no impact on prognosis.[24-26] Thus, patients with the most frequent lymph node metastases are young and have the best prognosis, while patients who have the fewest lymph node metastases are older and have a generally more guarded prognosis. Since the bulk of the patients with lymph node metastases are young and otherwise healthy with a good prognosis, the removal of lymphatic tissue of the neck should primarily be governed by the cosmetic and functional outcome. Therefore, neck dissections need to be considered as an adjunct to surgery of the thyroid gland and therefore should be performed to prevent repeated episodes of recurrent nodal disease in the neck for convenience and patient satisfaction in follow-up. Bilateral lymph node dissections are seldom required and should always be performed in a conservative manner.

RESULTS OF THE TREATMENT

The greatest recent advance in selecting therapy for patients with differentiated thyroid carcinoma has been the development of reliable and easily reproducible risk group definitions by both the Mayo Clinic and the Lahey Clinic. Over 85 per cent of patients are in the low-risk category in both series and these patients have a death rate of less than 2 per cent. High-risk patients constitute slightly over 10 per cent of cases but carry a mortality rate of close to 50 per cent. The death rate ratio of the low-risk to high-risk cases is between 1:23 and 1:26, which indicates a strikingly successful risk group separation. These studies and other literature indicate that the group of patients at high risk of a poor outcome from thyroid carcinoma can be easily defined. Understanding the biology of the disease, although appreciating the extremely favorable outcome in low-risk patients, helps to advocate the type of surgery necessary and to select postoperative treatments and follow-up procedures.

In young patients in the low-risk group, follow-up does not need to involve the use of radioactive iodine, extensive laboratory tests, or complicated or intrusive procedures. Physical examination of the cervical lymph node areas and the thyroid bed or residual thyroid gland is performed every six months for the first two years and then yearly thereafter. Recurrent cervical lymph node metastases occur in less than 5 per cent of cases and should be removed either with a functional neck dissection or as an individual node as circumstances warrant. Recurrences in the thyroid gland or the thyroid bed should generally be resected. Pulmonary metastases are uncommon and, if encountered, will usually respond to a combination of thyroid hormone and radioactive iodine (RAI) therapy. Obviously therapeutic radioactive iodine can only be given in the absence of normal thyroid tissue because of its strong avidity for iodine. Metastatic disease is much less efficient in iodine metabolism and will take up radioactive iodine only after the more efficient normal thyroid is eliminated surgically or by RAI therapy.

High-risk patients need to be followed more closely and may justify the use of RAI diagnostic scans periodically to search for occult metastatic disease and attempt therapeutic use of RAI if metastatic disease is found. Recurrence in the thyroid bed or neck area may well justify another surgical approach for an attempted resection but more commonly can be treated by radioactive iodine or external radiation if RAI is not picked up by the thyroid carcinoma.[27] Distant metastases in bones, lung, liver, and other locations should be treated by RAI therapeutically if uptake can be achieved on diagnostic scans. Some metastatic disease is efficient at taking up RAI but unfortunately the majority of metastases do not concentrate RAI sufficiently to eliminate the metastatic disease in high-risk patients. Thus, despite the use of RAI, the vast majority (95 per cent) of high-risk and older patients with distant metastases from thyroid carcinoma will eventually die of disease in a time period that ranges over a few years but may occasionally extend to as long as 10 years.

In contrast, papillary (and mixed papillary and follicular) carcinoma of the thyroid, when metastatic to lungs, can be treated with a higher rate of success with RAI; such patients have a better than 50 per cent chance of disease-free long-term survival.

Standard adjuvant treatment after surgery for thyroid carcinoma is to utilize thyroid stimulating hormone (TSH) suppression by use of exogenous thyroid hormone administration. Despite this convention and the assumption that thyroid carcinoma is initiated on the background of a disturbed TSH-thyroid hormone feedback mechanism, it is difficult to prove that routine adjuvant use of TSH suppression by thyroid hormone administration actually increases the cure rate. However, patients who are not on adequate dosages of thyroid hormone and who have metastatic disease, particularly in the low-risk group, may have a dramatic regression of disease when TSH is thoroughly suppressed by thyroid hormone administration. Patients with poor prognostic features in the high-risk group, or with metastatic disease, must be maintained on TSH suppression after complete thyroid gland ablation.[28]

BIOLOGIC IMPLICATIONS FROM TREATMENT RESULTS

The biology of differentiated thyroid carcinoma remains puzzling. However, with good prognosis and bad prognosis risk groups largely determined by age, it can be inferred that differentiated thyroid carcinoma, while appearing the same histologically, constitutes at least two basic varieties of disease. Differentiated thyroid carcinoma that arises in young individuals and without involvement of tissues outside the thyroid gland behaves in a relatively innocuous manner and requires only conservative tissue-sparing and technology-sparing treatment approaches. Thyroid cancers that occur in older patients, that are large or invading outside the thyroid gland, or with major capsular invasion, may justify a more aggressive and technologically sophisticated approach because of its poor outcome.[29, 30] Such patients should have removal of most if not all the opposite thyroid lobe at the first operation for efficiency of the later use of radioactive iodine. The deliberate resection of adjacent organs involved such as esophagus, larynx, or trachea, however, should not be performed at the initial operation since the efficiency of radioactive iodine in eliminating these areas of extension should be tested and the clinical progress of the disease may be very slow. In low-risk patients, less than 15 per cent will ever die of disease. Thus, after discovering extension into adjacent vital organs, the initial thyroid resection should not sacrifice these tissues. Indeed, functioning laryngeal nerves that are surrounded by carcinoma can and should be dissected out and preserved if possible. If a laryngeal nerve is nonfunctional, it may be sacrificed as part of the initial surgical procedure.

When recurrent disease involves trachea, larynx, and esophagus, later radical resections may occasionally need to be performed if RAI or external radiation has failed. Long-term survival after such radical resection of recurrence is almost entirely confined to younger low-risk patients.

MEDULLARY CARCINOMA

Medullary carcinoma that arises in the parafollicular C cells that are incorporated within the thyroid gland embryologically, after arising in the laryngeal pouches (ultimo-branchial bodies), is a separate and distinctive carcinoma. Eighty per cent of medullary carcinomas are sporadic in origin and occur as a single focus in one lobe of the thyroid without C cell hyperplasia in the residual gland. Roughly 20 per cent of medullary carcinomas occur in genetically predisposed families, either with other endocrine abnormalities or with medullary carcinoma alone (Mea 1, 2H, 2B, or FMC). Such medullary cancers are multifocal, bilateral, and associated with diffuse C cell hyperplasia in the thyroid gland. The familial background of the patient undergoing operation for a thyroid nodule is usually not well known prior to thyroidectomy. Therefore, the standard operative approach to medullary carcinoma should be total thyroidectomy. Some medullary carcinomas discovered at surgery may later be found to be the initial case in a familial or genetic cluster.

Medullary carcinomas have a high propensity for lymph node metastases and thus ipsilateral lymph node dissection should be considered in all clinical cases. This lymph node resection should be a functional dissection since the outcome is the same as if a radical dissection were performed. The long-term prognosis is poor if lymph node metastases are present, although the disease course may be very prolonged.

With preoperative needle aspiration cytology most cases of medullary carcinoma of the thyroid should be diagnosed preoperatively by their unique cytologic findings. Medullary carcinoma diagnosed by cytology should have preoperative calcitonin determination and a detailed family history obtained. However, routine calcitonin values should not be done for all patients with thyroid nodules. The median age of sporadic medullary carcinoma is over 40, whereas the median age of familial carcinomas tends to be much younger with screening of families. Indeed, in defined familial and genetic clusters of medullary carcinoma, calcitonin screening can be utilized for early detection at the stage of C cell hyperplasia before the appearance of carcinoma. Such calcitonin-screened patients may be operated on under the age of 10 years with the expectation of 100 per cent survival. Because of the success of screening of family members and reduction of mortality, every patient with medullary carcinoma should have an extensive family history taken and family members should be screened for calcitonin. The sporadic or familial nature of the disease can be strongly suggested by details of pathology (multifocal; C cell hyperplasia) but calcitonin screening still may be crucial.

Medullary carcinoma of the thyroid has a prolonged clinical course and a significant number of patients still die of disease after 10, 15, or even 20 years of follow-up. While after initial surgery patients can be followed by calcitonin screening, the implications of an elevated calcitonin after complete local and regional surgery are not completely understood. If the initial thyroid resection for the medullary carcinoma was inadequate, or lymph node dissection was not performed, and the postoperative thyrocalcitonin is elevated, further surgery on the thyroid or lymph node areas should be conducted. However, if complete surgical removal of the thyroid, the tumor, and the lymph node metastases has been achieved and the thyrocalcitonin is elevated postoperatively, it is not justified to do localization studies and metastatic work-up since such patients may have prolonged disease-free periods and live out a normal life span. Accurate localization techniques are not known. Carcinoembryonic antigen (CEA) elevations are also utilized in evaluating medullary thyroid cancer patients, and CEA elevations have shown correlation with outcome of the disease.

ADRENAL GLAND

With the advent of computed tomography (CT) and magnetic resonance imaging (MRI), adrenal masses are being seen with increasing frequency. It has been shown that adrenal masses less than 3 cm in diameter infrequently are carcinomas, while a high percentage (25 per cent or more) of lesions over 6 cm in diameter are malignant. This applies whether or not the adrenal masses are functioning. Thus, decisions about surgical removal of incidentally discovered adrenal tumors seen on CT or MRI scans (usually done for other reasons) are based on size and any other features suggestive of malignancy. Lesions less than 3 cm in diameter should be observed with repeated studies for evidence of growth. If stable in size, such small adrenal "incidentalomas" can be observed at less frequent intervals after the six- and 12-month repeat studies, but progressive growth demands excision. Adrenal masses over 6 cm in diameter should be surgically removed. For adrenal masses between 3 and 6 cm in diameter, either course of action may be selected based on other clinical factors and patient desires.

Many adrenal carcinomas are functional, producing hypercorticism, masculinization, or signs and symptoms of pheochromocytoma such as hypertension and the like. Obviously, adrenal tumors that are functionally active require surgical removal regardless of size. This process of careful preoperative preparation is required in cases of pheochromocytoma to prevent catastrophic hypertensive crises. Currently, with adequate drug preparation, removal of pheochromocytoma is very safe. Adrenal tumors that produce hypercorticism need to be prepared preoperatively and maintained postoperatively with steroids since the opposite adrenal gland has undergone prolonged suppression. Recovery of endocrine function occurs slowly and on average requires about one year to achieve homeostasis.

The basic surgical approach to adrenal surgery is governed by the size and function of the lesion, evidence of involvement of adjacent organs, and the possibility of bilaterality and extra-adrenal sites, all well evaluated by preoperative MRI and CT scans. While the transabdominal approach has been more widely used in the past and is still necessary when assessment of adjacent structures is required, more limited lateral, thoracodorsal, or even a posterior approach may be undertaken for small adrenal tumors. The surgical approach to adrenal tumors must be meticulous, particularly with pheochromocytomas. Since dangerous exacerbations of hypertension may occur if the patient is not thoroughly prepared, anaesthetic management must be sophisticated, thorough, and experienced.

Pheochromocytomas should be handled minimally during resection, if possible, and the blood supply interrupted early in the course of dissection.

Only a small minority of pheochromocytomas are malignant and thus wide en bloc removal of these tumors is not required. Unfortunately cure is relatively infrequent in the full-blown malignant adrenocortical carcinomas, and while vigorous attempts should be made to remove all local structures initially, local recurrence and metastatic disease occur frequently.

REFERENCES

1. Carcangiu, M.L., Zampi, G., Pupi, A., et al.: Papillary carcinoma of the thyroid: A clinicopathologic study of 241 cases treated at the University of Florence, Italy. Cancer 55:805–827, 1985.

2. Buckwalter, J.A., Thomas, C.G., and Freeman, J.B.: Is childhood thyroid cancer a lethal disease? Ann. Surg. *181:*632–639, 1975.
3. LaQuaglia, M.P., Corbally, M.T., Heller, G., et al.: Recurrence and morbidity in differentiated thyroid carcinoma in children. Surgery *104:*1149–1156, 1988.
4. Ceccarelli, C., Pacini, F., Lippi, F., et al.: Thyroid cancer in children and adolescents. Surgery *104:*1143–1148, 1988.
5. Cady, B., Rossi, R., Silverman, M., and Wool, M.: Further evidence of the validity of risk group definition in differentiated thyroid carcinoma. Surgery *98:*1171–1178, 1985.
6. Cady, B., and Rossi, R.: An expanded view of risk-group definition in differentiated thyroid carcinoma. Surgery *104:*947–953, 1988.
7. Belfiore, A., LaRosa, G.L., Padova, A., et al.: The frequency of cold thyroid nodules and thyroid malignancies in patients from an iodine deficient area. Cancer *60:*3096–3102, 1987.
8. Sambade, M.C., Goncalves, V.S., Dias, M., and Sobrinho-Simoes, M.A.: High relative frequency of thyroid papillary carcinoma in northern Portugal. Cancer *51:*1754–1759, 1983.
9. Goodman, M.T., Yoshizawa, C.N., and Kolonel, L.N.: Descriptive epidemiology of thyroid cancer in Hawaii. Cancer *61:*1272–1281, 1988.
10. Spitalnik, P.F., and Straus, F.H.: Patterns of human thyroid parenchymal reaction following low-dose childhood irradiation. Cancer *41:*1098–1105, 1978.
11. Cerletty, J.M., Guansing, A.R., Engbring, N.H., et al.: Radiation-related thyroid carcinoma. Arch. Surg. *113:*1072–1076, 1978.
12. Fjalling, M., Tisell, L-E., Carlsson, S., et al.: Benign and malignant thyroid nodules after neck irradiation. Cancer *58:*1219–1224, 1986.
13. McHenry, C., Jarosz, H., Calandra, D., et al.: Thyroid neoplasia following radiation therapy for Hodgkin's lymphoma. Arch. Surg. *122:*684–686, 1987.
14. Komorowski, R.A., Deaconson, T.F., Vetsch, R., et al.: DNA content in radiation-associated thyroid cancer. Surgery *104:*992–996, 1988.
15. Hall, T.L., Layfield, L.J., Philippe, A., and Rosenthal, D.L.: Sources of diagnostic error in fine needle aspiration of the thyroid. Cancer *64:*718–725, 1989.
16. Grant, C.S., Hay, I.D., and Gough, I.R., et al.: Long-term follow-up of patients with benign thyroid fine-needle aspiration cytologic diagnosis. Surgery *106:*980–985, 1989.
17. Brooks, J.R., Stranes, H.F., Brooks, D.C., and Pilkey, J.N.: Surgical therapy for thyroid carcinoma: A review of 1249 solitary thyroid nodules. Surgery *104:*940–945, 1988.
18. Donohue, J.H., Goldfien, S.D., Miller, T.R., et al.: Do the prognoses of papillary and follicular thyroid carcinomas differ? Am. J. Surg. *148:*168–173, 1984.
19. Cady, B., Sedgwick, C.E., Meissner, W.A., et al.: Changing clinical, pathologic, therapeutic, and survival patterns in differentiated thyroid carcinoma. Am. Surg. *184:*541–553, 1976.
20. Noguchi, S., Noguchi, A., and Murakami, N.: Papillary carcinoma of the thyroid. I. Developing pattern of metastasis. Cancer *26:*1053–1060, 1970.
21. Foster, R.S.: Morbidity and mortality after thyroidectomy. Surg. Gynecol. Obstet. *146:*423–429, 1978.
22. Schroder, D.M., Chambors, A., and France, C.J.: Operative strategy for thyroid cancer. Is total thyroidectomy worth the price? Cancer *58:*2320–2328, 1986.
23. Grant, C., Hay, I.D., Gough, I.R., et al.: Local recurrence in papillary thyroid carcinoma: Is extent of surgical resection important? Surgery *104:*954–962, 1988.
24. Hay, I.D., Grant, C.S., Taylor, W.F., and McConaley, W.M.: Ipsilateral lobectomy versus bilateral lobar resection in papillary thyroid carcinoma: A retrospective analysis of surgical outcome using a novel prognostic scoring system. Surgery *102:*1088–1094, 1987.
25. Zimmerman, D., Hay, I.D., Gough, I.R., et al.: Papillary thyroid carcinoma in children and adults: Long-term follow-up of 1039 patients conservatively treated at one institution during three decades. Surgery *104:*1157–1166, 1988.
26. Hoie, J., Stenwig, A.E., and Brennhovd, I.O.: Surgery in papillary thyroid carcinoma: A review of 730 patients. J. Surg. Oncol. *37:*147–151, 1988.
27. Rossi, R.L., Cady, B., Silverman, M.L., et al.: Surgically incurable well-differentiated thyroid carcinoma. Prognostic factors and results of therapy. Arch. Surg. *123:*569–574, 1988.
28. Cady, B., Cohn, K., Rossi, R.L., et al.: The effect of thyroid hormone administration upon survival in patients with differentiated thyroid carcinoma. Surgery *94:*978–983, 1983.
29. Clark, O.: Total thyroidectomy: The treatment of choice for patients with differentiated thyroid cancer. Ann. Surg. *3:*366–370, 1982.
30. Harness, J.F., Fung, L., Thompson, N.W., et al.: Total thyroidectomy: Complications and technique. World J. Surg. *10:*781–786, 1986.

11

MELANOMA

by Blake Cady, M.D.

Malignant melanoma has elicited great anxiety and fear because of its appearance in young people, as well as its rapid growth, delayed metastases, wide dissemination, and sometimes bizarre and even grotesque patterns of metastatic disease. Before 1948 the vast majority of patients diagnosed with malignant melanoma died, and that lethal heritage has contributed to the reputation of melanoma as a malignancy with poor prognosis. Beginning in 1948,[1] when major public education campaigns began, there has been a steady improvement in the clinical manifestation with decreases in the maximum diameter and the measured thickness of melanoma. Currently, well over 50 per cent of melanomas are of a very early stage.[1] Extensive clinical investigational studies in the 1960s and 1970s defined the clinical varieties of melanoma[2,3] and their antecedent pigmented lesions,[4-8] which have lead to early recognition,[9-11] definition of high-risk groups, and even prevention. The overall cure rate of melanoma patients seen in the late 1980s is at least 75 per cent and the prognosis of early lesions approaches 100 per cent cure rate.

However, the frequency of melanoma is markedly increasing with rates throughout the world that are four to seven times what they were only two or three decades ago.[12-15] The steady upward path of the incidence slope shows no signs of abating. In Queensland, Australia at least 1 per cent of the population develops melanoma by the age of 80.[14] This subtropical area of high-intensity sunlight into which a northern European Scotch-Irish population has moved probably represents the highest population susceptibility for melanoma. This area serves as a model for future concerns and clinical aspects of melanoma.[16] The Queensland melanoma project and other Australian melanoma studies have defined many of the epidemiologic aspects of melanoma as we currently understand them.[12,14]

ETIOLOGY AND EPIDEMIOLOGY

Melanoma incidence is related to sun exposure in susceptible populations.[12,14,16] The particular aspects of the solar spectrum are unclear but include visible, ultraviolet, and near infrared wavelengths. Thus, fair-skinned, blonde-haired, blue-eyed, and particularly red-haired people who are sunlight sensitive and tend to burn without tanning are at highest risk from sun exposure. In contrast, black-skinned populations of the equatorial areas do not develop melanoma of the pigmented skin, although melanoma is common in nonpigmented cutaneous areas and mucosal surfaces.[17] The movement of white populations into more sunlight-exposed areas such as the southwestern United States, northern Australia, and other subtropical areas, as well as vacation patterns that produce frequent exposure to high-intensity sunlight accompanied by marked changes in clothing style that expose a larger skin surface are the apparent reasons for the marked increase in melanoma incidence. It may well be that sunlight exposure in the early years of childhood is the most significant period of risk from ultraviolet tissue damage just as other developing organs (thyroid, breast) are more susceptible to etiologic agents such as radiation.[14] Particular patterns of exposure may also be important with intermittent more hazardous than continuous exposure and episodes of blistering sunburns more dangerous than more moderate exposures. In Africa, albinos have an extraordinary high rate of cutaneous cancer and indicate that the genetic background of the black races is not protective but that skin coloration from melanin disposition is. There is no indication that changes in the earth's protective ozone layer has anything to do with current melanoma incidence changes. There is every reason, however, to implicate changing clothing and vacation styles, and emigration patterns that reverse Darwinian selection processes that produced fair skin in regions of low-intensity sunlight for effective vitamin D production.[12–14, 16]

There is both a direct and indirect effect of sunlight exposure on the incidence of melanoma. Lentigo malignant melanoma occurs only on chronically sunlight-exposed areas, usually of the face, back of hands, and lower legs in women. Over 90 per cent of melanomas of the lower leg occur in women, presumably on the basis of the sun exposure below skirts. The majority of trunk, particularly back, melanomas occur in men, particularly in those who have outdoor occupations or recreations. On the other hand, superficial spreading melanoma occurs in sunlight-sensitive people usually in exposed areas but also in non-sunlight–exposed areas such as the breasts in women, the buttocks and feet in men and women, and the legs in men.

Genetics may play a role in the incidence of melanoma as families of melanoma patients carry a substantially increased risk usually on the basis of similar sunlight sensitivity but also from specific melanoma genetic inheritance in the dysplastic nevus syndromes.[6, 18] Even patients from races that include darker natural skin without sunlight sensitivity may be at increased risk if they have red-haired relatives.

PATHOLOGY

The principal achievement in prognostication and pathology in melanomas over the past several decades has been the determination of accurate measurements of thickness that directly correlate with prognosis. The original Clark level system[2] that evaluated thickness as a function of anatomic invasion of various skin layers has proved to be less accurate because of variations in skin thickness in different parts of the body. The measured micrometer thickness of melanoma, a technique described by Breslow,[3] can be performed with great accuracy by trained pathologists. The continuum of Breslow measurements and resulting prognosis seems to have "break points" that separate different general prognostic groups. Thus, patients with very thin melanomas have an extraordinarily favorable prognosis with a 99 per cent survival if the melanomas are less than 0.76 mm (or in some reports 0.85 mm) in thickness.[19] Thickness of 1.69 mm separates a good prognostic group (90 per cent survival) from a moderate prognostic group between 1.70 mm and 3.64 mm in thickness in which survival approximates 67 per cent overall.[20] Melanomas over 3.65 mm in thickness have a poor prognosis with survival expectations of about 35 per cent. Thus, accurate pathologic micrometer measurements of melanoma thickness are crucial in prognostication. However, although there is controversy about the exact "break points" in the thickness relationship to prognosis, there is an overall linear relationship between measured depth and curability for all melanoma types.

The millimeter thickness measurements clearly depend on an accurate vertical cut through the melanoma by the pathologist. Biopsies or pathologic sections that are cut obliquely may adversely affect the melanoma thickness measurement. Furthermore, a thickness measurement of other than the most prominent nodular portion of a melanoma may give unreasonably optimistic suggestions about prognosis. Accurate thickness measurements of ulcerated melanomas or some auto-regressed lesions are not possible and may account for the relatively poor prognosis of ulcerated lesions and some thinner lesions displaying significant areas of auto-regression. A wide variety of other histologic features of melanoma have been analyzed for correlations with prognosis. Currently, there are no histologic features that are universally accepted or analyzed that can be reliably utilized to more accurately prognosticate above and beyond the thickness measurements.[21] However, absence of inflammation, infiltration, and extreme undifferentiation, lack of pigment, poor nuclear grade, high mitotic rate, and presence of auto-regression with depigmentation all suggest a somewhat less favorable prognosis.[21]

Occasionally, specific histochemical stains must be utilized to accurately diagnose and separate melanoma from other very poorly differentiated malignant lesions. These sophisticated pathologic techniques should be resorted to whenever questions arise about the nature of the cutaneous primary lesion or lymph node metastases, or distant metastases with an unknown primary.

CLINICAL PRESENTATION

Melanomas occur in four distinctive clinical types, in each of which the thickness measurement is pertinent for prognostication.[1] The most common type is superficial spreading melanoma, which has a prolonged horizontal superficial growth phase that lasts up to many years before a vertical growth phase becomes demonstrable clinically by the appearance of a nodule. The physical characteristics of superficial spreading melanoma are variations of height, outline, and color. Superficial spreading melanomas are characterized clinically by red, white, and blue coloration. Red indicates an inflammatory reaction. Blue results from the Tyndall effect of deeper-lying pigment in which reflected light other than blue is filtered out so that blue wavelengths predominate in the visual appearance. White or grayish areas represent auto-regression of pigment-laden melanoma cells and absence of melanin. The variation in height represents the nodular vertical growth phase while the variation in outline represents the pattern of early irregular horizontal lateral growth that frequently leaves a "coast of Maine" appearance of variable pigmentation. Lesions may have the appearance of a miniature coral atoll with a depigmented "lagoon" and the advancing front of horizontally spreading pigment representing the island. As melanomas are detected earlier in their clinical evolution these clinical recognition features have become more subtle.

The median duration of time from the appearance of a pigmented lesion and the diagnosis of superficial spreading melanoma has been reported to be as long as six years. Thus, public and professional education campaigns for early recognition should be emphasized; these lesions can be detected at a very early phase in their clinical evolution in the overwhelming majority of cases by patients and careful nonprofessional observers. Visual educational material is extremely successful in teaching these clinical hallmarks of recognition, and the clinical diagnosis is highly accurate (95 per cent or better).

The second most common clinical manifestation of melanoma is the nodular variant. These lesions occur with a vertical growth phase from inception and have a much shorter growth period without all of the usual clinical hallmarks of early recognition. The colors of nodular melanomas tend toward black, dark brown, and purple, and there is little or no evidence of a preliminary horizontal growth phase surrounding the nodule. These nodules tend to be traumatized because of their vertical nodular pattern and may bleed and ulcerate early in their clinical evolution. Because of their pure vertical growth pattern nodular melanomas tend to have a worse prognosis overall, particularly when ulcerated, since the thickness measurement may not represent a full vertical dimension of the previous intact melanoma. However, thickness for thickness, the prognosis of nodular malignant melanoma is the same as that of superficial spreading melanoma.

Lentigo maligna melanomas occur only on chronically sunlight-exposed areas such as ears, face, backs of hands, and, occasionally, lower legs of women. The median age of patients diagnosed with lentigo maligna melanoma is approximately 70 years,[1] 20 years older than the median age of patients with superficial spreading or nodular melanoma. Furthermore, the median duration of a pigmented lesion prior to the clinical development of melanoma also ranges up to 20 years. Lentigo maligna melanoma arises from a flat brown or tan lesion (Hutchinson freckle or lentigo maligna), which is the very slowly evolving horizontal growth phase of in situ melanoma. Lentigo maligna melanomas are superficial and have a late onset of the vertical growth phase. They are treated earlier in their clinical progression to vertical growth usually because of the prominent location and larger size that promotes concern. Overall prognosis in lentigo maligna melanoma is far better because of the late development of vertical growth. However, level for level, the prognosis in lentigo maligna melanoma is the same as for superficial spreading or nodular melanoma. The color of lentigo maligna melanoma tends toward light tan, brown, white, and gray, but darker areas occur also. Lentigo maligna melanomas frequently require plastic surgical techniques for coverage and reconstruction to avoid unsightly scars in prominently visible areas of the face.

Acral lentiginous melanomas arise in the subungual, mucosal membrane, plantar, and palmar areas.[22, 23] They have a distinctive pathologic appearance and a slightly worse overall prognosis because of the delayed diagnosis and thicker occurrence. Although dark brown, purple, and black pigmentation tends to be prominent, acral lentiginous melanomas occasionally will have depigmented areas or be amelanotic.

Malignant melanomas also occur on the mucosal surfaces of the upper aerodigestive tract, conjunctiva, vagina, and anal areas.[24, 25] Junctional nevi in the upper aerodigestive tract mucosa of dark-skinned races seem to predispose to mucosal melanomas. In Nigeria, mucosal lesions are the most common presentation of melanoma, and palmar and particularly plantar melanomas are the common occurrence in blacks.

The evolution of pigmented nevi to malignant melanoma is not clearly defined and obviously occurs rarely because of the enormous numbers of nevi and the relatively few melanomas. Probably less than one in 100,000 pigmented nevi ever develops into a melanoma. However, pigmented nevi of increased risk can be well defined: congenital hairy nevi, nevi present at birth or nevi that arise in the prepubertal years in children, and dysplastic nevi. Most nevi occur after puberty and increase in number during the early adult years. Thereafter they decrease in number and disappear by a process of auto-regression, so that by late adulthood there may be only half as many nevi present than at the age of 21. The particularly well-defined clinical and pathologic entity of dysplastic nevi is a precursor lesion for malignant melanoma.[5, 6, 8] Dysplastic nevi are seen at the periphery of many melanomas, and in other skin areas of patients with melanoma. They also occur in family members of genetic syndromes of malignant melanoma and dysplastic nevi. In addition, individual dysplastic nevi have been shown to evolve into malignant melanoma in patients under close observation with photodocumentation. Thus dysplastic nevi are not only precursor lesions but a marker for increased susceptibility to melanoma. Patients and family members with dysplastic nevi have a higher incidence of the development of malignant melanoma. Dysplastic nevi are characterized clinically by diameter greater than 1 cm, irregular patterns of color and border outline with pigment "streaming" into surrounding skin, and colors that are light tan to brown. They frequently occur in patients with a total nevus count of over 25 and with nevi in unusual locations such as buttocks, breasts, and lower abdomen.

The clinical and histologic differential diagnosis of melanoma includes not only active junctional nevi, dysplastic nevi, and pigmented basal cell carcinoma, but also spindle cell or Spitz nevi.[26] These latter lesions were sometimes called "juvenile melanomas," a serious misnomer since such lesions occur in adults as well as children and are not malignant. Spindle cell nevi may represent difficult diagnostic problems for the pathologist as histologically they may closely resemble melanoma. To the clinician, spindle cell nevi tend to be less of a concern since they are lighter and uniform in color, regular in outline, and are of uniform height. They have no history of change in appearance in parameters such as size, outline, or color. Thus, any lesion that is reported by a pathologist to be a melanoma, which clinically did not seem suspicious, should elicit a request for slide consultation and consideration of spindle cell nevi or other lesions.

Other differential diagnostic problems arise with pigmented basal cell carcinomas, which frequently have the array of colors and irregular borders seen with superficial spreading melanomas. Cellular blue nevi have no growth or change, uniform outline and height, and color that is uniformly deep blue to purple. Careful history will reveal that the lesion has been present and unchanged for many years.

BIOLOGY

Each clinical variety of melanoma has a unique biologic behavior pattern with significant periods of in situ or thin superficial horizontal growth (except nodular varieties) without significant risk of dissemination followed by a later vertical growth in a nodule in one area that progressively increases the risk of cell dissemination and distant metastases as the thickness increases. Melanomas spread systemically by both lymphatic and hematogenous routes since many patients with negative lymph nodes will have distant metastases; survival free of distant metastases occurs in a significant proportion of patients with positive regional lymph nodes.[27] In a proportion of patients with lymph stasis after prophylactic regional node dissection, "satellitosis" or growth of melanoma cells in subdermal lymphatics develops, which confirms the lymphatic dissemination of melanoma. Melanoma cells thus reside in some situations without progressive growth for long periods of time, even many years, in organs and such subdermal sites. "Satellitosis" and regional subdermal nodular growth has been reported many years and even decades after the primary melanoma source of the malignant cells has been excised. When melanoma metastasizes distantly, the most common organs involved are lungs, liver, bone, brain, distant nonregional lymph nodes, and skin and subcutaneous tissues. However, widely disseminated malignant melanoma may involve any organ in the body; cardiac and splenic metastases, virtually unheard of in other human cancers, are not uncommon.

There is a suggestion that a very delayed appearance of metastases may occur in clinically early, thin primary melanomas.[19] Thus, longer periods of follow-up may be required to fully evaluate the curability of thinner melanomas. Even in thicker melanomas, there are significant decreases in apparent cure between 5 and 10 years and after 10 years from original therapy.

DIAGNOSTIC WORK-UP

Since melanomas for the most part today are diagnosed at an early stage, palpable regional lymph nodes are relatively uncommon, and systemic metastases at presentation are rare. Thus, extensive diagnostic searches for metastatic disease are unwarranted in the usual presence of melanoma. Even if asymptomatic distant metastases were found, no curative therapies are available and the local melanoma resection is still required to be performed for palliation and local control. Since currently radical local surgery is not widely practiced in the treatment of primary melanoma, and regional prophylactic node dissections are not usually performed, there seems little justification in embarking on an extensive diagnostic search for asymptomatic metastatic disease prior to local therapy. Thus, bone scans, liver scans, and extensive searches by the use of computed tomography (CT) or magnetic resonance imaging (MRI) are unjustified. Routine blood tests and a chest x-ray are all that is necessary prior to melanoma excision. Obviously, symptoms suggestive of metastases, such as headache or abnormal liver function tests, should lead to a directed search for dissemination. Cases in which regional node metastases occur, particularly if multiple nodes are involved, should be considered for extensive diagnostic work-up; however, even in these cases it is not mandatory.

ISSUES IN MELANOMA MANAGEMENT

The two major current issues in the surgical management of malignant melanoma regard the extent of local resection and the timing and extent of lymphatic resection for lymph node metastases.

Local Resection

The original recommendation for melanoma resection margins was based on a single lesion observed in one patient seen in the early 1900s. Furthermore, that lesion was a metastatic nodule in a cutaneous location and not even a primary melanoma! The suggestions from that report that recommend a 5 cm local tissue margin were continued through the surgical literature for decades without question. This arbitrary 5 cm margin for soft tissue sacrifice around melanomas has been completely modified in the last decade; smaller resection margins are deemed appropriate for the excision of the usual cutaneous malignant melanoma. Arbitrary 3 cm margins, or at least two lesional diameters[1] (considering the horizontal measurement of melanoma) to the nearest excision margin are both advocated as the basis for the extent of local excision of skin and subcutaneous fat. These result in irreducible rates of local recurrence. It is apparent from studies by Breslow[28] that even narrower margins (1 cm) are acceptable for melanomas less than 0.76 mm in thickness, since they essentially never recur locally. A recent European randomized prospective trial found no local recurrence difference comparing 1 cm and 3 cm resection margins for melanomas 1 mm or less in thickness.[20] However, for thicker melanomas margins of 2 cm, 3 cm, or 4 cm, or variable margins based on measured diameter of the melanoma, all seem to give equivalent and extremely low risk of local recurrence (less than 3 per cent).[1] An ongoing prospective randomized clinical trial comparing 2 cm and 4 cm margins is currently being conducted in the United States in a multi-institutional setting and should provide a further definitive answer to this particular choice regarding adequacy of local excision margins in thicker melanomas.

It has become apparent in a recent report[1] that a local recurrence does not by itself impair survival but is related to, or is a reflection of, poor outcome because of basic prognostic factors of the primary melanoma. Thus, compromising local margins, which is frequently necessary when melanomas are located on cosmetically prominent or functionally significant areas such as the face, ears, or hands, is acceptable provided these patients are observed carefully in postoperative follow-up and local recurrences promptly excised if they occur. Local recurrence rates of 15 per cent or more are recorded when margins are inadequate. However, when margins are adequate, local recurrence does not exceed 2 or 3 per cent and is not further reduced by more extensive or radical local surgery.[30]

Closure

The ability to close melanoma excision sites primarily or with local rotation flaps in contrast to coverage with split thickness skin grafts has been the major step in simplifying and reducing the scope of surgical treatment of melanoma. It is also the primary advantage of utilizing more limited local resections. There is no evidence that the covering of a melanoma excision site primarily or with local rotation flaps in any way reduces the survival or increases the local recurrence rate compared with skin graft application when similar excision margins are compared.[1]

Another issue in local treatment is the value of excising the superficial muscular fascia beneath the melanoma. Although until recently such removal was dogma in melanoma excisions, this has been shown to provide no added advantage and is no longer considered necessary in melanoma excision. The concept of surgical "block" excision of melanomas, however, remains valuable despite the reduced scope of the tissue sacrifice. The surgical resection should encompass adequate skin and subcutaneous tissue down to (or including) the muscular fascia so that a block of tissue is removed with vertical sides to ensure that adequate margins are obtained not only of the skin but also of the subcutaneous tissue. Removal of superficial muscular fascia while not necessary may be performed to ensure that the block excision concept is carried out and to improve the adherence of skin grafts or local skin flaps that may heal more readily to muscle than fascia.

Only a few places on the body require compromised margins routinely (ears, face, nose) or the routine use of skin grafts (lower leg, hands, feet).

Lymph Node Dissection

The other major therapeutic controversy in melanoma continues to revolve around the need for "prophylactic" lymph node dissection of regional draining nodal basins in the absence of palpable enlargement. Proponents of prophylactic nodal dissections cite markedly increased incidences of disease-free survival in retrospective studies, whereas opponents of prophylactic dissection cite the biologic and clinical studies that suggest that lymph node metastases are "indicators but not governors" of survival[27] and the failure to show better survival results in prospective randomized trials[29] comparing routine node dissection versus observation and later therapeutic dissection. In breast and other cancers it is apparent that regional lymph node treatment does not alter prognosis.[27] This latter assumption, of course, presupposes a similarity in basic biologic behavior of metastases and spread between breast cancer and melanoma that seems apparent to us but is arguable by others.

Palpable regional lymph nodes require resection whenever they appear in the absence of distant metastases. These regional lymph node dissections are generally done as radical resections because of the high likelihood of multiple nodes being positive in malignant melanoma as well as the high propensity for local tissue implantation and recurrence that is so characteristic of melanoma. If prophylactic lymph node dissections are not selected as the option at the time of the original treatment of melanoma, it is essential to examine the patient frequently (every three months for instance) so that lymph node metastases, which become palpable, can be resected promptly. Since the incidence of lymph node metastases in melanomas less than .76 mm in thickness is no more than 1 per cent, even proponents of prophylactic lymph node dissection do not suggest resection in cases with such thin melanomas. In melanomas between .76 mm and 1.5 mm (or between .85 mm and 1.69 mm in thickness), the incidence of positive lymph nodes ranges between 5 and 10 per cent, and in melanomas between 1.70 mm and 3.65 mm in thickness the incidence of positive nodes is about 25 to 33 per cent, while the incidence of distant metastases initially is low. Thus, most proponents of prophylactic node dissection confine their prophylactic dissections to primary melanomas between 1.5 mm and 3 or 4 mm in thickness.[32]

There would be less resistance to performing prophylactic lymph node dissection in melanoma if the complications of the operation were not significant, particularly in the inguinal area. Following radical regional lymph node dissections in the groin for lower extremity melanomas the incidence of significant lymphedema of the leg is at least 25 per cent and the incidence of measurable but less significant edema is probably at least another 25 per cent. Disabling edema unfortunately occurs in a small proportion of these patients. Delayed wound healing and skin edge necrosis is common in groin dissection and lymph collections occur commonly. In addition, the occurrence of "satellitosis" is virtually unheard of when lymph node dissections are not performed in the regional drainage basins. The incidence of complications following axillary or cervical dissections is not as high but still occurs. Arm edema following modified axillary dissection appears in at least 15 per cent of patients and is higher if a radical axillary dissection is performed. However, only occasionally will the arm edema be of disabling nature. When neck dissections are performed, shoulder disability occurs if the spinal accessory nerve is not preserved; this nerve preservation should always be attempted. Otherwise, lymphatic resection complications concern cosmetic appearance, which is clearly of secondary nature, but still important, particularly if significant survival advantage cannot be displayed for prophylactic resection.

The final conclusions about the usefulness and appropriateness of "prophylactic" regional lymph node dissection will be obtained from the large multi-institutional American prospective trial comparing prophylactic dissection versus observation and later therapeutic node dissection. While patient accrual in this trial has been rapid, results will not be available for several years.

Amputation

Digit amputation of a greater or lesser extent is the surgery of choice of subungual melanoma since a cutaneous margin of resection cannot be achieved otherwise. These can usually be performed in a cosmetically and functionally satisfactory manner.

Major limb amputations are seldom necessary except for neglected or recurrent melanoma that manifests in such a way that no other method of resection can provide a reasonable or even compromised margin of removal.

Limb Perfusion

The isolated perfusion of extremities with chemotherapeutic agents, with or without regional hyperthermia in an attempt to increase local control and cure of melanomas, has a long and varied history.[33] Retrospective studies and recent control trials indicated some increased survival by such limb perfusions. However, this therapy remains highly controversial partly because of significant expense and toxicity (vascular, neural, cutaneous). The concept that more extensive local therapy will increase cure rates in melanoma when death occurs only from systemic, not local or regional disease, is biologically difficult to explain, especially since other data indicate that the extent of local resection and timing of nodal resections does not control outcome.[34]

Isolated limb perfusion is an effective therapy for extremity satellitosis or in-transit metastases and extensive local recurrence of an extremity. However, these problems are far less common today than many years ago because of the less frequent use of prophylactic lymph node dissections and the markedly earlier clinical occurrence of extremity melanomas with high cure rates and infrequent local recurrence. The value of primary limb perfusion for adjuvant treatment of primary melanoma remains to be resolved in future studies. However, in our opinion, primary limb perfusion is unlikely to contribute to cure although it may reduce local recurrence rates and prevent extensive regional recurrences.

Adjuvant Therapy

The history of adjuvant therapy in melanoma is replete with exciting initial reports that have failed to be substantiated over time or are under considerable scrutiny.[35] A variety of immunotherapy modalities of a nonspecific nature has been reported to cause regression in occasional patients with metastatic melanoma, and some have been tested as adjuvant therapy.[36] These immunologic agents have included vaccinia vaccine, rabies vaccine, BCG, interferon, and now interleukin 2 with lymphocyte activated killer (LAK) cells and tumor infiltrating lymphocytes (TIL). These treatments have been associated with demonstrable regression in a few cases of metastatic or recurrent disease. Because of the regular demonstration of auto-regression in superficial spreading melanoma and the occasional reports of spontaneous regression of distant metastases, the immunology and immunotherapy of melanoma has always attracted wide attention and research interest. All previous attempts of nonspecific immunotherapy have been abandoned after clinical trials because of the lack of effect in treating visceral metastases. The current enthusiasm for interleukin 2 is the latest chapter in the so far fruitless search for immunologic therapies in melanoma. Interleukin 2, however, has been combined with lymphocyte activated killer (LAK) cells or tumor infiltrating lymphocytes (TIL) so that more specificity of immunologic therapy may be achieved. Regression rates of 25 or 30 per cent are currently reported in trials of interleukin 2 and LAK cells. Further trials with these more specific immunologic maneuvers are under way and the results will be available in the future. If continual effectiveness occurs, trials of such therapy as an adjuvant to primary resection may be undertaken, but extremely high cost, both physiologic and financial, will be clear impediments to widespread use.

Numerous chemotherapeutic drugs used after surgical resection have produced no therapeutic benefit when compared with no such therapy in adjuvant trials. There are no trials currently under way utilizing chemotherapeutic agents, indicating the complete frustration with attempts at systemic prophylaxis of micrometastases by the use of chemotherapy. Thus, no adjuvant therapies are currently of value for melanoma patients even at high risk of metastases.

FOLLOW-UP AND THERAPY OF RECURRENCE

Because of the lack of major effect of routine systemic modalities (chemotherapy or immunotherapy) in the treatment of recurrent or disseminated melanoma, surgery remains the treatment of choice whenever possible in melanoma recurrences. Local recurrences, which may appear after inadequate previous excision margins, are easily handled by further local resections. Since inadequate margins are usually a function of operating on cosmetically or functionally difficult areas of the face, scalp, hands, feet, and digits, the surgery of the local recurrence may also be compromised for cosmetic or functional purposes. Isolated local recurrence in the scar of the previous melanoma excision may portend a bad outcome or poor prognosis but is not the cause of such poor outcome. When the recurrence is obviously caused by the previous incomplete local excision, outcome may be quite satisfactory. However, local recurrence in the presence of a previous adequate local resection usually is associated with poor prognostic features in the original melanoma such as high mitotic rate, extreme thickness, depigmentation, or local primary satellitosis. In such cases the overall prognosis is poor but not caused by the local recurrence; local recurrence is a manifestation of the poor prognostic features. Nevertheless, local recurrences should be treated appropriately and early to prevent growth to dimensions that would make local surgical removal difficult.

IN-TRANSIT METASTASES—"SATELLITOSIS"

Dermal metastases or subcutaneous nodular metastases lying between the primary excision site on an extremity and the regional nodal drainage basin present a difficult management problem and connote a poor prognosis. Such clinical manifestations of recurrent disease are less common than in previous years with much earlier clinical presentation, far higher cure rates, and far fewer prophylactic regional lymph node resections. When satellitosis appears after local resection, a diagnostic survey should be obtained to determine if distant metastases are also present. If the satellitosis is an isolated phenomena, therapy of some sort should be undertaken with the expectation of a reasonable regional control. Depending on the size and extent of the various lesions the satellitosis or subcutaneous nodules can be managed surgically by limited individual resection of the nodules, by wide sacrifice of skin and subcutaneous tissues, or by regional limb perfusion with chemotherapeutic agents and hyperthermia. Frequently, with minimal in-transit disease, repeated limited surgical excisions can provide simple and satisfactory control. Long-term control rates with hyperthermic chemotherapeutic perfusions are also reported to be high. This therapy can also be repeated in the event of failure or further satellitosis. Almost all types of therapy for such in-transit disease are associated with approximately a 20 per cent long-term survival.

REGIONAL LYMPH NODE METASTASES

Regional lymph node enlargement following local resection of melanomas in the absence of a previous prophylactic lymph node dissection should be treated by a lymphatic resection at the time the node metastases become palpable. Such therapeutic node dissections in the absence of systemic distant metastases play a significant role in the regional control of melanoma and may be associated with long-term survival rates of 25 per cent or more. If only one or two lymph node metastases are detected, the prognosis for long-term survival may be 50 per cent or more.[37, 38] When a single lymph node metastasis occurs, particularly after a long disease-free interval, the prognosis may be not too dissimilar from that of patients with negative lymph nodes. However, when patients have multiple lymph node metastases or a short disease-free interval, prognosis is poor but not hopeless by any means. Non-regional lymph node metastases, which become palpable in the absence of systemic distant metastases, should likewise be resected for palliation. However, these metastases obviously carry an extremely poor long-term prognosis since they imply systemic dissemination and not just regional disease.

When regional lymph nodes become palpable during the follow-up of patients without prophylactic dissections, open node biopsies are not required. One can either proceed directly to a nodal resection or do a preliminary needle aspiration biopsy to prove disease. Open biopsy may reduce the opportunity to perform a lymphatic resection with clear margins and predispose to local wound implantation and recurrence.

Subcutaneous Nodules

Distant non-regional subcutaneous metastases are a frequent pattern of recurrent disease in malignant melanoma. Satisfactory palliation of such patients can be achieved by repeated local excisions, which may spare the patient the anxiety of observing continued growth of known metastatic disease. Such distant subcutaneous metastatic disease may be associated with a relatively prolonged disease course with survival duration of many months to a few years.

Visceral Metastases

Occasional patients with isolated pulmonary metastases that are few in number may achieve long-term disease-free survival by pulmonary resection.

Such patients obviously require careful selection, but long-term survival rates of 25 per cent have been reported in highly selected cases.[39] Patients with brain metastases that are solitary may have significant palliation for many months by judicious neurosurgical resection and radiation therapy. Visceral metastases, however, are generally associated with an extremely poor prognosis, and hepatic resections, even for apparently solitary metastasis, are not usually justified. Gastrointestinal tract metastases that cause bleeding or obstruction should be resected for palliation.

FUTURE CONSIDERATIONS

In no human cancer is the potential for control by public education and early detection more likely than in malignant melanoma. The clinical recognition features of variations in height, outline, and color are so characteristic that the clinical diagnosis of melanoma is accurate in at least 95 per cent of cases. Education campaigns including short television public service announcements to alert the public to these early recognition signs may produce enormous benefits in terms of early detection and increased survival rate. Observant lay people can make relatively accurate estimations with such proper education. Currently, well over 50 per cent of patients with malignant melanoma appear at a very early clinical stage with expected survival rates of over 95 per cent. Only a small fraction of patients appear with advanced neglected primary melanoma. At a time when the incidence of melanoma continues to increase rapidly and the number of deaths from melanoma continues to be a significant clinical problem, the gains from public education campaigns regarding the hazards of overexposure to ultraviolet radiation in susceptible races, both naturally and in tanning salons, may yield significant benefits. It should be expected that in another decade only a small fraction of patients with malignant melanoma will die of disease, recognizing that the overall prognosis in melanoma has increased from a 30 per cent cure rate to an 80 per cent cure rate between 1945 and 1985, largely through the effect of early detection resulting from professional and public education.

REFERENCES

1. Bagley, F.H., Cady, B., Lee, A., and Legg, M.A.: Changes in clinical presentation and management of malignant melanoma. Cancer 47:2126–2134, 1981.
2. Clark, W.H., Jr., Ainsworth, A.M., Bernardino, E.A., et al.: The developmental biology of primary human malignant melanomas. Semin. Oncol. 2:83–103, 1975.
3. Breslow, A.: Thickness, cross-sectional area and depth of invasion in prognosis of cutaneous melanoma. Ann. Surg. 172:902–908, 1970.
4. Elder, D.E.: Dysplastic nevus syndrome—biological significance. Semin. Oncol. 15:529–540, 1988.
5. Elder, D.E., Goldman, L.I., Goldman, S.C., et al.: Dysplastic nevus syndrome: A phenotypic association of sporadic cutaneous melanoma. Cancer 46:1787–1794, 1980.
6. Greene, M.H., Clark, W.H., Tucker, M.A., et al.: High risk of malignant melanoma in melanoma-prone families with dysplastic nevi. Ann. Intern. Med. 102:458–465, 1985.
7. Hendrickson, M.R., and Ross, J.C.: Neoplasms arising in congenital giant nevi. Morphologic study of seven cases and a review of the literature. Am. J. Surg. Pathol. 5:109–135, 1981.
8. Cooke, K.R., Spears, C.F.S., Elder, D.E., and Greene, M.H.: Dysplastic naevi in a population-based survey. Cancer 63:1240–1244, 1989.
9. Tucker, M.A., and Bale, S.J.: Clinical aspects of familial cutaneous malignant melanoma. Semin. Oncol. 15:524–528, 1988.

10. Rivers, J.K., Kopf, A.W., Vinokur, A.F., et al.: Clinical characteristics of malignant melanomas developing in persons with dysplastic nevi. Cancer 65:1232–1236, 1990.
11. Koh, H.K., Caruso, A., Gage, I., et al.: Evaluation of melanoma/skin cancer screening in Massachusetts. Preliminary results. Cancer 65:375–379, 1990.
12. English, D.R., and Armstrong, B.K.: Identifying people at high risk of cutaneous malignant melanoma: Results from a case-control study in Western Australia. Br. Med. J. 296:1285–1288, 1988.
13. Gallagher, R.P., Elwood, J.M., and Yang, C.P.: Is chronic sunlight exposure important in accounting for increases in melanoma incidence? Int. J. Cancer 44:813–815, 1989.
14. Glass, A.G., and Hoover, R.N.: The emerging epidemic of melanoma and squamous cell skin cancer. JAMA 262:2097–2140, 1989.
15. Roush, G.C., Schymura, M.J., and Holford, T.R.: Patterns of invasive melanoma in the Connecticut tumor registry. Is the long-term increase real? Cancer 61:2586–2595, 1988.
16. Loggie, B.W., and Eddy, J.A.: Solar considerations in the development of cutaneous melanoma. Semin. Oncol. 15:494–499, 1988.
17. Lewis, M.G., and Johnson, K.: The incidence and distribution of pigmented naevi in Ugandan Africans. Br. J. Derm. 80:362–366, 1968.
18. Bale, S.J., Dracopoli, N.C., Tucker, M.A., et al.: Mapping the gene for hereditary cutaneous malignant melanoma-dysplastic nevus to chromosome 1_p. N. Engl. J. Med. 320:1367–1372, 1989.
19. Woods, J.E., Soule, E.H., and Creagan, E.T.: Metastasis and death in patients with thin melanomas (less than 0.76 mm). Ann. Surg. 198:63–69, 1983.
20. Drzewiecki, K.T., Frydman, H., Anderson, K., et al.: Malignant melanoma. Changing trends in factors influencing metastasis-free survival from 1964 to 1982. Cancer 65:362–366, 1990.
21. Ronan, S.G., Han, M.C., and Das Gupta, T.K.: Histologic prognostic indicators in cutaneous malignant melanoma. Semin. Oncol. 15:558–565, 1988.
22. Patterson, R.H., and Helwog, E.B.: Subungual malignant melanoma: A clinical-pathologic study. Cancer 46:2074–2087, 1980.
23. Krementz, E.T., Reed, R.J., Coleman, W.P., et al.: Acral lentiginous melanoma, a clinico-pathologic entity. Ann. Surg. 195:632–645, 1982.
24. Rapini, R.P., Golitz, L.E., Greer, R.O., et al.: Primary malignant melanoma of the oral cavity. A review of 177 cases. Cancer 55:1543–1550, 1985.
25. Ross, M., Pezzi, C., Pezzi, T., et al.: Patterns of failure in anorectal melanoma. A guide to surgical therapy. Arch. Surg. 125:313–316, 1990.
26. Weedon, D., and Little, J.H.: Spindle and epithelioid cell nevi in children and adults. A review of 211 cases of the Spitz nevus. Cancer 40:217–224, 1977.
27. Cady, B.: Lymph node metastases. Indicators, but not governors of survival. Arch. Surg. 119:1067–1072, 1984.
28. Breslow, A., and Macht, S.D.: Optimal size of resection margin for thin cutaneous melanoma. Surg. Gynecol. Obstet. 145:691–692, 1977.
29. Veronesi, U., Cascinelli, N., Adamus, J., et al.: Thin stage I primary cutaneous malignant melanoma. Comparison of excision with margins of 1 or 3 cm. N. Engl. J. Med. 318:1159–1162, 1988.
30. Urist, M.M., Balch, C.M., Soong, S., et al.: The influence of surgical margins and prognostic factors predicting the risk of local recurrence in 3445 patients with primary cutaneous melanoma. Cancer 55:1398–1402, 1985.
31. Cascinelli, N., Vaglini, M., Bufalino, R., and Morabito, A.: Bans. A cutaneous region with no prognostic significance in patients with melanoma. Cancer 57:441–444, 1986.
32. Balch, C.M., Soong, S., Milton, G.W., et al.: Changing trends in cutaneous melanoma over a quarter century in Alabama, USA, and New South Wales, Australia. Cancer 52:1748–1753, 1983.
33. Edwards, M.J., Soong, S-J., Boddie, A.W., et al.: Isolated limb perfusion for localized melanoma of the extremity. A matched comparison of wide local excision with isolated limb perfusion and wide local excision alone. Arch. Surg. 125:317–321, 1990.
34. Sim, F.H., Taylor, W.F., Pritchard, D.J., and Soule, E.H.: Lymphadenectomy in the management of Stage I malignant melanoma: A prospective randomized study. Mayo Clin. Proc. 61:697–705, 1986.
35. Veronesi, U., Adamus, J., Augert, C., et al.: A randomized trial of adjuvant chemotherapy and immunotherapy in cutaneous melanoma. N. Engl. J. Med. 301:913–916, 1982.
36. Mastrangelo, M.J., Schultz, S., Kane, M., and Berd, D.: Newer immunologic approaches to the treatment of patients with melanoma. Semin. Oncol. 15:589–594, 1988.
37. Callery, C., Cochran, A.J., Roe, D.J., et al.: Factors prognostic for survival in patients with malignant melanoma spread to the regional lymph nodes. Ann. Surg. 96:69–75, 1982.
38. Coit, D.G., and Brennan, M.F.: Extent of lymph node dissection in melanoma of the trunk or lower extremity. Arch. Surg. 124:162–166, 1989.
39. Overett, T.K., and Shiu, M.H.: Surgical treatment of distant metastatic melanoma. Indications and results. Cancer 56:1222–1230, 1985.

12

SOFT TISSUE SARCOMAS

by Michael D. Stone, M.D., and Blake Cady, M.D.

Soft tissue sarcomas are malignant tumors arising in the extraskeletal connective tissues of the body. The word sarcoma is derived from the Greek "sarkoma" meaning fleshy growth. The soft tissues at risk for sarcoma development include those parts of the body between the epidermis and the visceral organs and include muscles, tendons, fibrous tissue, fat, and synovial tissue. These connective tissues originate in the primitive mesenchyme, which is, in turn, a component of the embryonal mesoderm. Although malignant tumors of the epithelium are referred to as carcinomas, malignant tumors of the mesothelium and of the vascular and lymphatic endothelium are included in the category of sarcomas. Sarcomas therefore constitute a heterogeneous group of neoplasms.

The American Cancer Society has estimated that 5800 new soft tissue sarcomas will be diagnosed in 1991 in the United States. Soft tissue sarcomas represent 0.5 per cent of all cancers. The annual age-adjusted incidence is 2 per 100,000, and the estimated yearly death rate is 3,100.[1]

EPIDEMIOLOGY

At the present time, our understanding of the epidemiology of soft tissue sarcomas is limited. There are, however, several clinical situations that are associated with sarcoma. Sarcomas affecting radiation fields have been described after radiation for breast cancer and Hodgkin's disease. These are most commonly fibrosarcomas and osteosarcomas. It is difficult to determine the exact risk of the development of such sarcomas. Kim et al identified only 13 cases of fibrosarcoma of the chest wall in the world literature in women previously managed by mastectomy and radiation therapy for breast cancer.[2] The median time of development of sarcomas after radiation is 11 years.[3] Halperin et al have calculated a 0.9 per cent risk of sarcoma occurring in five-year survivors of Hodgkin's disease.[4]

Lymphangiosarcoma may occur in the lymphedematous arm after axillary node dissection for breast cancer (Stewart-Treves syndrome). Neurofibrosarcoma is noted in 15 per cent of patients with neurofibromatosis.[5] Patients with Gardner's syndrome are known to be at risk for desmoid tumors within the abdominal cavity. Thorotrast, a radiologic contrast agent used until the 1950s, and polyvinyl chloride have been associated with angiosarcomas and other malignancies of the liver and biliary tracts.

As many as 30 per cent of patients with soft tissue sarcomas give a history of recent injury to the area of the tumor, and examination of the site may lead to the diagnosis of underlying sarcoma. Given the temporal relationship, it is highly unlikely that such trauma is causally related to the sarcoma. Desmoid tumors of the abdominal wall are known to occur in young women after childbirth, frequently in the cesarean section scar. Scars at other sites have also been identified as the site of development of subsequent sarcomas, but there is no clear etiologic role. There is no clear genetic predisposition to the development of soft tissue sarcomas.

PATHOLOGY

Site

Because of their origin in connective tissue, soft tissue sarcomas may occur anywhere in the body. Approximately 46 per cent of these tumors are found in the lower extremity. Three quarters of the latter are at or above the knee. The upper extremity is the site of approximately 13 per cent of soft tissue sarcomas. Slightly less than one-third of these tumors are located in the trunk, and, of these, 40 per cent are within the retroperitoneum. Nine per cent of sarcomas are located in the head and neck[6] (Table 12–1).

Histologic Types

Pathologic classification of soft tissue tumors is now based on the putative cell of origin of each tumor, as suggested by Enzinger and Weiss.[7] The most important components of pathologic classification are the tissue type, whether benign or malignant, and the histopathologic grade of malignant tumors. The classification described by Enzinger and Weiss is based on 17 different tumor categories ranging from fibrous, adipose, and muscle tumors, to

TABLE 12–1. SOFT TISSUE SARCOMAS BY SITE (ACOS SURVEY, 1987)

Sites		
Head and Neck	406	9%
Trunk	872	19%
Retroperitoneum	568	12%
Upper Extremity	594	13%
Lower Extremity	2,110	46%
Total	4,550	

From Lawrence, W., Donegan, W.L., Natarajan, N., et al.: Adult soft tissue sarcomas. A pattern of care survey of the American College of Surgeons. Ann. Surg. 205:349–359, 1987.

tumors of uncertain histogenesis and tumors that cannot be further classified. Between 10 and 20 per cent of sarcomas fit into the latter category. Pathologists may disagree on the histologic type in one-third of the cases.[8] The low incidence of sarcomas and their capacity to dedifferentiate from their cell of origin contribute to the difficulty competent pathologists may have in specification of the histopathologic type of a given tumor (Table 12–2).

Any of the soft tissues can have both benign and malignant tumors. Pathologic differentiation between the two is obviously crucial. Reactive lesions such as proliferative fasciitis and the early stages of myositis ossificans may grossly resemble sarcomas. Some parts of tumors may appear more or less malignant than other areas. With a previously excised "benign" tumor, the apparent transformation and recurrence as a malignant sarcoma is a rare event, and almost always results from inadequate pathologic sampling of the original tumor. One exception is the occasional transformation of neurofibromas to malignant schwannomas in patients with neurofibromatosis.

There are tumors of soft tissues that appear histologically malignant and have the capability of aggressive local invasion but rarely metastasize. Examples of these tumors are desmoid tumors, dermatofibrosarcoma protuberans, and well-differentiated liposarcomas. The importance of differentiating these locally aggressive but nonmetastasizing tumors is obvious given the potentially enormous differences in therapy.

Grade

A reproducible and universally accepted grading system for soft tissue sarcomas does not currently exist. Nonetheless, histologic grade is widely accepted as the most important indicator of the biologic behavior of soft tissue sarcomas.[7, 9–11] Approximately one-third of soft tissue sarcomas are low grade.[8] Low-grade sarcomas tend to grow locally and invade aggressively but metastasize in only 14 per cent of cases.[12] High-grade tumors, on the other hand, are much more likely to metastasize to distant sites, most commonly to the lung.

A number of grading schemes have been developed, employing two, three, or four grades. The most commonly used system classifies sarcomas as low, intermediate, and high grade, depending on some or all of the following criteria: mitotic rate, nuclear morphology, degree of cellularity,

TABLE 12–2. PARTIAL LIST OF COMMON HISTOPATHOLOGIC TYPES OF SOFT TISSUE SARCOMAS

Histopathology	
Alveolar soft part sarcoma	Leiomyosarcoma
Angiosarcoma	Liposarcoma
Dermatofibrosarcoma protuberans	Malignant fibrous histiocytoma (MFH)
Desmoid tumor	Malignant peripheral nerve tumor (schwannoma)
Extraskeletal chondrosarcoma/ osteosarcoma	Rhabdomyosarcoma
Fibrosarcoma	Synovial cell sarcoma

cellular anaplasia or pleomorphism, presence of necrosis, amount of surrounding stroma, and vascularity (Table 12–3). Differentiation of tumors on the basis of these criteria is semi-quantitative at best. It therefore is no surprise that pathologists disagree on grade in more than one-third of cases.[9] The degree of necrosis has been suggested as the single best histopathologic parameter predicting both time of recurrence and overall survival of patients.[13]

These difficulties in pathologic assessment of more than 50 types of soft tissue neoplasms of differing grades and variable metastatic potential may be intimidating to the general surgeon (Fig. 12–1). Fortunately, two factors simplify the understanding of sarcoma management. First, more than 75 per cent of sarcomas at all sites are of six histologic types (Fig. 12–2). Second, sarcomas of differing histopathologies, but of the same grade, have a similar natural history (Fig. 12–3). Therefore, it is reasonable to evaluate and discuss management of these tumors as a single group, recognizing that there are occasional differences in behavior between histologic subtypes.

It is incumbent upon the surgeon to assist the pathologist in accurate diagnosis by providing information regarding the age and sex of the patient, the site and size of the tumor, and whether the patient has had prior treatment. For all sarcomas, the surgeon should review biopsy and resection slides with the pathologist and then obtain a statement about grade even if the pathologist cannot specify the cell type. On review of resection specimens, the pathologist should provide a description of the proximity of the tumor to important structures such as bones, vessels, nerves, and margins. Given the difficulties of defining certain aspects of the pathology of these tumors, surgeons and pathologists who see them infrequently should have a low threshold for arranging pathologic consultations in medical centers with special experience in the diagnosis and management of soft tissue sarcomas when there is doubt about their nature.

Management of soft tissue sarcoma should be carried out in a stepwise manner as follows: (1) clinical and radiologic imaging evaluation and diagnosis, (2) biopsy and histopathologic diagnosis, (3) treatment selection(s) and planning, (4) pathologic evaluation of the surgical specimen and determination of stage, (5) adjuvant therapy to prevent local recurrence, and (6) adjuvant therapy for occult metastatic disease.[14]

TABLE 12–3. GUIDELINES FOR HISTOLOGIC GRADING OF SOFT TISSUE SARCOMAS

Grading Criteria	
Low Grade	*High Grade*
Good differentiation	Poor differentiation
Hypocellular	Hypercellular
Much stroma	Minimal stroma
Hypovascular	Hypervascular
Minimal necrosis	Much necrosis
Less than 5 mitoses per 10 hpf	More than 5 mitoses per 10 hpf

Modified from Hajdu, S.I.: Pathology of Soft Tissue Tumors. Philadelphia, Lea & Febiger, 1979.

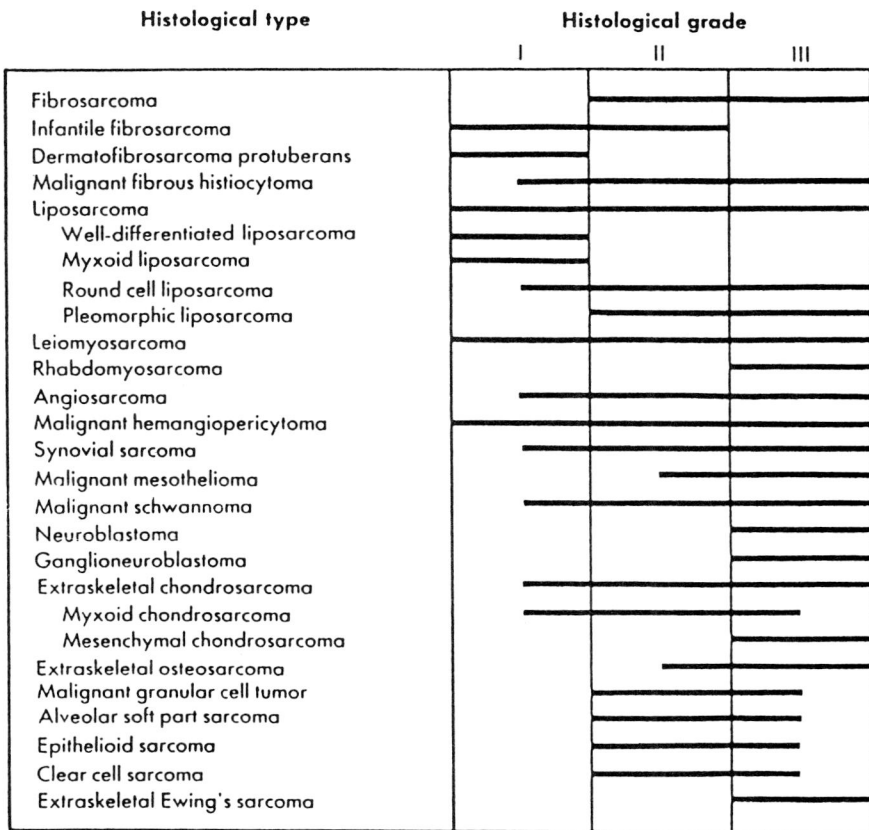

Figure 12–1. Range of grading for soft tissue sarcomas by histologic type. (From Enzinger, F.M., and Weiss, S.W.: Soft Tissue Tumors, 2nd ed. St. Louis, C.V. Mosby, 1988, p. 9.)

CLINICAL PRESENTATION AND EVALUATION

A sarcoma typically occurs as a painless mass. Because sarcomas arise in soft, compressible tissues, patients may remain asymptomatic until the tumor is considerably larger than the anatomic place of origin. A few patients may experience pain that results from either hemorrhage or necrosis within a tumor or compression of peripheral nerves. Sarcomas are usually small when located superficially. When occurring over bony prominences, they may be more easily detected. Lesions in fleshy areas such as the buttock and thigh may reach larger proportions, and retroperitoneal sarcomas may be huge before clinical detection by the patient or physician.

There are no reliable physical signs or historic data that distinguish between benign and malignant soft tissue lesions. A history of a mass of long-standing duration does not exclude the possibility of sarcoma. Liposarcomas, for example, may grow slowly and occur in this manner. Therefore, all soft tissue masses that persist should be biopsied. Small (less than 3 cm) soft tissue lumps that have been present and unchanged for many years may be followed; however, lesions larger than this as well as any enlarging tumors should be biopsied.

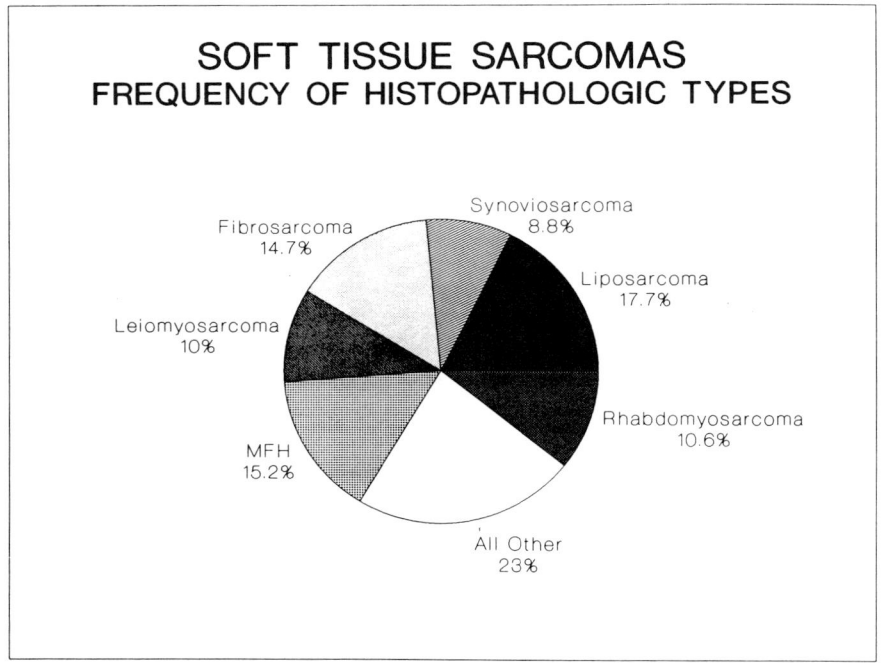

Figure 12–2. Histologic types of soft tissue sarcomas at all sites. Data compiled from five series from 1977 to 1990. Actuarial overall survival for high-grade sarcomas of the extremity by histologic type. There is no significant difference in survival.

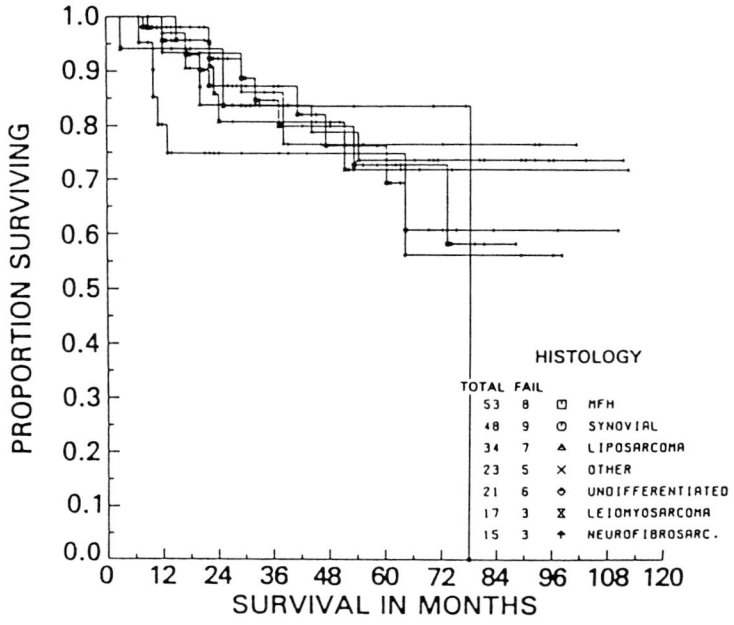

Figure 12–3. Overall survival is similar for high-grade sarcomas of different histologic subtypes. (From Potter, D.A., Kinsella, T., and Glatstein, E.: High-grade soft tissue sarcomas of the extremities. Cancer 58:190–205, 1986.)

Clinical evaluation of the patient should include a comprehensive medical history with specific attention to any history of familial disorders such as Gardner's syndrome, neurofibromatosis, and exposure to radiation. Examination of the tumor itself should include assessment of its attachment to deep or superficial structures, its relationship to prior biopsy site, functional status of the body part or extremity, and the presence of prior injury or concurrent medical disease that might affect treatment by surgery or radiation. For extremity sarcomas, proximity to bone, joints, major nerves, and blood vessels is obviously important. Evaluation of tumors at other sites requires consideration of involvement of other visceral organs, including the gastrointestinal and urinary tracts for trunk lesions and important structures of the head and neck for lesions in that area.

Radiology

Routine x-rays of soft tissue sarcomas are of little clinical value. Their use should be limited to those patients in whom there is clinical suspicion of bone erosion by tumor. In this setting, bone radiographs are more useful than bone scans, which are not routinely used for detection or management of soft tissue sarcomas. The incidence of true bone invasion is low and increased radionuclide uptake in bone adjacent to a soft tissue sarcoma may merely indicate tissue reaction secondary to tumor proximity. In a study from Memorial Hospital, the sensitivity of both bone scanning and plain radiographs for detecting pathologically confirmed invasion of bone by soft tissue sarcomas was 100 per cent.[15] The specificity of plain films was also 100 per cent. However, false-positive bone scans were obtained in seven of 12 patients, for a specificity of 42 per cent. The false impression of bone invasion may lead to unnecessary amputation in patients who may be candidates for limb sparing multimodality therapy.

Computerized tomography (CT) and, more recently, magnetic resonance imaging (MRI) are the most useful modalities for evaluation of soft tissue sarcomas. Contrast-enhanced CT scanning allows visualization of major vascular, gastrointestinal, and genitourinary structures, providing important information for surgical and radiation treatment planning. However, on CT scans, tumors of muscle origin may be difficult to differentiate from surrounding normal muscular tissues. MRI appears to offer better delineation between tumor and surrounding muscle. MRI also allows the tumor to be viewed in coronal and sagittal views as opposed to only the transaxial view of the CT scan. Specific muscle compartments may be easily outlined and this information may facilitate surgical planning (Fig. 12–4). In a prospective study, MRI and CT were equally accurate in assessing proximity of the tumor to major neurovascular and skeletal structures, the major determinants of resectability.[16]

Currently, neither MRI or CT is sufficiently refined to determine whether a soft tissue tumor is benign or malignant. MRI allows for better assessment of muscle and compartment involvement and is the procedure of choice for extremity lesions. CT scans may offer better resolution of intraabdominal viscera and may be preferable for intraabdominal and retroperitoneal lesions. It is not necessary for patients to undergo both CT scan and MRI.

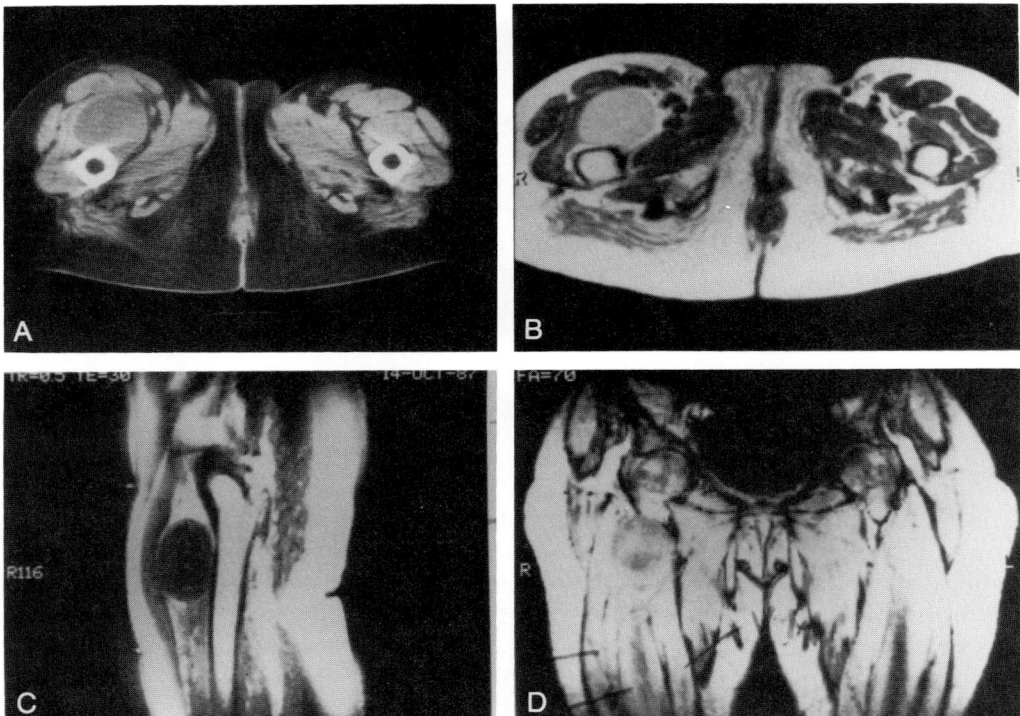

Figure 12–4. *A,* CT scan image of low-grade liposarcoma of the upper thigh. *B,* MRI of same patient. Determination of bone or vascular invasion and, therefore, resectability is not improved. *C,* Sagittal MRI shows proximity to bone and better delineates muscle group involvement. *D,* Coronal image further delineates muscle group involvement.

Arteriography offers little in the way of diagnostic information that cannot be obtained by either CT scan or MRI. Its use should be limited to patients in whom vascular resection and reconstruction is necessary, and to patients who are candidates for intraarterial chemotherapy for unresectable tumors.

Only 4 to 11 per cent of patients with soft tissue sarcoma show obvious clinical metastases.[17] Approximately 80 per cent of metastases are discovered in the lung, pleura, or mediastinum, and are detectable by chest radiographs. Therefore, all patients with soft tissue sarcoma should undergo chest radiography. Conventional linear tomography identifies more pulmonary nodules than plain radiographs, most of which prove to be metastases. Chest CT is again more sensitive, detecting twice as many lesions as linear tomography. However, only half of these lesions prove to be metastases.[18] Since sarcomas generally occur in patients who are young and rarely have coexisting pulmonary disease, and new pulmonary nodules are almost always metastases in this age group,[19] serial chest CT scans are superior to linear tomography.[20] For patients with a small or low-grade extremity lesion, a routine chest x-ray is adequate. When knowledge of the presence of pulmonary metastases would alter surgical treatment, as in patients about to undergo major ablative procedures such as hindquarter amputation, a chest CT scan is appropriate. Patients who participate in adjuvant chemotherapy protocols should also undergo chest CT scanning. It should also be kept in mind that solitary pulmonary nodules may represent primary lung cancers in older patients, particularly in those with a history of smoking.

Biopsy

Many benign and malignant lesions may mimic sarcoma (Table 12–4), and it is impossible to determine whether soft tissue masses are benign or malignant by either palpation or imaging studies. With the exception of hematoma and inflammatory cysts, all of the lesions discussed require surgical treatment. Therefore, the next step in the surgical management of soft tissue masses is a biopsy.

The objectives of biopsy are (1) to obtain enough tissue to identify the histologic type of the tumor, (2) to determine whether the lesion is benign or malignant, (3) to determine the histologic grade of a malignant lesion, and (4) to obtain these data with minimal tumor disruption and contamination of normal surrounding tissues. The first three objectives are important for planning a surgical approach to the lesion, the extent of dissection, and the use of adjuvant preoperative, or intraoperative radiotherapy. Minimizing tumor disruption and tissue contamination are crucial because of the well-known propensity for sarcomas to implant and recur locally. Biopsy may be performed by incisional, excisional, punch, or needle techniques. The optimal biopsy technique for a particular tumor is determined by the size and location of the mass, and the relative importance of the above objectives given the clinical situation (Fig. 12–5).

Aspiration cytology, because of limited sampling and difficulty in differentiating the cellular elements of reactive and benign neoplasms from those of malignant neoplastic lesions, has a limited role in the primary diagnosis of soft tissue sarcomas. Core needle biopsy is simple and may be performed in the office setting under local anesthesia. Contamination of surrounding tissue planes is minimal when only one pass is made into the tumor. The primary disadvantage of this technique is that a small, potentially nonrepresentative sample is obtained. Determination of histologic type, grade, or even whether the lesion is malignant may not be possible. Multiple needle passes should be avoided as the amount of tissue retrieved will still be small, and the risk of local recurrence may be increased by difficulties in encompassing all needle tracts in the surgical or radiation fields. The skin puncture site may heal and become unnoticeable prior to the time of definitive surgical treatment. Therefore, the skin puncture site and needle tract must be placed

TABLE 12–4. DIFFERENTIAL DIAGNOSES OF SOFT TISSUE TUMORS

Hematoma	Benign peripheral nerve tumor
Chronic abscess	Nodular fascitis
Myositis ossificans	Fibromatosis
Hemangioma	Metastatic tumor
Lymphangioma	Lymphoma
Lipoma	Chloroma
Ganglion	Bone sarcoma

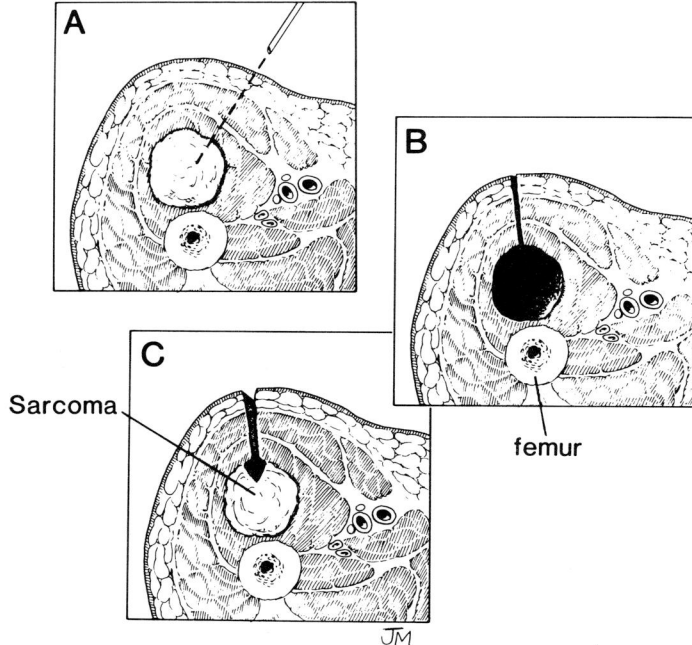

Figure 12–5. *A,* Core needle biopsy provides a limited amount of tissue for histologic evaluation. The needle tract must be completely excised at the time of definitive resection. *B,* Enucleation of sarcomas leaves prongs of tumor behind; therefore, a large volume of tissue and multiple planes are contaminated by tumor cells. *C,* Incisional biopsy should provide an adequate tissue sample with minimal contamination.

so as to be readily included in an elliptic incision appropriate for later wide excision, if the mass is proved to be a sarcoma.

Needle biopsy is very useful when the objective is to confirm the diagnosis in the setting of suspected metastatic or locally recurrent sarcoma, and in the setting of an unresectable intrathoracic or intraabdominal sarcoma, which would otherwise require a thoracotomy or laparotomy for diagnosis.

Punch biopsy may be easily performed under local anesthesia in the office for small, superficial ulcerated lesions. It is the appropriate technique for endoscopic sampling of gastrointestinal, genitourinary, or respiratory tract sarcomas. Punch biopsies provide small samples and are subject to the same limitations as needle biopsies. Multiple punches may be obtained to allow diagnosis of the histologic type and, occasionally, the determination of grade.

Excisional biopsy or tumor "enucleation" provides a large sample, i.e., the entire tumor for determination of malignancy, histologic type, and grade. They may be simple and easily performed under local anesthesia for small, superficial masses. However, sarcomas typically have a surrounding pseudocapsule of compressed normal tissue. Prongs of tumor invade through the pseudocapsule, and local excision by enucleation in the plane of the pseudocapsule will leave behind microscopic foci of sarcoma. The extent of tumor contamination of normal tissue planes will vary with the depth of the biopsy and the size of the sarcoma. A deep biopsy cavity will be contaminated along several or all planes, making wide resection more difficult or inadequate and increasing the risk of subsequent local recurrence. Excisional biopsies should be restricted to superficial lesions less than 3 cm in diameter.

Incisional biopsy is simple to perform under local anesthesia and is the procedure of choice for most sarcomas. The incision should be placed directly over the tumor mass to facilitate its inclusion in an elliptical resection incision should the tumor be determined to be a sarcoma. Careful dissection, without elevation of skin flaps, is necessary to minimize contamination. It should be easy to obtain a 1 × 1 × 1 cm tissue sample, which should be adequate for pathologic determination of malignancy, histologic type, and grade. Intraoperative consultation with the pathologist and obtaining frozen sections may be appropriate to ensure that an adequate piece of tissue has been obtained. However, treatment decisions should not be made on frozen section specimens. Hemostasis must be meticulous. Dissection of hematoma along tissue planes may result in contamination of extensive areas after incisional biopsy. Bleeding raw tumor should be cauterized with the electrocautery for hemostasis. Drains are usually not needed and should be avoided. When absolutely necessary, drains should be brought out through the incision and not through remote stab wounds, which will need to be excised at the time of definitive resection.

For extremity masses, the biopsy incision and the long access of the elliptical wide incision should be oriented longitudinally along the limb (Fig. 12–6). For truncal lesions, the incision should parallel the underlying muscle fibers. Wide excision of horizontally based biopsy incisions on an extremity may result in inadequate soft tissue for closure or coverage of the defect. Skin grafts or local flaps may be required to close such defects.

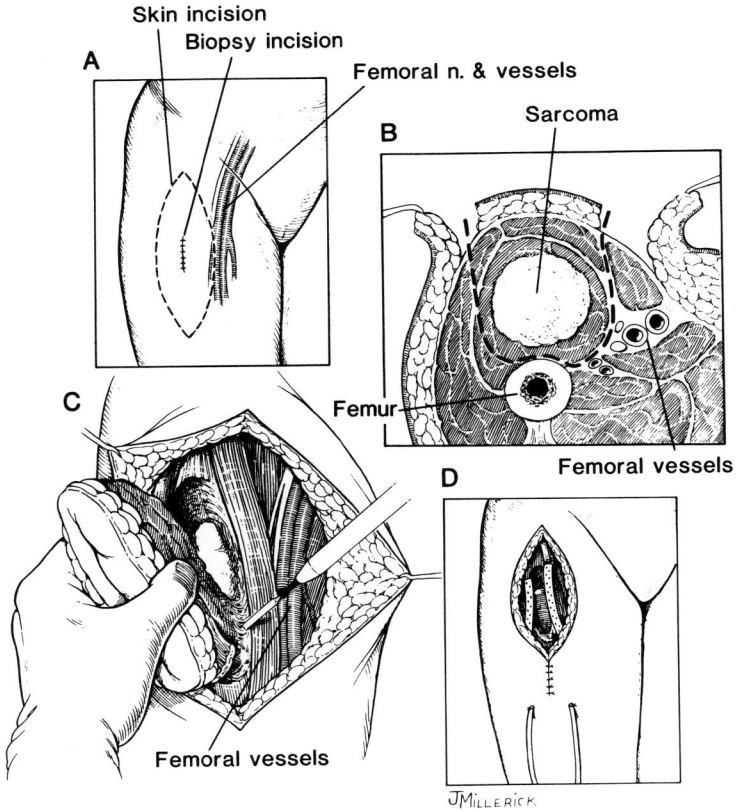

Figure 12–6. *A,* An elliptical skin incision should be oriented longitudinally over the underlying muscles in the extremities. *B,* The tumor should be removed completely with a rim of normal soft tissue. *C,* Dissection is performed with the electrocautery and is guided by careful palpation and inspection. The tumor itself should not be entered or directly visualized during this procedure. *D,* The flaps are closed over closed suction drains.

TABLE 12–5. AMERICAN JOINT COMMITTEE ON CANCER STAGING SCHEME FOR SOFT TISSUE SARCOMAS (1988)

TNMG Classification		
T: Primary tumor	T_1	<5 cm diameter
	T_2	>5 cm diameter
N: Regional lymph nodes	N_0	Not involved
	N_1	Involved (proved)
M: Distant metastases	M_0	None
	M_1	Present
G: Histologic grade	G_1	Low grade
	G_2	Intermediate grade
	G_3	High grade

Staging

Several staging systems for soft tissue sarcoma have been proposed and are based on prognostic factors derived from retrospective studies. All staging systems are based primarily on histologic grade, the most important prognostic indicator of survival. The staging system for soft tissue sarcomas of the American Joint Committee on Cancer is based on three histologic grades (G), tumor size (T), status of regional lymph nodes (N), and whether distant metastases are present (M) (Table 12–5).[21] The utility of this system is clear, as survival decreases with increasing stage (Table 12–6). However, the inclusion of lymph node status may be unnecessary as nodal metastases from sarcomas are uncommon, and other prognostic factors such as site (proximal or distal) are omitted.

A simplified alternative has been suggested by Hajdu based on experience at Memorial Hospital, using two histologic grades, tumor size, and relationship of the tumor to the deep fascia (superficial or deep) (Table 12–7).[22,23] The usefulness of this system is evident from the five-year survival figures associated with increasing stage (Table 12–8).

Staging information is important for treatment planning, as patients at high risk for death from disease should be included in adjuvant systemic therapy protocols. Similar prognostic data have been developed for local

TABLE 12–6. PROGNOSIS OF SOFT TISSUE SARCOMAS ACCORDING TO STAGE (AJCC STAGING SCHEME: SOFT TISSUE SARCOMA, 1988)

Stage Criteria and 5-Year Survival			
Stage I:	IA	$G_1\ T_1\ N_0\ M_0$	83%
	IB	$G_1\ T_2\ N_0\ M_0$	72%
Stage II:	IIA	$G_2\ T_1\ N_0\ M_0$	59%
	IIB	$G_2\ T_2\ N_0\ M_0$	53%
Stage III:	IIIA	$G_3\ T_1\ N_0\ M_0$	42%
	IIIB	$G_3\ T_2\ N_0\ M_0$	26%
Stage IV:	IVA	$N_1\ M_0$	23%
	IVB	M_1	—

The major determinants are grade and tumor size (greater than or less than 5 cm).

TABLE 12–7. SOFT TISSUE SARCOMAS: PROGNOSTIC FACTORS

Feature	Favorable	Unfavorable
Size	Small	Large
Site	Superficial	Deep
Histologic Grade	Low	High

Modified from Hajdu, S.I.: Histologic diagnosis and grade of soft tissue sarcomas. *In* Shiu, M.H., and Brennan, M.F. (Eds.): Surgical Management of Soft Tissue Sarcoma. Philadelphia, Lea & Febiger, 1989, p. 13.

recurrence, indicating the importance of age, grade, recurrent disease, inadequate surgical margins, and histologic type.[24]

TREATMENT

Evolution of Current Concepts

The surgical treatment of soft tissue sarcomas has changed considerably over the last fifty years. In the 1940s and 1950s, local excision with little or no margin was commonly used and was associated with an unacceptably high local recurrence rate of 50 to 90 per cent, followed by distant metastases and death. It was recognized that the frequency of local control by surgery alone was directly proportional to the extent of surgical resection, and thereby to the degree of anatomic and functional loss.[25–27] This experience led to the adoption of more radical compartment resections and amputation, which was associated with improvement of local control rates to more than 80 per cent.[14] By the early 1970s, it was apparent that survival rates at five and 10 years from radical resection remained quite poor at 20 to 50 per cent, despite the improved local control achieved.[28]

Interest in multimodality therapy for soft tissue sarcomas of adults was stimulated in the 1960s by experience with rhabdomyosarcoma in children. The use of adjuvant chemotherapy and radiation therapy, along with less radical surgery, was associated with an improvement in survival from less than 10 per cent to 60 to 70 per cent.[29] High local recurrence rates of approximately 50 per cent seen with wide excision of adult sarcomas compared with approximately 10 per cent with amputation strongly sug-

TABLE 12–8. STAGING OF SOFT TISSUE SARCOMA

	Grade	Size	Depth	5-Year Survival
Stage 0	Low	<5 cm	Superficial	100%
Stage 1	Low	<5 cm	Deep	
	Low	>5 cm	Superficial	92%
	High	<5 cm	Superficial	
Stage 2	Low	>5 cm	Deep	
	High	<5 cm	Deep	64%
	High	<5 cm	Deep	
Stage 3	High	>5 cm	Deep	21%

From Hajdu, S.I.: Pathology of Soft Tissue Tumors. Philadelphia, Lea & Fegiber, 1979.

gested the need for adjuvant local therapy if function-preserving resections were to be a reality. In addition, high distant recurrence rates, despite the excellent local control afforded by amputation, indicated the need for adjuvant therapy for occult distant micrometastases.

Early reports of radiation therapy for sarcomas indicated that these tumors were relatively radioresistant.[30] Responses were unpredictable and short-lived when obtained. As experience with the application of high dosages of radiotherapy to sarcomas was obtained, multiple series suggested that satisfactory local control of sarcomas, that otherwise would have required amputation, could be achieved by combining function-preserving resections with radiation.[31-34] Despite the apparent benefits of radiation therapy when applied to more conservative excisions, limb preservation for extremity sarcomas was not widely accepted in the mid 1970s. At that time, Rosenberg et al at the National Cancer Institute began a prospective randomized trial of amputation versus limb-sparing surgery plus radiation in patients with high-grade–extremity sarcomas. All of these patients also received adjuvant chemotherapy postoperatively. At a median follow-up of greater than nine years, no significant differences were found in disease-free or overall survival. In the limb-sparing group, four of 27 patients had lesions that recurred locally versus none of 17 patients in the amputation group having recurrent lesions. This difference is not significant.[35] Local control, disease-free survival, and overall survival were similar in the two groups (Fig. 12–7). Conservative function and limb-sparing therapy with surgery and radiation is now an accepted and preferred treatment of most soft tissue sarcomas.

Local Treatment

The objectives of local treatment for soft tissue sarcomas are (1) the complete eradication of local disease, (2) prevention of local recurrence, (3) prevention of distant recurrence, and (4) preservation of tissue and function.

Surgery

The extent of surgery is determined by the size, depth, and anatomic relationships of the tumor, the propensity of sarcomas to extend microscopically beyond visible or palpable boundaries, the anatomic and functional loss that will result from a wide resection, and the availability of effective radiation therapy to mitigate the extent of resection. The prime technical objective in sarcoma surgery is to achieve negative surgical margins, regardless of the extent of the procedure. The types of surgical procedures possible for soft tissue sarcomas include enucleation, limited margin excision, wide excision, and radical resection, including muscle group or compartmental excision and amputation.

Enucleation of a sarcoma by dissection within the pseudocapsule and "shelling out" the tumor may be tempting, because of its ease, to the surgeon inexperienced in sarcoma surgery. The pseudocapsule represents compressed normal tissue, through which microscopic fingers of malignant tumor invade surrounding tissue. This technique leaves gross tumor behind, guarantees local recurrence, and should never be the sole treatment.

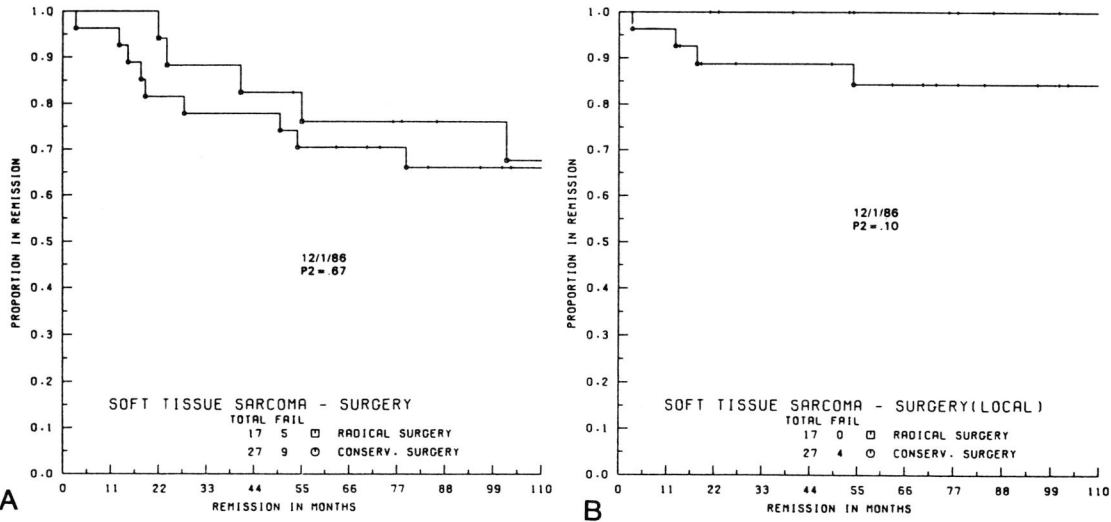

Figure 12–7. Prospective randomized trial comparing amputation versus limb conserving surgery, plus radiation in patients with high-grade extremity sarcomas. A, Disease-free survival. B, Local control. No statistically significant difference is seen. (From Chang, A.E., Rosenberg, S.A., Glatstein, E.J., and Antman, K.H.: Sarcomas of soft tissues. In DeVita, V.T., Hellman, S., and Rosenberg, S. (eds.): Cancer: Principles & Practice of Oncology, 3rd ed, vol. 2. Philadelphia, J.B. Lippincott, 1989, p. 1374.)

Limited margin excision or local excision involves removal of the tumor with little or no margin around the pseudocapsule, and is associated with a local recurrence rate of 50 to 90 per cent.[25] This type of resection may be useful as part of a limb-sparing treatment plan with radiotherapy in patients with tumors in proximity to vital organs, bones, or major neurovascular structures.

Wide excision involves the resection of a sarcoma along nonanatomic planes with a margin of surrounding normal tissue in all directions. No standard margin distance can be specified as adequate because the extent of microscopic extent of sarcomas is quite variable. Some sarcomas may extend long distances along fascial planes or have skip areas.[36] This type of resection is associated with a local recurrence rate of 50 per cent.[17] For low-grade sarcomas, wide excision alone is adequate therapy. Wide excision of all gross tumor with adjuvant radiation therapy is appropriate for local treatment of high-grade sarcomas.

Radical resection requires the removal of all tissue in the anatomic compartment occupied by the tumor. Muscle group or compartment resections are radical resections typically applied to tumors contained within muscle compartments. This type of resection involves dissection along a fascial plane at least one uninvolved anatomic structure away from the tumor, and should include the removal of the origin and insertion of all muscles within that compartment. Excellent local control, similar to that seen with amputation, may be achieved.[37, 38]

Such extensive surgery does not obviate the prime surgical objective—negative margins around the tumor. Radical surgery alone, leaving any positive margins, results in universal local failure.[37] It is difficult to apply this type of resection to sarcomas bridging across defined compartments, and to those located in areas of sparse surrounding soft tissue, such as the groin, popliteal space, and upper extremity.[14] Sarcomas such as these are better treated either by amputation when necessary (see further on), or limb-preserving surgery with radiation therapy. Muscle group excisions have little use in modern sarcoma therapy.

Extremity amputation for local control of sarcoma should be limited to those tumors not otherwise treatable by surgery plus radiotherapy because of extensive circumferential involvement of the limb, invasion of a joint, or invasion of major neurovascular structures beyond the reach of reconstruction. Amputation should be viewed as a means of obtaining a wider margin than that possible with less radical surgery. The surgeon must keep in mind the propensity of these tumors to spread inconspicuously along fascial planes and within muscle bundles that may cross the joint above or below the tumor. An amputation at any level that allows only a narrow margin is inappropriate and likely to result in recurrence in the stump. Complete eradication of the tumor often requires amputation above the joint proximal to the tumor. Earlier diagnosis and the development of limb-preserving therapies has relegated the use of amputation to less than 10 per cent of cases now seen.[6]

TREATMENT OF REGIONAL NODES

Metastases to regional lymph nodes are found in approximately 5 per cent of patients.[39] Node metastases are more common with embryonal rhabdomyosarcoma (12 per cent), synovial cell sarcoma (17 per cent), and epithelioid sarcoma (48 per cent).[40] The presence of node metastases early in the clinical course of patients with sarcoma is a very poor prognostic sign, which indicates a high probability of distant micrometastases, local recurrence, and early death.[24, 39] Therefore, elective regional node dissection is not warranted for adult patients with sarcoma. Along the same lines, curative treatment is improbable in patients with gross regional node disease. Suspicious nodes should be excised for pathologic confirmation of metastatic disease, and treatment should be geared toward prevention and/or palliation of local tumor complications such as pain or ulceration.

Treatment: Technical Considerations

For most sarcomas, the appropriate surgical procedure is wide excision of all gross tumor. The extent of surgery must be determined beforehand by careful examination and review of MRI or CT scans. An elliptical skin incision should be used, encompassing any previous incisions and drainage tracts. Thick, subcutaneous skin flaps are raised to allow wide resection around the tumor if at all possible. Thin flaps may result in wound complications if adjuvant radiotherapy is used. Early identification of structures that are to be preserved, such as major neurovascular bundles or bone, should be accomplished early in the dissection, allowing further, rapid dissection along their surface. A wide margin of normal tissue around the tumor should be removed, consistent with preservation of reasonable function of the part (see Fig. 12–6). The line of dissection should be carefully palpated and visualized throughout the procedure. The electrocautery is preferable for this dissection, except when close to major neurovascular structures. The actual tumor should not be entered or even visualized during the procedure.

After the tumor has been removed, meticulous hemostasis should be achieved. The surgical field and the specific location of the tumor should be carefully marked with clips if radiation therapy is being considered. Skin approximation should be airtight over closed suction drains to speed healing of the flaps to the tumor bed. Drains should be brought out through distal stab wounds. Should the tumor recur locally, resection of these drain tracts will be necessary. Drain incisions proximal to the field may necessitate a higher amputation level if that procedure is required.

Pathologic Evaluation

The surgeon must ensure that the specimen is properly evaluated pathologically by orienting the specimen for the pathologist. Careful gross anatomic evaluation of the tumor and surrounding structures must be carried out at the time of resection. A thorough assessment of the surgical margins for tumor involvement, including evaluation of muscle, bone, nerve, and vascular structures at the edge of amputation specimens, should be performed. The location and relationships of positive margins must be clearly determined to direct further resection, if possible.

Radiation Therapy

Radiation therapy has been used alone for treatment of soft tissue sarcomas with varying success. Dosages in excess of 6500 centigray (cGy) appear to be necessary for local control. In the Massachusetts General Hospital experience, of 26 patients treated with dosages greater than 6500 cGy 61 per cent were free of local relapse at four years follow-up.[41] Only two of 28 patients treated with dosages less than 6500 cGy were alive and free of disease for more than two years. Local control rates are also affected by tumor size, and range from 88 per cent for lesions less than 5 cm to 33 per cent for lesions greater than 10 cm.[42] On the other hand, sarcomas smaller than 5 cm are also easily and successfully treated by surgery alone.

It is clear that radiation therapy in dosages of 6000 cGy or more can eradicate microscopic foci of tumor.[31-33] Local control and five-year disease-free survival rates achievable by conservative excision plus preoperative or postoperative radiation therapy are shown in Table 12–9. Local control is comparable to that seen with radical resections including amputation. Although the series are not truly comparable, the local recurrence data are similar for preoperative and postoperative radiation therapy. Whether one approach is better remains unclear. Functional results have generally been excellent in these trials. The major morbidity has been that of local wound problems related to radiation of skin flaps.

Preoperative radiation has several theoretic advantages over postoperative therapy. These include (1) the eradication of tumor cells, thereby preventing implantation in the wound, (2) tumor cells are better oxygenated preoperatively and are more susceptible to radiation effects, (3) the radiation

TABLE 12–9. RADIATION THERAPY AND SURGERY FOR SOFT TISSUE SARCOMAS: COMBINED SURGERY AND RADIATION THERAPY

	N	FU (Years)	Local Recurrence (%)	5-year DFS (%)
Preoperative Radiation				
MGH[4x]	90	1–18	17	74
M.D. Anderson[2x]	27	5+	7	56
Florida[3x]	19	1–5	5	58
Total	136		13	68
Postoperative Radiation				
MGH[1x]	123	1–12	12	65
M.D. Anderson[31]	300	2–7	22	68
NCI[50]	129	1–8	8	60
UCSF[32]	29	2+	10	68
Total	581		17	65

MGH = Massachusetts General Hospital; Florida = University of Florida; NCI = National Cancer Institute; UCSF = University of California, San Francisco.

treatment volume of the tumor alone is less than the postoperative treatment volume, which includes all dissected tissues and drain tracts, (4) conservative resection may be easier after shrinkage from radiation, and (5) unresectable tumors may be made resectable by radiation therapy. The disadvantages of preoperative radiation therapy are the risk of compromising wound healing and the possibility of incomplete tumor response potentially resulting in a positive resection margin in an area that cannot be further irradiated.

As part of a multimodality treatment plan for sarcomas, radiotherapy is most commonly given in the postoperative period. The advantages of postoperative radiation are (1) the wound is healed prior to the initiation of therapy, (2) the tumor bed can be marked with clips by the surgeon, (3) the surgical specimen can be evaluated to determine those areas where the margins are most narrow, which should continue to be treated when the radiation field is shrunk, and (4) there are experimental data suggesting that radiation treatment of microscopic sarcoma is more effective than treatment of gross disease.[43] Disadvantages of postoperative radiation include the potential for delay in therapy because of wound complications. In addition, residual tumor cells may be rendered hypoxic by surgery, making them less susceptible to radiation. The treatment volume may be increased by the need to include all dissected tissues as well as drainage tracts.

Brachytherapy

Intraoperative or postoperative brachytherapy refers to the application of radioactive sources within or close to the tumor. With this technique, tumors may be directly implanted with iodine-125 seeds. More commonly, for sarcomas, hollow plastic catheters are placed percutaneously into the bed of the resection site. Wires containing iridium-192 sources are then loaded through the catheters postoperatively for four to five days providing a dosage of approximately 4500 cGy. In 1984, Shiu studied a series of 33 patients with locally advanced soft tissue sarcomas treated with surgery plus brachytherapy at Memorial Hospital.[34] More than half of these patients had been advised to undergo amputation. At a median follow-up of 36 months, none of 17 patients with previously untreated sarcomas suffered local tumor recurrence after combined therapy. Subsequently, a prospective randomized trial of resection of all gross tumors plus brachytherapy versus resection alone was carried out at the same institution. All patients with high-grade sarcomas also received adjuvant chemotherapy.[44] At a median follow-up of 16 months, two of 52 patients receiving brachytherapy developed local recurrences compared with nine of 65 patients in the group not receiving brachytherapy (p = 0.06). For high-grade lesions, a significant improvement in local control was seen for patients receiving brachytherapy (no recurrences in 41 patients) compared with those treated by surgery alone (five recurrences in 47 patients; p = 0.03) (Fig. 12–8).

Theoretic advantages to brachytherapy include the potential to provide a high dosage at the tumor bed with maximal sparing of adjacent normal tissues because of the rapid dosage fall off; the possibility of use in selected patients who have received previous external beam radiation therapy in the same area; and the completion of therapy within two weeks after surgery compared with the six to eight weeks required for postoperative radiation therapy. This technique has not gained wide acceptance because of the special equipment and expertise required, and the substantial wound problems associated with high dosages of radiation.

Intraoperative Radiation Therapy

Intraoperative radiation therapy (IORT) involves the use of a single high dose of electron beam or orthovoltage therapy at the time of surgery, delivered directly to the tumor bed. Surrounding structures can be moved out of the field of radiation and protected with lead shields. IORT has predominantly been used for retroperitoneal sarcomas. Although the frequency of radiation enteritis is reduced in such patients receiving IORT, a small randomized trial showed no disease-free or overall survival benefit in

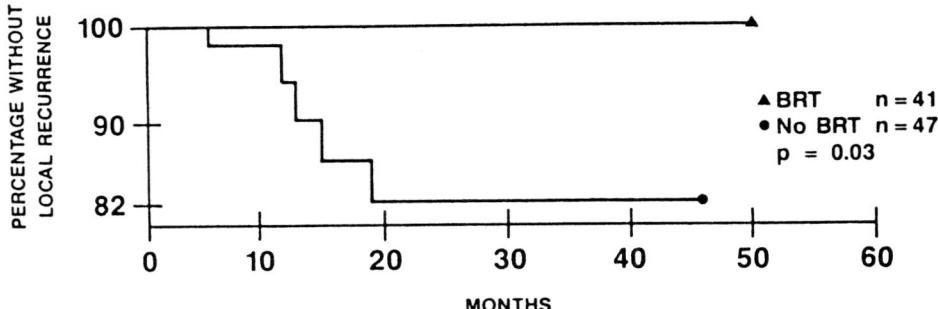

Figure 12–8. Freedom from local recurrence in patients with high-grade sarcomas. Prospective randomized trial of surgery plus brachytherapy (BRT) versus surgery alone. A significant improvement in local control is seen with the addition of brachytherapy. (From Brennan, M.F., Hilaris, B., Shiu, M.H., et al.: Local recurrence in adult soft tissue sarcoma. A randomized trial of brachytherapy. Arch. Surg. *122*:1289–1293, 1987.)

patients receiving IORT compared with those receiving postoperative external beam therapy.[45] Therefore, it is not possible to define a specific role for IORT for the treatment of soft tissue sarcomas.

The success in controlling local disease by radiation and surgery should not divert surgeons from their primary technical objective: providing an adequate resection margin when possible. Radiation is not a substitute for inadequate, poorly planned, or poorly executed surgery. Conservative treatment plans are most effective in achieving local control when adequate negative margins are achieved by the surgeon.[24] Nonetheless, adjunctive radiation therapy may improve functional results by reducing the necessity of wide margins, thereby preserving tissue. Eighty-five per cent of patients undergoing conservative resection and radiotherapy for extremity sarcomas can be expected to maintain functional limbs.[31]

Most of the data available on conservative resection and radiation therapy relate to high-grade tumors. At the present time, there is little evidence to indicate any benefit in local recurrence for low-grade tumors, which can be adequately excised. The risk of metastatic disease with low-grade sarcomas is approximately 14 per cent and is not altered by any type of adjuvant therapies, local recurrence, or the adequacy of surgical margins.[12]

Adjuvant Chemotherapy

Unfortunately, many patients with soft tissue sarcomas will develop metastatic disease, predominantly in the lungs, despite adequate local control. Most of these patients with metastatic disease have high-grade sarcomas and, for this patient group, effective adjuvant systemic therapy is needed. Attempts to demonstrate benefit from adjuvant chemotherapy have been plagued by a number of factors. Sarcomas are relatively uncommon tumors. Few institutions have been able to accrue a substantial number of cases necessary to perform adequate studies. Patients have usually been treated with a variety of combinations of chemotherapy, surgery, and radiation therapy, increasing the number of variables to be evaluated. Pathologists frequently do not agree with each other on the histologic type or grade of sarcomas, making comparison of results between studies difficult or inappropriate. Prognosis varies with different sites, further reducing the number of comparable patients within a particular series.

Despite these difficulties, several themes are common to both retrospective and prospective studies of adjuvant chemotherapy. Doxorubicin (Adriamycin) is the single most effective agent with overall response rates of 25 to 40 per cent in advanced disease. Although it has been combined in a number of trials with other drugs, it is not clear that combinations of chemotherapeutic agents are better than doxorubicin alone. A number of retrospective studies using historic controls suggested that disease-free survival was improved by adjuvant chemotherapy containing doxorubicin.[46] Recent prospective randomized studies indicate that historic survival data are considerably lower than those that can be expected now, and are inappropriate controls.

There are now at least nine prospective randomized trials of adjuvant chemotherapy for soft tissue sarcomas (Table 12–10). The drug common to all studies is doxorubicin. Most of these studies have included only interme-

TABLE 12–10. PROSPECTIVE RANDOMIZED TRIALS OF ADJUVANT CHEMOTHERAPY FOR SOFT TISSUE SARCOMAS

Author/ Institution		Year	N	Grade	Site	Chemo-therapy	FU (Months)	% DFS Treated/ Control	% Survival Treated/ Control
Baker, A.	NCI	1988	67	High Int	Ext	A, C, M (HD)	60	75/53*	82/60
Picci	IOR Bologna	1987	77	High Int	Ext	A		68/41*	87/67
Benjamin	MDAH	1987	43	High	Ext	A, C, V, Amd	60	60/35*	75/61
Bramwell	EORTC	1988	358	All	All	CYVADIC	36	67/52*	79/74
Alvegard	Scand	1986	139	High	Ext	A		55/52	44/40
Edmonson	Mayo	1985	61	All	All	Amd, VC/ VA, DTIC	60	82/63	91/77
Wilson	DFCI/ ECOG/ MGH	1986	75	High Int	All	A	48	74/62	68/66
Eilber	UCLA	1986	114	High	Ext	A	30	78/74	
Baker, L.	Intergroup Sarcoma Committee	1987	41	High Int	All	A	24	77/50	72/62

* p < 0.05
NCI = National Cancer Institute; MDAH = M.D. Anderson Hospital; EORTC = European Organization for Research on Treatment of Cancer; IOR = Instituto Ortopedico Rizzoli; Scand = Scandinavian Sarcoma Group; DFCI = Dana-Farber Cancer Institute; ECOG = Eastern Cooperative Oncology Group; MGH = Massachusetts General Hospital; UCLA = University of California at Los Angeles; Mayo = Mayo Clinic.

A = Adriamycin; C = cyclophosphamide; M = Methotrexate; HD = High dose; Amd = dactinomycin; V = vincristine; DTIC = dacarbazine; CYVADIC = cyclophosphamide, vincristine, Adriamycin, dacarbazine.

diate or high-grade lesions. Some have included patients who were treated preoperatively. The types of surgery in these studies were variable. Follow-up in several studies is short.

The results are mixed. Four studies have shown a statistically significant improvement in disease-free survival. The remainder have shown a slight, but not statistically significant, improvement in disease-free survival. Only the National Cancer Institute study has shown an improvement in overall survival. This suggests that adjuvant chemotherapy may delay the time to evidence of metastasis without altering the overall course. The major toxicity of doxorubicin has been a significant incidence of cardiomyopathy.

There is no evidence for benefit from adjuvant chemotherapy for nonextremity sarcomas. At the present time, the benefit of adjuvant chemotherapy for treatment of patients with soft tissue sarcomas remains unresolved. A number of trials are ongoing and adjuvant chemotherapy for high-grade soft tissue sarcomas should only be administered within these prospective clinical trials.

Intraarterial Infusion Therapy

Preoperative intraarterial infusion of doxorubicin with and without synchronous radiation therapy has been reported.[47,48] This therapy has been applied to patients with very large tumors for preoperative shrinkage, and as preoperative adjuvant therapy in patients with smaller tumors. Disease-free survival has been comparable to that seen with postoperative adjuvant therapy. Histologic evidence of tumor necrosis is noted after doxorubicin infusion alone and seems to be enhanced by the combination of synchronized radiotherapy. There is no comparative data that show any benefit of this technique over postoperative or no adjuvant chemotherapy.

FOLLOW-UP AND RECURRENCE

Follow-up of patients with soft tissue sarcoma is based on the temporal and anatomic patterns of and the ability to treat recurrent tumors. Eighty per cent of local recurrences occur within the first two years after treatment, and almost all are apparent by five years (Fig. 12–9).[28, 37, 49] Local recurrence is not uncommon depending upon the location of the primary and the nature of primary treatment. Sarcomas of the head and neck are prone to local recurrence because of difficulties obtaining adequate margins. As noted previously, lymph node metastases are uncommon. The lungs are virtually always the first site of dissemination for patients with extremity sarcoma. The liver becomes more important for patients with intraabdominal tumors (Table 12–11). Approximately 80 per cent of all recurrences become evident within five years.[6]

Patient follow-up should include frequent early reexaminations of the local regional site every three months for the first two years, every six months for the next two years, and yearly thereafter. For sarcomas located in deep fleshy locations, CT scans or MRI of the local area may be appropriate. Tumors previously located in superficial locations can be further evaluated for recurrence by careful physical examination.

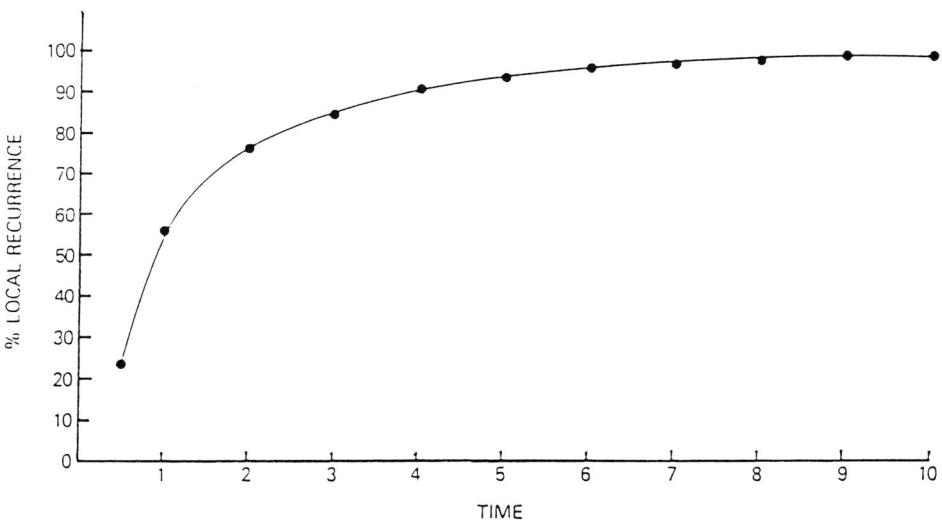

Figure 12–9. Temporal pattern of local recurrence among those tumors that will recur. (From Cantin, J., McNeer, G.P., Chu, F.C., and Booher, R.J.: The problem of local recurrence after treatment of soft tissue sarcoma. Ann. Surg. *168:*47–53, 1968.)

TABLE 12–11. SITES OF INITIAL RECURRENCE FROM SOFT TISSUE SARCOMA

	Total No.	Adjuvant Chemotherapy	No Adjuvant Chemotherapy
Isolated pulmonary	56	26	30
Isolated local	21	10	11
Bone	4	1	3
Retroperitoneum	1	1	0
Liver	3	2	1
Mesentery	1	0	1
Epidural	2	1	1
Subcutaneous	3	1	2
Lymph nodes	1	0	1
Lung + bone	2	1	1
Diffuse abdominal sarcomatosis*	6	3	3
Local + lung + bone	1	0	1
Lung + lymph nodes	2	0	2
Lung + liver + local + subcutaneous	1	0	1
Local + lung	1	1	0
Local + lymph nodes	1	0	1
Peritoneal wall + lymph nodes	1	1	0
Total	107	48	59

*Diffuse abdominal sarcomatosis is defined as widespread, multiple-organ, intraabdominal disease with greater than three discontinuous lesions.

From Potter, D.A., Glenn, J., Kinsella, T., et al.: Patterns of recurrence in patients with high grade soft tissue sarcomas. J. Clin. Oncol. 3:353–366, 1985.

Isolated locally recurrent disease is amenable to further surgical treatment. In the National Cancer Institute experience, 20 of 21 isolated local recurrences were resectable with three-year disease-free and overall survival rates of 59 and 69 per cent (Fig. 12–10). Similar results have been recorded from Memorial Hospital where the five-year survival rate was 45 per cent.[28, 50] Therapy for recurrent sarcomas of any grade consists of surgical resection of disease with the addition of radiotherapy in those patients not previously treated. A wide resection of all tissue planes previously dissected is necessary. Amputation may be appropriate for some patients as described previously.

Pulmonary resection for sarcoma metastases to the lung is now widely accepted. A plain chest x-ray should be obtained every six months for the first two years. Patients previously evaluated by chest CT scans are best followed by serial scans because the development of a new nodule in these patients almost always represents metastatic disease. The finding of nodules suspicious of metastatic disease on plain chest x-ray warrants further evaluation with the CT scan because multiple nodules may be present.

The criteria for resection of pulmonary metastases include (1) the patient must be medically fit for thoracotomy, (2) the local disease must be controlled or controllable, (3) there must be no other effective therapy, and (4) there should be no extra pulmonary metastatic sites. Approximately 70 to 80 per cent of patients with isolated pulmonary metastases may be rendered free of disease after surgery.[51] Approximately 25 to 30 per cent of patients will survive five years. Patients with fewer than four nodules, tumor doubling

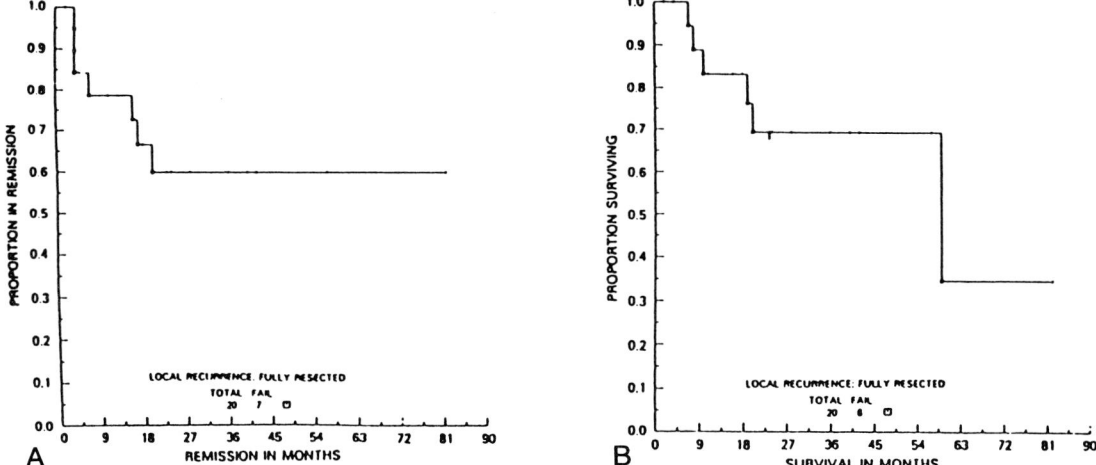

Figure 12–10. *A,* Disease-free and *B,* Overall survival in patients with high-grade sarcomas after resection of local only recurrence. (From Potter, D.A., Glenn, J., Kinsella, T., et al.: Patterns of recurrence in patients with high-grade soft tissue sarcomas. J. Clin. Oncol. *3:*353–366, 1985.)

time of greater than 20 days, and disease-free interval greater than six months appear to have improved rates of survival.[52] Mortality from pulmonary resection for sarcoma is negligible and morbidity is low because these lesions are frequently located peripherally and are amenable to wedge resection.

RETROPERITONEAL SARCOMAS

Sarcomas of the retroperitoneum are a subset of soft tissue sarcomas for which all aspects of management are more difficult and challenging. The anatomic location makes biopsy difficult. Only one-third of retroperitoneal masses will be sarcomas, indicating the potential benefit of diagnosis prior to definitive therapy.[53] The options include needle biopsy, which provides a small piece of tissue that may be inadequate for diagnosis and grading and may also allow the seeding of malignant cells along the needle tract. Open biopsy also increases the risk of local tumor implantation due to the spillage of cells at the time of surgery. Nonetheless, an open intraoperative biopsy should always be performed if the lesion is unresectable or if an alternative malignant process, such as lymphoma or germ cell tumor, are suspected. Every attempt should be made to minimize spillage of tumor cells. It may be reasonable to resect a tumor without prior biopsy if the patient has symptoms of obstruction or hemorrhage and would be treated surgically regardless of the diagnosis. In general, major ablative procedures such as pancreaticoduodenectomy or abdominoperineal resection should not be undertaken without histologic confirmation.

Most retroperitoneal sarcomas are quite large, averaging more than 20 cm in diameter (Table 12–12), and are locally invasive over an extensive area. Consequently, it is uncommon for these tumors to be resected with

TABLE 12-12. RETROPERITONEAL SARCOMAS: SIZE

Diameter	Number of Patients	
	Pathologic	*Clinical*
<5 cm	0	1
5-10 cm	8	9
>10 cm	61	59

The mean diameter is approximately 20 cm.
Most retroperitoneal sarcomas achieve very large dimensions prior to diagnosis and treatment.
From Jaques, D.P., Coit, D.G., and Brennan, M.F.: Soft tissue sarcomas of the retroperitoneum. *In* Shiu, M.H., and Brennan, M.F. (Eds.): Surgical Management of Soft Tissue Sarcoma. Philadelphia, Lea & Febiger, 1989. p. 161.

negative microscopic margins, and a true wide resection is extremely rare. Resection of other intraabdominal organs may be necessary. Complete resection is possible in approximately 50 per cent of cases.[26] Published survival data approximate 40 to 70 per cent at five years with lesions that are completely resected.[16]

Additional treatment is clearly necessary for these patients. However, despite its widespread use, in a randomized trial, adjuvant chemotherapy provided no advantage in disease-free or overall survival, and the toxicity in the chemotherapy arm was substantial.[54] Radiation therapy is limited by toxicity to surrounding structures and, therefore, adequate dosages are difficult to deliver and therapeutic benefit is therefore compromised. Intraoperative radiation therapy has been used with the objectives of providing a higher dosage but reducing the risk of radiation enteritis. With IORT, structures can be moved out of the field of radiation or protected by lead shields. However, a small trial comparing IORT and external beam radiation therapy showed no benefit in disease-free survival, local control, or control within the field of radiation itself.[45]

Reported five-year survival rates following treatment of retroperitoneal sarcomas vary from 16 to 37 per cent. Complete resection, which is possible in approximately 50 per cent of cases, is associated with a five-year survival of 40 to 70 per cent (Table 12–13).[53] Very few patients whose tumors are left unresected survive five years. Patients treated by partial resection have a five-year survival of approximately 40 per cent (Fig. 12–11).[55] This apparent improvement may be illusory as the latter patients typically have less disease.

TABLE 12-13. RESECTABILITY OF SOFT TISSUE SARCOMAS IN MULTIPLE SERIES

Series	No. Pts	Completely Resected	Partially Resected	Unresectable
Braasch	37	40%	20%	40%
Cody	68	66%		
Jaques	86	50%	40%	10%
Karakousis	68	40%	10%	50%
McGrath	47	38%	38%	24%
Storm	54	61%	9%	30%

Modified from Jaques, D.P., Coit, D.G., and Brennan, M.F.: Soft tissue sarcomas of the retroperitoneum. *In* Shiu, M.H., and Brennan, M.F. (Eds.): Surgical Management of Soft Tissue Sarcoma. Philadelphia, Lea & Febiger, 1989, p. 165.

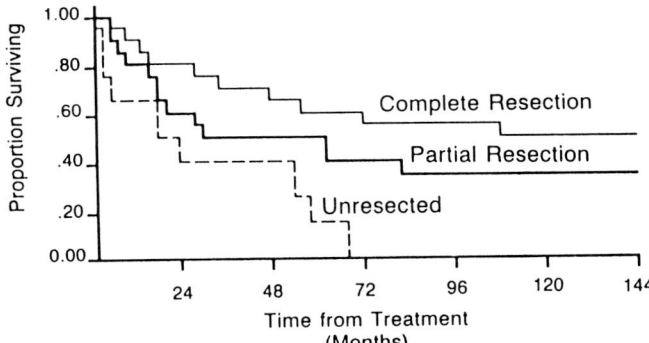

Figure 12–11. Actuarial survival of patients with retroperitoneal sarcomas after complete resection, partial resection, or nonresection. (From Jaques, D.P., Coit, D.G., and Brennan, M.F.: Soft tissue of the retroperitoneum. *In* Shiu, M.H., Brennan, M.F. (Eds.): Surgical Management of Soft Tissue Sarcoma. Philadelphia, Lea & Febiger, 1989, p. 166.)

REFERENCES

1. Boring, C.C., Squires, T.S., and Tong, T.: Cancer Statistics, 1991. CA *41:*19–36, 1991.
2. Kim, K., Tidrick, R.T., Skeel, R.T., et al.: Fibrosarcoma of the chest wall following mastectomy in radiation therapy for mammary carcinoma. Breast, Diseases of the Breast *6:*26–30, 1980.
3. Kim, J.H., Chu, F.C., Woodard, H.Q., et al.: Radiation induced soft tissue and bone sarcoma. Radiology *129:*501–508, 1978.
4. Halperin, E.C., Greenberg, M.S., and Suit, H.D.: Sarcoma of bone and soft tissue following treatment of Hodgkin's disease. Cancer *53:*232–236, 1984.
5. Smith, J.: Post-radiation sarcoma of bone in Hodgkin's disease. Skeletal Radiol. *16:*524–532, 1987.
6. Lawrence, W., Donegan, W.L., Natarajan, N., et al.: Adult soft tissue sarcomas. A pattern of care survey of the American College of Surgeons. Ann. Surg. *205:*349–359, 1987.
7. Enzinger, F.M., and Weiss, S.W.: Soft Tissue Tumors. St. Louis, C.V. Mosby, 1983, pp. 6–9.
8. Presant, C.A., Russell, W.O., Alexander, R.W., et al.: Soft tissue and bone sarcoma peer review: The frequency of disagreement in diagnosis and the need for second pathology opinions. The Southeastern Cancer Study Group experience. J. Clin. Oncol. *4:*1658–1661, 1986.
9. Lack, E.E., Steinberg, S.M., White, D.E., et al.: Extremity soft tissue sarcomas: Analysis of prognostic variables in 300 cases and evaluation of tumor necrosis as a factor in stratifying higher grade sarcomas. J. Surg. Oncol. *41:*263–273, 1989.
10. Costa, J., Wesley, R.A., Glatstein, E., et al.: The grading of soft tissue sarcomas. Results of a clinical histopathologic correlation in a series of 163 cases. Cancer *53:*530–541, 1984.
11. Trojani, M., Contesso, G., Coindre, J.M., et al.: Soft tissue sarcomas of adults: Study of pathologic prognostic variables and definition of histopathological-creating system. Intl. J. Cancer *33:*37–42, 1984.
12. Donahue, J.H., Collin, C., Friedrich, C., et al.: Low grade soft tissue sarcomas of the extremities. Analysis of risk factors for metastasis. Cancer *62:*184–193, 1988.
13. Costa, J., Wesley, R.A., Glatstein, E., et al.: The grading of soft tissue sarcomas. Results of a clinical histopathologic correlation in a series of 163 cases. Cancer *53:*530–541, 1984.
14. Shiu, M.H., and Hajdu, S.I.: Management of soft tissue sarcoma of the extremity. Semin. Oncol. *8:*172–179, 1981.
15. Shiu, M.H., and Brennan, M.F.: Clinical features in diagnosis of soft tissue sarcoma. *In* Shiu, M.H., and Brennan, M.F. (Eds.): Surgical Management of Soft Tissue Sarcoma. Philadelphia, Lea & Febiger, 1989, pp. 23–38.
16. Demas, B.E., Heelan, R.T., Lane, J., et al.: Soft tissue sarcomas of the extremities: Comparison of MR and CT in determining the extent of disease. AJR *150:*615–620, 1988.
17. Rosenberg, S.A., and Glatstein, E.J.: Perspectives on the role of surgery and radiation therapy in the treatment of soft tissue sarcomas of the extremities. Semin. Oncol. *8:*190–200, 1981.
18. Chang, A.E., Schaner, E.G., Conkel, A.M., et al.: Evaluation of computed tomography in the detection of pulmonary metastases: A prospective study. Cancer *43:*913, 1979.
19. Roth, J.A.: Treatment of metastatic cancer to lung. *In* DeVita, V.T., Jr., Hellman, S., and Rosenberg, S. (Eds.): Cancer Principles and Practice of Oncology, 3rd ed. Philadelphia, J.B. Lippincott, 1989, pp. 2261–2275.
20. Pass, H.I., Dwyer, A., Makuch, R., and Roth, J.A.: Detection of pulmonary metastases in

patients with osteogenic and soft tissue sarcomas: The superiority of CT scans compared with conventional linear tomograms using dynamic analysis. J. Clin. Oncol. *3:*1261–1265, 1985.
21. Bears, O.H., Henson, D.E., Hutter, R.U.P., and Myers, M.H. (Eds): American Joint Committee on Cancer Manual for Staging of Cancer, 3rd edition, Philadelphia, J.B. Lippincott, 1988, pp. 127–129.
22. Hajdu, S.I.: Differential Diagnosis of Soft Tissue and Bone Tumors. Philadelphia, Lea & Febiger, 1985.
23. Shiu, M.H., and Brennan, M.F.: Staging of soft tissue sarcoma. *In* Shiu, M.H., and Brennan, M.F. (Eds.): Surgical Management of Soft Tissue Sarcoma. Philadelphia, Lea & Febiger, 1989, pp. 39–44.
24. Collin, C., Godbold, J., Hajdu, S.I., et al.: Localized extremity soft tissue sarcoma: Analysis of factors affecting survival. J. Clin. Oncol. *5:*601, 1987.
25. Fine, G., Ohorodnik, J.M., Horn, R.C., Jr., et al.: Soft tissue sarcomas: Their clinical behavior and course and influencing factors: *In* Seventh National Cancer Center Conference Proceedings. Philadelphia, J.B. Lippincott, 1973, pp. 873–882.
26. Gerner, R.E., Moore, G.E., and Pickren, J.W.: Soft tissue sarcomas. Ann. Surg. *181:*803–808, 1975.
27. Markhede, G., Angervall, L., and Stener, B.: A multivariate analysis of the prognosis after surgical treatment of malignant soft tissue tumors. Cancer *49:*1721–1733, 1982.
28. Shiu, M.H., Castro, E.B., Hajdu, S.I., et al.: Surgical treatment of 297 soft tissue sarcomas of the lower extremity. Ann. Surg. *182:*597, 1975.
29. Kilman, J.W., Clatworthy, H.W., Jr., Newton, W.A., et al.: Reasonable surgery for rhabdomyosarcoma. A study of 67 cases. Ann. Surg. *178:*346, 1973.
30. McNeer, G.P., Cantin, J., Chu, F., et al.: Effectiveness of radiation therapy in the management of sarcoma of the soft somatic tissues. Cancer *22:*391, 1968.
31. Lindberg, R.D., Martin, R.G., Romsdahl, M.M., and Barkley, H.T., Jr.: Conservative surgery in postoperative radiotherapy in 300 adults with soft tissue sarcomas. Cancer *47:*2391–2392, 1981.
32. Leibel, S.A., Tranbaugh, R.F., Wara, W.N., et al.: Soft tissue sarcomas of the extremities: Survival and patterns of failure with conservative surgery and postoperative irradiation compared to surgery alone. Cancer *50:*1076–1083, 1982.
33. Suit, H.D., Proppe, K.H., Mankin, H.F., and Wood, W.C.: Preoperative radiation therapy for sarcoma of soft tissue. Cancer *47:*2269–2274, 1981.
34. Shiu, M.H., Turnbull, A.D., Nori, D., et al.: Control of locally advanced extremity soft tissue sarcoma by function saving resection and brachytherapy. Cancer *53:*1385–1392, 1984.
35. Rosenberg, S.A., Tepper, J., Glatstein, E., et al.: The treatment of soft tissue sarcomas of the extremities. Prospective randomized trial of (1) limb sparing surgery plus radiation therapy compared with amputation and (2) the role of adjuvant chemotherapy. Ann. Surg. *196:*305–315, 1982.
36. Shiu, M.H., and Brennan, M.F.: Principles of surgical management. *In* Shiu, M.H., Brennan, M.F. (Eds): Surgical Management of Soft Tissue Sarcoma. Philadelphia, Lea & Febiger, 1989, pp. 64–76.
37. Simon, M.A., and Enneking, W.F.: The management of soft tissue sarcomas of the extremities. J. Bone Joint Surg. (Am.) *58:*317, 1976.
38. Bowden, L., and Booher, R.J.: The principle and technique of resection of soft parts sarcoma. Surgery *44:*963, 1958.
39. Weingrad, D.N., and Rosenberg, S.A.: Early lymphatic spread of osteogenic and soft tissue sarcomas. Surgery *84:*231–240, 1978.
40. Chase, D.R., and Enzinger, F.M.: Epithelioid sarcoma. Am. J. Surg. Pathol. *9:*241–263, 1985.
41. Suit, H.D.: Sarcomas of soft tissue. *In* The 3rd Annual Current Approaches to Radiation Oncology, Biology, and Physics. San Francisco, University of California, 1983, pp. 138–141.
42. Tepper, J.E., and Suit, H.D.: Radiation therapy of soft tissue sarcomas. Cancer *55:*2273–2277, 1985.
43. Todoroki, T., and Suit, H.D.: Effective fractionated irradiation prior to conservation and radical surgery on therapeutic gain in spontaneous fibrosarcoma of the C-3H mouse. J. Surg. Oncol. *31:*279–286, 1986.
44. Brennan, M.F., Hilaris, B., Shiu, M.H., et al.: Local recurrence in adult soft tissue sarcoma. A randomized trial of brachytherapy. Arch. Surg. *122:*1289–1293, 1987.
45. Kinsella, T.J., Sindelar, W.F., Lack, E., et al.: Preliminary results of a randomized study of adjuvant radiation therapy in resectable adult retroperitoneal soft tissue sarcomas. J. Clin. Oncol. *6:*18–25, 1988.
46. Greenall, M.J., McGill, G.B., Dacoste, J.J., et al.: Chemotherapy for soft tissue sarcoma. Surg. Gynecol. Obstet. *162:*193, 1986

47. Karakousis, C.P., Lopez, R., Catane, R., et al.: Intra-arterial adriamycin in the treatment of soft tissue sarcomas. J. Surg. Oncol. *13:*21, 1980.
48. Morton, D.L., Eilber, F.R., Townsend, C.M., Jr., et al.: Limb salvage from a multidisciplinary treatment approach for skeletal and soft tissue sarcoma to the extremity. Ann. Surg. *184:*268–278, 1976.
49. Cantin, J., McNeer, G.P., Chu, F.C., and Booher, R.J.: The problem of local recurrence after treatment of soft tissue sarcoma. Ann. Surg. *168:*47–53, 1968.
50. Potter, D.A., Glenn, J., Kinsella, T.J., et al.: Patterns of recurrence in patients with high grade soft tissue sarcomas. J. Clin. Oncol. *3:*353–366, 1985.
51. Martini, N., McCormack, P.M., Bains, M.S., et al.: Surgery for solitary and multiple pulmonary metastases. NY State J. Med. *78:*1711–1713, 1978.
52. Roth, J.A., Putnam, J.B., Wesley, M.N., et al.: Differing determinants of prognosis following resection of pulmonary metastases from osteogenic and soft tissue sarcoma patients. Cancer *55:*1361–1366, 1985.
53. Jaques, D.P., Coit, D.G., and Brennan, M.F.: Soft tissue sarcoma of the retroperitoneum in surgical management of soft tissue sarcoma. *In* Shiu, M.H., and Brennan, M.F. (Eds.): Surgical Management of Soft Tissue Sarcoma. Philadelphia, Lea & Febiger, 1989, pp. 157–169.
54. Glenn, J., Sindelar, W.F., Kinsella, T.J., et al.: Results of multimodality therapy of resectable soft tissue sarcomas of the retroperitoneum. Surgery *97:*316–324, 1985.
55. Jaques, D.P., Coit, D.G., Hajdu, S.I., and Brennan, M.F.: Management of primary and recurrent soft tissue sarcoma of the retroperitoneum. Ann. Surg. *212:*51–59, 1990.
1x. Suit, H.D., Mankin, H.J., Wood, W.C., et al.: Pre-operative, intraoperative, and postoperative radiation in the treatment of soft tissue sarcoma. Cancer *55:*2659–2667, 1985.
2x. Lindberg, R.: Treatment of localized soft tissue sarcomas in adults at M.D. Anderson Hospital and Tumor Institute (1960–1981). Cancer Treatment Symposium *3:*59–65, 1985.
3x. Enneking, W.F., and McAuliffe, J.A.: Adjunctive preoperative radiation therapy in treatment of soft tissue sarcomas: A preliminary report. Cancer Treatment Symposium *3:*37–42, 1985.
4x. Suit, H.D., Mankin, H.J., Schiller, A.L., et al.: Results of treatment of sarcoma of soft tissue by radiation and surgery at Massachusetts General Hospital. Cancer Treatment Symposium *3:*43–47, 1985.
5x. Hajdu, S.I.: Histologic diagnosis and grade of soft tissue sarcomas. *In* Shiu, M.H., and Brennan, M.F. (eds.): Surgical Management of Soft Tissue Sarcoma. Philadelphia, Lea & Febiger, 1989, p. 13.

13

UROLOGIC CARCINOMA

PROSTATE CANCER
by Paul A. Church, M.D.

INCIDENCE AND EPIDEMIOLOGY

Prostate cancer continues to present both diagnostic dilemmas and therapeutic challenges to the clinician. Prostatic carcinoma is the most common malignancy in men over 50 years of age. It is clear that the overall prevalence of occult prostatic malignancy far exceeds its overt clinical detection and morbidity. Autopsy studies have shown carcinoma of the prostate in 10 to 46 per cent of men dying from other causes.[1,2] The incidence increases with age and may approach 80 per cent by the ninth decade of life.[3] Furthermore, unsuspected carcinoma is not an infrequent finding (10 per cent) in tissue removed with a clinical diagnosis of benign prostatic hyperplasia.

In the United States, prostate cancer appears to be surpassing lung neoplasms as the most common cancer in men over 50 years of age. However, as a cause of cancer deaths, it ranks third in this age group. American Blacks have the highest incidence of prostatic carcinoma, while Orientals have the lowest. Epidemiologic studies indicate that both genetics and environment may influence the expression of prostatic carcinoma. When prostatic cancer does occur in younger men, it may appear to have a more aggressive and lethal behavior. This observation is influenced by few competing causes of death and a longer risk period for tumor progression. Recent analyses indicate that prognosis directly relates to grade, stage, and treatment, rather than to age.[4]

The etiology of prostate cancer is unknown. Efforts to find a link between prostatic cancer and sexual practices or sexually transmitted diseases have been inconclusive. Age and functioning testes play a crucial role in the development of prostate cancer; it rarely occurs before the age of 50, and it has not been observed in eunuchs. Although some studies have suggested an increased risk for prostatic malignancy in men with benign prostatic hyperplasia, it seems more likely that these two conditions develop independently in the aging male population.

The occurrence of occult carcinoma and the discrepancy between prevalence and morbidity have led some observers to postulate that there are different subsets of prostatic carcinoma with markedly different histologic behavior. However, the work of McNeal suggests an explanation for tumor progression based on size and loss of differentiation.[5] In this theory, the vast majority of prostatic tumors are at least moderately differentiated initially and expand slowly as predicted by long doubling times. Loss of differentiation directly correlates with increasing tumor volume. The ability to metastasize probably develops as a tumor reaches a "critical mass" and areas of poorly differentiated cells appear. A change in tumor kinetics then leads to an acceleration in disease progression.

DIAGNOSIS

In its earliest stages, carcinoma of the prostate is asymptomatic. The majority of prostatic neoplasms are diagnosed in more advanced stages. Voiding symptoms often develop in these more advanced cancers, although patients with early lesions may present with complaints referable to associated benign prostatic hyperplasia. Diagnosis may result from analysis of specimens removed during prostatectomy for bladder outlet obstruction and presumed benign prostatic enlargement. Some patients will have symptoms and signs of metastatic disease, such as weight loss, anemia, and bone pain.

For many years, digital rectal examination (DRE) and needle biopsy have been the standard "tools" for detection of prostatic malignancy.[6] For early diagnosis, the clinician must maintain a high index of suspicion for subtle changes in gland texture and consistency, since the classic finding of stony-hard nodularity is often present only after local advancement and extracapsular spread have already occurred. Approximately 75 per cent of carcinomas develop in the posterior, "peripheral" zone and, therefore, are most accessible to transrectal detection.

Transrectal ultrasound (TRUS) is emerging as a valuable tool in the early detection of small prostatic neoplasms. TRUS can detect lesions less than 1 cm in diameter and lesions that are not palpable by DRE.[7, 8] Preliminary reports suggest that TRUS may be more sensitive than DRE in the detection of prostatic cancer.[9] Our institution is presently involved in a multicenter, national study (National Prostate Cancer Detection Project) to address the overall usefulness of TRUS as a "screening tool" for early detection of prostate cancer. In our preliminary experience with this study, the addition of TRUS to routine digital examination has more than doubled the detection rate of small carcinomas, primarily by discovering nonpalpable, peripherally located tumors.

Following initial   ction by DRE or TRUS, a biopsy must be done to confirm the diagnosis. Needle biopsies are commonly performed either transperineally or transrectally.

Spring-loaded biopsy devices and smaller needles have reduced pain and discomfort, allowing biopsies to be performed with little or no anesthesia. Ultrasound guidance of biopsies has improved the sampling of small prostatic lesions. Transrectal fine needle aspiration (FNA) has also gained acceptance for diagnosing prostatic carcinoma. The sensitivity of FNA may be greater than conventional core biopsies for detection of malignancy, probably by the sampling of more areas. The skills of an experienced cytopathologist are necessary to accurately interpret aspirates.

GRADE AND STAGE

Histologic grading of prostatic carcinoma has prognostic significance and may therefore influence the choice of therapy. The grade of the neoplasm tends to directly correlate with the clinical behavior, the risk of metastatic disease, and overall prognosis. Descriptively, prostatic adenocarcinoma can be classified as well, moderately, or poorly differentiated. The commonly used Gleason grading system is an effort to further quantitate the degree of differentiation and heterogeneity of prostatic cancer by assigning a "score" between two (well) and ten (poor). The Mostofi system uses grades between I and III based on glandular architecture and individual cellular characteristics.

Efforts to identify more accurate predictors of biologic behavior and prognosis have focused on nuclear DNA content and nuclear shape analysis. Ploidy studies of prostate tumor cells have revealed that diploid carcinomas have a more favorable prognosis than tetraploid or aneuploid tumors. Tumor ploidy may correlate better with patient survival than with histologic grade and thereby prove to be useful in selecting therapy in certain subgroups of patients with prostatic carcinoma.[10] Studies of nuclear shape, including indicators such as "roundness factor" have shown a high correlation between nuclear irregularity and progression of disease. Nuclear shape analysis may allow stratification of patients with prostatic cancer into prognostic categories and predict outcome better than other indicators.[11] Currently, the clinical utility of nuclear shape analysis is limited by its labor-intensive methodology.

A staging evaluation is necessary prior to decisions regarding management. The work of McNeal and Stamey has shown that tumor volume and grade have predictive value for estimating risk of metastatic disease.[12] Invasion and penetration of the prostatic capsule occur first in the local advancement of prostatic neoplasm. Extension to the seminal vesicles and bladder neck may occur before the onset of disseminated disease. The obturator lymph nodes tend to be the initial sites of metastatic spread. Later, other pelvic and other retroperitoneal nodes are involved, followed by osseous dissemination, and much less commonly, visceral metastases.

The Whitmore-Jewett classification of prostatic cancer is the most commonly used system in the United States. The staging system proposed by the Union Internationale Contre Le Cancer (UICC), sometimes called the TNM System, uses the T category to define the extent of primary tumor, the N to indicate lymph nodes status, and M to designate distant metastases. The stages of prostate cancer are described in Table 13–1. There is ample evidence to show that disease does not always progress in stepwise sequence from stage A to stage D. Stage A neoplasms are undetected by rectal examination. These cancers have proved to be especially challenging and

TABLE 13–1. STAGING OF PROSTATIC CANCER

Whitmore-Jewett System	UICC	Description
A1	T_{0a}	Microscopic focal tumors, generally fewer than 5 foci or less than 5% area
A2	T_{0b}	Microscopic but diffuse cancer; includes all high-grade microscopic tumors
B1	T_{1a}, T_{1b}	Palpable nodule <2 cm in size or confined to one lobe of prostate
B2	T_{1c}, T_2	Palpable nodule >2 cm in size or involving both lobes of prostate
C	T_3, T_4	Palpable tumor that extends beyond prostatic capsule to involve seminal vesicles or lateral pelvic wall
D0	$T_{0-4}, N-, M-$	Elevated acid phosphatase level, without other evidence of disease beyond prostate or periprostate region
D1	$T_{0-4}, N+, M-$	Lymph node metastasis without evident extrapelvic disease
D2	$T_{0-4}, N+, M+$	Metastatic disease outside the pelvis, usually to bone

From Smith, J.A., Jr., and Middleton, R.G.: Clinical Management of Prostatic Cancer. Year Book Medical Publishers, Inc., 1987.

controversial since their behavior may be even more aggressive than clinically apparent carcinomas. Stage A cancers are subdivided into A1 and A2 categories to reflect important differences in clinical behavior and prognosis. For similar reasons, the stage B cancers are also subdivided to take into consideration the important factor of tumor volume.

The distinction between tumor contained within the "capsule" of the prostate (stages A and B) and tumor extension beyond the confines of the gland (stage C) is crucial in selecting patients for appropriate therapy. While involvement of the bladder neck, seminal vesicles, and periprostatic tissue clearly portends a worse outcome, the prognostic significance of microscopic capsular invasion or apical extension within the gland is unsettled and is undergoing active investigation.

The pelvic lymph nodes are most often involved in regional spread of disease (stage D1). Bone metastases are the most common site for distant involvement (stage D2) while visceral metastases occur late and are usually recognized in autopsies or end-stage lesions.

Clinical staging is performed by palpation and endoscopic/cystoscopic assessment, imaging studies, and determination of serum markers. A carefully performed digital rectal examination will provide initial information regarding the local extent and size of the lesion, although "understaging" is common. Cystoscopy may be helpful for assessment of the bladder outlet and the possibility of bladder neck or trigonal involvement. Transrectal ultrasonography may be useful for local staging, providing information about size and extent of the lesion. TRUS does not permit assessment of nodal status, which can best be done with CT scanning or MRI. Pelvic lymphadenopathy suspicious of metastatic disease can be visualized by CT or MRI, and percutaneous aspiration biopsy can be performed if clinically indicated. A radionucleotide bone scan is the most sensitive method for detection of skeletal metastases. Selective radiographs can be used in conjunction with bone scans. Approximately 80 per cent of patients with osseous metastases have osteoblastic lesions, while pure lytic lesions occur in 5 per cent and mixed lesions are seen in 15 per cent.

For many years, acid phosphatase has been a useful serum marker in staging and following patients with carcinoma of the prostate. Elevation of acid phosphatase is very suggestive of extracapsular disease. Changes in acid phosphatase levels in patients with known metastatic disease tend to correlate with tumor activity and response to treatment. The enzyme acid phosphatase is not unique to prostatic tissue, but prostatic isoenzymes (PAP) have been identified and can be assayed. Despite efforts to refine the assay and improve its clinical value, newer assays tend to be less specific for prostatic cancer and prone to more false positives. Acid phosphatase determination is not an effective screening test for prostatic malignancy, since it is generally normal in patients with localized disease, and may be elevated in benign prostatic conditions.

Prostate specific antigen (PSA) is a glycoprotein different than PAP found only in benign and malignant prostate tissue. Elevated PSA occurs in roughly 80 per cent of prostate cancer patients, rising with increasing tumor volume,[13] but elevations are also common in benign prostatic conditions such as benign prostatic hypertrophy (BPH). In lower-stage disease, PSA appears to be substantially more sensitive than acid phosphatase. It may prove to be of some value in early diagnosis, especially when correlated with findings on TRUS. However, like PAP, it cannot stand alone as a screening test for early malignancy, because false negatives occur and, more importantly, because elevations are common with benign prostatic disease. Perhaps the greatest value of PSA is in monitoring patients after initial therapy, as it correlates even better with disease activity than PAP.[14] It is especially useful in patients after radical prostatectomy, in whom there should be no detectable PSA; i.e., a "0" level. In regards to following patients with known carcinoma of the prostate, serial PSA determinations are a useful adjuvant in monitoring disease activity and response to treatment.

TREATMENT AND MANAGEMENT

Decisions regarding treatment of prostatic carcinoma depend on grade and stage of the lesion, the age of the patient, and the overall medical condition of the patient, including the presence of comorbid diseases. In men with life expectancies of 5 to 10 years and malignancy confined to the prostate, radical prostatectomy or radiation therapy are the two forms of definitive therapy recognized to have curative potential. Controversy still exists over which treatment modality produces the best long-term results, although 10-year survival rates appear comparable with either form of management.[15] Most comparisons suffer from the shortcomings of nonrandomized studies that tend to introduce both selection and treatment biases. Furthermore, survival data alone only indirectly address disease-free survival and genuine eradication of malignancy. In the only prospective randomized study, radical prostatectomy appeared to be more effective than megavoltage radiation in achieving disease control.[16]

Radical prostatectomy offers an excellent opportunity for disease control when the neoplasm is confined to the prostate. Unlike simple prostatectomy, in which the adenoma is enucleated, radical prostatectomy entails complete excision of the prostate with capsule, seminal vesicle, and adjacent vesical neck. A surgical anastomosis must be created between bladder neck and the severed end of the urethra distal to the prostatic apex. Radical prostatectomy may be accomplished by either the retropubic or perineal approach, but the retropubic route has become much more popular because the anatomy is more familiar to contemporary urologic surgeons and because it offers the opportunity to include a simultaneous staging pelvic lymphadenectomy.

The major disadvantages of traditional radical prostatectomy have been the risks of urinary incontinence (2 to 15 per cent) and impotence (90 to 100 per cent). These "quality of life issues" have often led patients and their physicians to choose less effective forms of treatment for prostatic neoplasm.

Perhaps the most significant advance in the surgical treatment of carcinoma of the prostate has been the development of the "potency-sparing," or "nerve-sparing," technique for radical prostatectomy. The success of this modification of the retropubic approach depends on preservation of the autonomic nerves that innervate the corpora cavernosa, which are responsible for erectile function. In 1982 Walsh and Donker delineated the course of these nerves and demonstrated that they travel outside of the prostatic capsule.[17] In traditional radical prostatectomies, these nerves appeared to be injured during steps in mobilization of the prostate and dissection of the prostate from the rectum. Subsequently, Walsh showed how the operative technique could be modified to prevent damage to these branches of the pelvic plexus that control erections.[18] Another essential component to the success of nerve-sparing operations was the development of techniques for improved hemostasis by better control of the "dorsal vein complex," overlying the anterior surface of the prostate and urethra. Applying these techniques, radical prostatectomy may be performed with significantly less blood loss, fewer intraoperative complications, improved continence, and preservation of potency in the majority of men with localized disease.

The nerve-sparing prostatectomy involves division of the lateral fascia surrounding the prostate closer to the capsule. This has raised questions regarding the adequacy of surgical margins and the risk of compromising the cancer removal. There is evidence from pathologic studies of radical prostatectomy specimens that capsular penetration occurs early in the region of the neurovascular bundle on the side of the lesion. Walsh and others have critically addressed this issue and came to the conclusion that, when applied appropriately, there is no evidence to indicate that the modifications compromise the cancer margins.[19] The primary objective of surgery is always to remove all tumor, with preservation of potency a secondary consideration. When extraprostatic extension of the neoplasm occurs, the dissection should be intentionally expanded to include the more lateral nerve-bearing fascia. Sexual function may be preserved even when the nerve bundles are sacrificed on just one side.[20]

External beam radiation therapy is commonly used for stages A, B, and C prostatic carcinoma. While it is clear that a certain proportion of prostatic cancers are sensitive to radiation (and therefore are potentially curable by this noninvasive modality), there is currently no way of testing individual tumors for radiosensitivity, so as to predict their response to treatment. Survival after radiation therapy correlates directly with tumor grade, volume, and stage. Generally, a linear accelerator is used to deliver a dosage of about 7000 cGy to the prostate itself, often accompanied by an extended field dosage of 5000 cGy to part of the pelvis or regional lymph nodes.

Patients with significant coexistent medical problems and older patients with life expectancies of less than 10 years may elect radiation therapy over radical prostatectomy as definitive treatment of localized carcinoma of the prostate. Five- and 10-year survival rates are similar to those reported for surgically treated groups of patients,[21] although the disease-free survival appears to be significantly less after radiation therapy. As a conservative alternative to radical prostatectomy, radiation therapy may be particularly appropriate for men who are not suitable surgical candidates or who are unwilling to accept the potential complications of impotence or urinary incontinence. Moreover, radiation therapy is probably the treatment of choice for stage C disease in which extraprostatic extension makes surgical extirpation difficult or impossible.

With contemporary radiation therapy, there should be a low incidence of complications and morbidity. Potential side effects include radiation cystitis and proctitis, as well as urethral stricture formation. The management of these troublesome complications can be challenging and frustrating for both patient and physician. Incontinence that results from therapy is rare, and the incidence of impotence ranges from 30 to 50 per cent.

Interstitial radiation therapy is another treatment modality for localized carcinoma of the prostate, although there seems to be declining interest in this alternative in favor of radical prostatectomy. The theoretic advantage of interstitial therapy is the delivery of higher dosages of radiation to the tumor area than would be possible with external beam alone. Most isotope implantations are performed operatively through a retropubic approach, incorporating a staging lymphadenectomy, but the use of percutaneous ultrasound guided implants is also being evaluated. The most common isotopes used for interstitial prostate radiation are iodine-125, gold-198, and iridium-192. Gold-198 and iridium-192 implantations are commonly combined with supplemental external radiation.

All interstitial isotopes are intended to deliver supralethal dosages of ionizing radiation to the prostatic tumor while sparing the surrounding uninvolved tissues. They may be applicable to cases of larger tumor volume in which radical prostatectomy would not be appropriate. Interstitial implantation can generally be accomplished with less blood loss than prostatectomy, and there is no risk of urinary incontinence. The incidence of postoperative impotence also appears to be rather low.

A major drawback of interstitial therapy is the potential for urinary retention when postoperative prostatic edema aggravates underlying anatomic obstruction. Uneven distribution of seeds and imprecise calculations of dosage (dosimetry) also represent potential problems with interstitial radiation. Serious delayed complications of radiation effect, such as proctitis and development of prostatorectal fistula, have been reported. Several studies have shown a disturbingly high incidence of persistent malignancy locally after radiation therapy.[22, 23] Although the percentage of positive prostate biopsies decreases with time elapsed from therapy, two years later the incidence of positive biopsies may be 40 to 60 per cent, including prostates that appear to be normal on rectal examination. Furthermore, although the clinical significance of positive postirradiation biopsies has been questioned, there is mounting evidence that patients with persistent tumor have a much higher chance of disease progression and a worse prognosis.[24] This whole issue has raised more doubts about the overall efficacy of radiation therapy for carcinoma of the prostate.

Transurethral resection is not used for definitive, curative therapy for localized prostatic carcinoma. It does have a role in the palliation of bladder outlet obstruction, arising either from neoplasm or from associated benign adenoma. Some urologists favor at least limited resection prior to radiation therapy in selected cases in which obstruction and retention may be aggravated by the course of treatment. Others have suggested that resection may actually promote the dissemination of neoplasm from the prostate.

Once disseminated neoplastic disease occurs, "hormone therapy" aimed at androgen ablation can be initiated to control disease and palliate symptoms. Approximately 80 to 85 per cent of patients with metastatic prostatic carcinoma will respond to androgen deprivation. Under physiologic conditions, testicular androgen biosynthesis is stimulated by pituitary luteinizing hormone (LH) secretion. The pituitary release of LH is, in turn, under the control of hypothalamic gonadotropin-releasing factor (LHRF), which generally exerts its effect in a pulsatile manner. There is a negative feedback mechanism involving testosterone inhibition of hypothalamic-releasing factor. The testes are responsible for 90 to 95 per cent of circulating androgen, with the remainder being primarily adrenal in origin. There are currently four general methods for achieving androgen ablation: (1) surgical castration/orchiectomy, (2) inhibition of androgen synthesis, (3) disturbance of the hypothalamic-pituitary control mechanisms over testosterone production, and (4) antagonism of androgen action at a cellular level.

The salutary effect of castration on prostatic cancer was discovered in 1941 by Huggins and Hodges.[25] Bilateral orchiectomy is a simple and very effective method to produce rapid androgen ablation. There is no activation of secondary androgen sources after orchiectomy and serum testosterone levels remain at "castrate" levels. Orchiectomy is a low-risk surgical procedure that can be performed with local or regional anaesthesia. Some patients will reject orchiectomy because of the psychologic trauma associated with castration.

Another method of producing androgen deprivation is provided by a group of agents that interfere with production of testosterone from cholesterol by inhibition of enzymes in the synthesis chain. Aminoglutethimide and ketoconazole, the antifungal agent, will block enzymatic pathways, and have been used clinically for this purpose. Adrenal steroidogenesis can also be affected, especially with aminoglutethimide, and replacement therapy with glucocorticoids and mineralocorticoids may be necessary. These problems, as well as other disturbing side effects such as lethargy, weakness, and depression, limit the clinical usefulness of these therapies.

For years, the most common method for achieving androgen deprivation by interference with the hypothalamo-pituitary axis was with estrogen therapy. Estrogens will suppress the release of LH from the pituitary in both sexes. Estrogens may also have a direct effect on the prostate gland, but there is no clear evidence to substantiate a clinical action in humans.

Diethylstilbestrol (DES) has been the most commonly used estrogen for hormone therapy of carcinoma of the prostate. When originally used in dosages of 5 mg per day, a higher incidence of cardiovascular-related deaths was observed, reducing the survival advantage gained in the estrogen group by reduced cancer mortality. Other studies have shown equivalent effectiveness comparing 1 mg per day to 5 mg per day in preventing cancer deaths and progression of disease.[26] However, DES in daily dosages of 1 mg or less does not uniformly suppress plasma testosterone to castrate levels. Reliable suppression is achieved in dosages of 3 mg per day or greater, which is probably the rationale behind the acceptance of the 3 mg per day DES regimen as the optimal therapy.

Another group of drugs that act on a hypothalamo-pituitary level are the agonist analogues of gonadotropin-releasing hormone. These agents, which are sometimes referred to as "super-agonists," initially result in increased LH production but then lead to total suppression of LH and consequently testosterone. This effect simulates surgical castration, and continues for the length of therapy. LHRH analogs do not have the side effects of estrogens, but there may be a clinical "flare-up" of disease associated with the initial stimulatory effect on the pituitary. However, the overall efficacy is similar to surgical castration or estrogen therapy.

The antagonists of androgen action on a cellular level are often known as "anti-androgens." Flutamide is a nonsteroidal blocking agent that inhibits the nuclear binding of androgen at a cellular level. Experience with flutamide for monotherapy in stage D prostate cancer is somewhat limited, at least in the United States, but existing data seem to support substantial antitumor activity similar to more conventional "first line" agents. The real clinical utility of flutamide currently surrounds its use in "combined androgen blockade."

The rationale for combined or total androgen blockade is that therapeutic response can be enhanced by elimination of all androgens, even those of adrenal origin, being presented to hormone-dependent tumor cells. Past experience with medical and surgical adrenal ablation for treatment of patients relapsing after previous hormone therapy had rarely shown any significant survival benefit. However, the availability of new drugs in therapies capable of blocking the effects of both testicular and adrenal androgen led to new studies to test the results of total androgen deprivation as initial therapy for patients with stage D2 disease. Labrie and coworkers found a greater response rate in patients with metastatic disease treated simultaneously with a combination of LHRH analog and flutamide.[27] A well-controlled multigroup study found a similar improvement in effectiveness with combination therapy in patients with disseminated, previously untreated prostate cancer.[28] Compared to the group receiving LHRH analog alone, the patients treated with both LHRH analog and flutamide showed small, but statistically significant improvements in time to disease progression and overall survival. Additional investigation will build upon this data base and attempt to define some groups of patients with stage D2 carcinoma who will benefit the most from combination therapy. At this time, it appears that total androgen blockage with surgical or medical (LHRH analog) castration and flutamide is superior treatment for metastatic disease (D2).

Another unresolved controversy in the treatment of prostatic carcinoma is the timing of the hormonal therapy. While advanced symptomatic disease demands prompt initiation of hormone therapy, it is not so clear that early endocrine manipulation provides any survival advantage for stage C and early stage D disease. Support for delayed hormone therapy was fueled by the results of an important Veteran's Administration cooperative study, which suggested that there were no adverse affects on survival from delayed therapy. Proponents contend that delaying the undesirable side effects associated with most endocrine therapies, such as impotence, improves overall quality of life in asymptomatic individuals. On the other hand, there are arguments favoring prompt initiation of hormonal therapy, including early recognition of non-responders who would then be better candidates for additional therapy, and data suggesting that radical prostatectomy and immediate endocrine therapy delays disease progression in selected patients.[29]

Chemotherapy has not proved to be very effective for advanced prostatic carcinoma. Objective response rates are generally less than 15 per cent but are difficult to accurately assess because of limitations in measurable disease parameters in most cases of metastatic carcinoma of the prostate. The most active single agents appear to be cyclophosphamide, cisplatin, doxorubicin, 5-fluorouracil, and estramustine phosphate. Results with combination drug therapy have failed to show significant superiority in controlled clinical trials.

Chemotherapy is often used in settings of progressive disease unresponsive to standard hormonal manipulation. These patients, treated late in the course of their disease, often have a large tumor burden and concurrent debilitating effects from disseminated disease, such as weight loss and anemia. It is attractive to consider chemotherapy as an adjuvant in earlier stage, advanced disease. However, in the absence of demonstrated benefits from early chemotherapy, it is questionable whether patients should be subjected to the side effects and potential complications of cytotoxic therapy.

REFERENCES

1. Andrews, G.S.: Latent carcinoma of the prostate. J. Clin. Pathol. 2:197, 1949.
2. Rich, A.R.: On the frequency of occurrence of occult carcinoma of the prostate. J. Urol. 33:215, 1935.
3. Hirst, A.E., Jr., and Bergman, R.T.: Carcinoma of the prostate in men 80 or more years old. Cancer 7:136, 1954.
4. Benson, M.C., Kaplan, S.A., and Olsson, C.A.: Prostate cancer in men less than 45 years old: Influence of stage, grade, and therapy. J. Urol. 137:888–890, 1987.
5. McNeal, J.E., Bostwick, D.G., Kindrachuk, R.A., et al.: Patterns of progression in prostate cancer. Lancet 1:60–63, 1986.
6. Guinan, P., Bush, I., Ray, V., et al.: The accuracy of the rectal examination in the diagnosis of prostate carcinoma. N. Engl. J. Med. 303:499–503, 1980.
7. Chodak, G.W., Wald, N., Parmer, E., et al.: Comparison of digital examination and transrectal ultrasonography for the diagnosis of prostate cancer. J. Urol. 135:951–954, 1986.
8. Lee, F., Littrup, P.J., and McLeary, R.D.: Needle aspiration and core biopsy of prostate cancer: Comparative evaluation with biplane, transrectal US guidance. Radiology 163:515–520, 1987.
9. Lee, F., Littrup, P.J., Kumasaka, G.M., et al.: The use of transrectal ultrasound in the diagnosis, guided biopsy, staging, and screening of prostate cancer. Radiographics 7:642–644, 1987.
10. Stephenson, R.A., James, B.C., Gay, H., et al.: Flow cytometry of prostate cancer: Relationship of DNA content to survival. Cancer Res. 47:2504–2509, 1987.
11. Epstein, J.I., Berry, S.I., and Eggleston, J.C.: Nuclear roundness factor: A predictor of progression in untreated stage A-II prostate cancer. Cancer 54:1666–1671, 1984.
12. Stamey, T.A., McNeil, J.E., Freiha, F.S., et al.: Morphometric and clinical studies on sixty-eight consecutive radical prostatectomies. J. Urol. 139:1235, 1988.
13. Stamey, T.A., Yang, N., Hay, A.R., et al.: Prostatic specific antigen as a serum marker for adenocarcinoma of the prostate. N. Engl. J. Med. 317:909, 1987.
14. Ercole, C.J., Lange, P.H., Mathisen, M., et al.: Prostate specific antigen and prostatic acid

phosphatase in the monitoring and staging of patients with prostatic cancer. J. Urol. *138*:1101–1184, 1987.
15. Prostate Cancer—Consensus Conference: The management of clinically localized prostate cancer. JAMA *258*:2727–2730, 1987.
16. Paulson, D.F., Lin, G.H., Hinshaw, W., and Stephanie, S.: Radical surgery versus radiotherapy for adeno-carcinoma of the prostate. J. Urol. *128*:502–504, 1982.
17. Walsh, P.C., and Donker, P.J.: Impotence following radical prostatectomy: Insight into etiology and prevention. J. Urol. *128*:492–497, 1982.
18. Walsh, P.C., Lepor, H., and Eggleston, J.C.: Radical prostatectomy with preservation of sexual function: Anatomical and pathological considerations. Prostate *4*:473–485, 1983.
19. Eggleston, J.C., and Walsh, P.C.: Radical prostatectomy with preservation of sexual function: Pathological findings in the first 100 cases. J. Urol. *134*:1146–1148, 1985.
20. Walsh, P.C., Epstein, J.I., and Lowe, F.C.: Potency following radical prostatectomy with wide unilateral excision of the neurovascular bundle. J. Urol. *138*:823, 1987.
21. Hanks, G.E.: Radical prostatectomy or radiation therapy for early prostate cancer, two roads to the same end. Cancer *61*:2153, 1988.
22. Freiha, F.S., and Bagshaw, M.A.: Carcinoma of the prostate: Results of post-irradiation biopsy. Prostate *5*:19, 1984.
23. Schellhammer, P.F., El-Mahdi, A.M., Higgins, E.M., et al.: Prostate biopsy after definitive treatment by interstitial iodine-125 implant or external beam radiation therapy. J. Urol. *1*:137, 897–901, 1987.
24. Scardino, P.T.: The prognostic significance of biopsies after radiotherapy for prostate cancer. Semin. Urol. *1*:237–242, 1983.
25. Huggins, C., and Hodges, C.U.: Studies on prostatic cancer: I. The effects of castration, of estrogen, and of androgen injection on serum phosphatases in metastatic carcinoma of the prostate. Cancer Res. *1*:293, 1941.
26. Byar, D.P.: The Veteran's Administration Cooperative Urological Research Group's studies of cancer of the prostate. Cancer *32*:1126–1130, 1973.
27. Labrie, F., DuPont, A., Lacourciere, Y., et al.: Combined treatment with flutamide in association with medical or surgical castration. J. Urol. *135*:71A, 1986.
28. Crawford, E.D., Eisenberger, M., McCleod, D., et al.: A controlled trial of leuprolide with and without flutamide in prostatic carcinoma. N. Engl. J. Med. *321*:419–424, 1989.
29. Zinke, H., Utz, D.C., Benson, R.C., et al.: Bilateral pelvic lymphadenectomy and radical retropubic prostatectomy for stage C adeno-carcinoma of prostate. Urology *24*:534–539, 1984.

RENAL CELL CARCINOMA
by Robert C. Eyre, M.D.

Renal cell carcinoma (RCC), also termed hypernephroma, is a malignant tumor that arises from the proximal convoluted tubular cells of the kidney. It is often referred to as "the internist's tumor" because it may occur with a variety of symptoms seemingly unrelated to the urinary tract, including fever, gastrointestinal, neurologic, hematologic, and biochemical abnormalities. The "classic triad" of flank pain, gross hematuria, and a palpable mass occurs in only 10 per cent of patients, and usually represents an advanced stage of the disease. Individually, these three symptoms are seen in up to 50 per cent of patients. Because of its frequently obscure presentation, any patient with unexplained constitutional symptoms or laboratory abnormalities (elevated erythrocyte sedimentation rate, anemia, erythrocytosis, or hepatic dysfunction) merits an evaluation of the genitourinary tract.

INCIDENCE AND EPIDEMIOLOGY

Renal cell carcinoma accounts for approximately 85 per cent of all primary malignant tumors of the kidney. Others include transitional cell tumors that occur in the renal pelvis (about 15 per cent), rare juxtaglomerular cell tumors, and squamous carcinomas. Because of its rich vascular supply, the kidney is a favored site for metastatic involvement from lung, breast, and thyroid cancers, as well as lymphomas. The incidence of RCC in the United States is 3.5 per 100,000 population per year, or about 18,000 new cases annually. Males are affected twice as often as females, usually during the sixth and seventh decades of life. More than two-thirds of patients with von Hippel-Lindau's disease will develop renal cell carcinomas (frequently multiple or bilateral). Recent research has demonstrated a loss of specific genetic loci on the short arm of chromosome 3 in patients with RCC.[1]

Cigarette smoking increases the risk of developing RCC, and patients in certain occupations involving exposure to cadmium, aromatic hydrocarbons, asbestos, and lead are believed also to be at increased risk.

DIAGNOSIS AND STAGING

The diagnosis of RCC is made radiologically. Intravenous pyelography may demonstrate a renal mass, calyceal distortion, or diminution of renal function. The solid or cystic nature of the mass should then be determined by ultrasonography (US). Complex cysts should be further defined by computerized tomography (CT), as they may contain malignant tumors in 2 to 7 per cent of cases. Diffuse or stippled calcification in the area of the kidney on a plain abdominal film is highly suggestive of RCC, and is seen in 2 to 35 per cent of tumors. Solid masses are further evaluated and staged clinically by CT, which provides information regarding tumor extension into the perinephric fat, psoas muscle, regional lymph nodes, renal vein, inferior vena cava, and adrenal glands with greater than 90 per cent accuracy. The CT scan has also been found to be useful in differentiating angiomyolipomas and oncocytomas from RCC. The plane between a renal tumor and contiguous organs may be hard to define by CT or US; thus, right-sided tumors may appear to involve the liver or hepatic flexure of the colon, while left-sided tumors may seem to be adherent to the spleen or splenic flexure of the colon. At surgery, one usually finds these planes to be intact without local tumor invasion.

In the past, arteriography was commonly used in the diagnostic evaluation of renal masses. However, since the advent of US and CT, the indications for invasive angiography have become more selectively limited to solitary kidneys and complex cases in which preoperative knowledge of the vascular anatomy is important to the surgical management. Because of the unique vascular anatomy within the renal parenchyma, RCC may grow into sinusoids and be propagated in the direction of venous outflow. Thus, tumor extension into the renal vein is frequently encountered, and extension into the inferior vena cava is seen in 5 per cent of tumors. This occurs most often with right-sided tumors since the right renal vein is shorter. Signs of venous or caval obstruction by tumor thrombus may include lower extremity edema, new onset of a varicocele on either side, or dilated abdominal wall venous collateral vessels. Symptoms related to left renal vein obstruction are unusual because of potential collateral drainage through the gonadal, adrenal, and lumbar branches. Clinical suspicion of venous occlusion should be high when there is nonfunction of the involved kidney by IVP or CT. If venous obstruction is ruled out, a diffuse infiltrative process within the parenchyma or collecting system such as transitional cell carcinoma, lymphoma, or metastatic disease should be considered.

While CT and US can usually determine the extent of vena caval tumor thrombus, an inferior vena cavagram may be necessary to precisely define it. Superior vena cavography should be done if the cephalad extent cannot be seen well from below. Recently we have used noninvasive MRI angiography to determine thrombus extent if the CT has been equivocal. Preoperative knowledge of the cephalad extent of tumor thrombus is essential for surgical planning, and will be discussed further on.

We believe that there is a very limited role for preoperative needle biopsy of a renal lesion. The tumors are often hypervascular, and hemorrhage may occur. A significant percentage of cells within a tumor may appear quite benign histologically, thus a fine-needle aspirate (as opposed to core biopsy) may be misleading. Appropriate indications for percutaneous renal biopsy are limited to those cases in which therapeutic decisions will clearly be determined by the results, such as elderly patients in whom comorbid disease might preclude nephrectomy, lesions felt to be metastatic to the kidney from a previous primary malignant site or from lymphoma, or lesions felt to be benign angiomyolipomas or oncocytomas by CT.

Urine cytology may provide diagnostic information in differentiating renal cell from transitional cell lesions; however, renal cell tumors will yield positive cytologies in under 10 per cent of cases.[2]

Once the clinical diagnosis of renal cell carcinoma is made, the extent of regional and distant organ involvement should be determined. Favored sites of metastatic spread include the regional lymphatics, lung, liver, bone, brain, ipsilateral adrenal gland, and contralateral kidney. In addition to the abdominal CT, chest tomography or CT and a liver chemistry profile should be performed. A radionuclide bone scan is obtained if the alkaline phosphatase is elevated. Any patient with neurologic symptoms should have a brain evaluation by nuclear scan, CT, or MRI. One must also assess contralateral renal function, as a compromised state might alter the traditional treatment of radical nephrectomy. Twenty-five to 30 per cent of patients will have disseminated metastases at the time of diagnosis, with a median survival of four months and few one-year survivors. Nephrectomy is rarely indicated for this group except for palliation of severe symptoms, particularly hemorrhage.

The most widely used staging system is that of Flocks, as modified by Robson (Fig. 13–1).[3] Surgical and pathologic staging of the specimen have major implications regarding survival. One limitation of this staging system is the incorporation of patients with vena caval extension or regional lymphatic involvement into the same prognostic group. Recent data critically examining the issue of vena caval involvement in the absence of lymphatic metastases have shown that complete surgical removal of tumor thrombus is associated with a survival similar to stage I disease.[4] Invasion of the wall of the vena cava is rare, and is associated with a dismal prognosis. It is our impression that in recent years many renal tumors are being diagnosed at

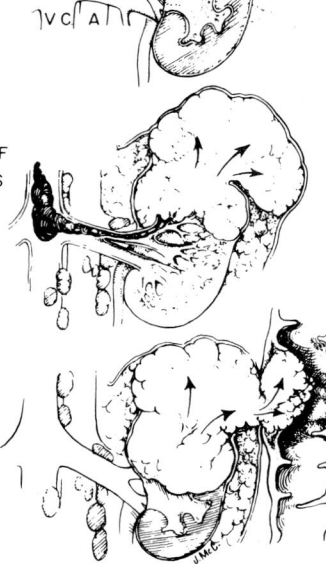

STAGING OF RENAL CELL CARCINOMA

STAGE I
TUMOR WITHIN CAPSULE

STAGE II
TUMOR INVASION OF PERINEPHRIC FAT (CONFINED TO GEROTA'S FASCIA)

STAGE III
TUMOR INVOLVEMENT OF REGIONAL LYMPH NODES AND/OR RENAL VEIN AND CAVA

STAGE IV
ADJACENT ORGANS OR DISTANT METASTASES

Figure 13–1. Staging of nephrocarcinoma as proposed by Holland, in accord with schemes of Robson, Murphy, and Flocks and Kadesky. (From Holland, J.M.: Cancer of the kidney—natural history and staging. Cancer 32:1030, 1973. Reproduced with permission of author and publisher.)

an earlier, asymptomatic stage by CT or US studies performed for other indications. It is interesting to speculate whether this trend toward earlier diagnosis will have a favorable impact on overall survival statistics for patients with RCC.[5]

SURGICAL MANAGEMENT

The only effective therapy for localized renal cell carcinoma is radical nephrectomy (en bloc removal of the kidney, ipsilateral adrenal gland, Gerota's fat and fascia, and regional lymphatics) with early ligation of the vascular pedicle. Several surgical approaches have been described; the surgeon should choose one that will allow complete and safe exposure based on the size and location of the tumor and the patient's body habitus. A thoracoabdominal approach should be used for large upper pole lesions or in patients with a solitary ipsilateral pulmonary metastasis, which should be resected.

For most tumors, we use an eleventh rib supracostal, extrapleural approach or a modified chevron incision. It is not necessary to resect a rib segment for exposure. Very large tumors require a thoracoabdominal approach. We use a split ring attachment to the Bookwalter retractor that can be adjusted for individual body habitus, which provides superior exposure (Fig. 13–2).

In the past few years, several studies have addressed the possibility of performing more conservative surgery for selected renal tumors. Novick et al.[6] found that enucleation of well-encapsulated tumors (as defined by CT and angiography) was associated with a 6 per cent local recurrence rate and a 90 per cent three-year survival. Appropriate indications for renal-sparing surgery might include patients with solitary kidneys or those with multiple tumors. Robey has demonstrated no difference in patient survival at five or nine years when leaving the ipsilateral adrenal gland in situ for localized carcinoma.[7] We occasionally spare the adrenal gland when removing lower pole tumors.

In the rare instance of bilateral synchronous renal cell carcinomas, one must determine which kidney is most suitable for partial nephrectomy based on tumor location and vascular supply (on arteriogram). The partial nephrectomy should be performed first in order to allow renal function to stabilize,

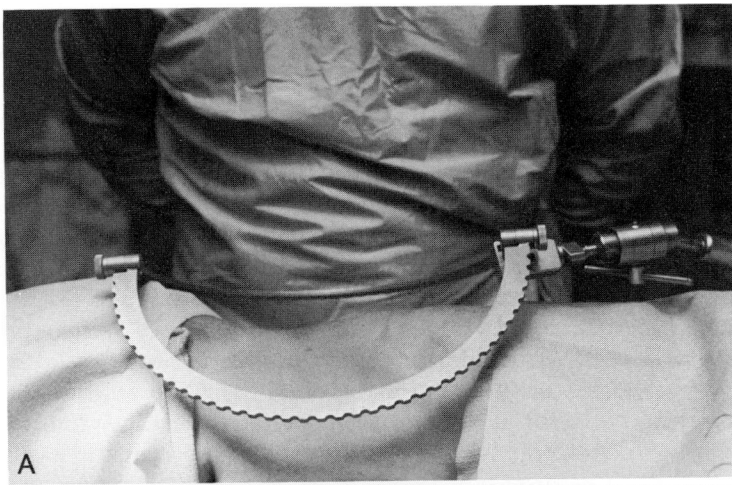
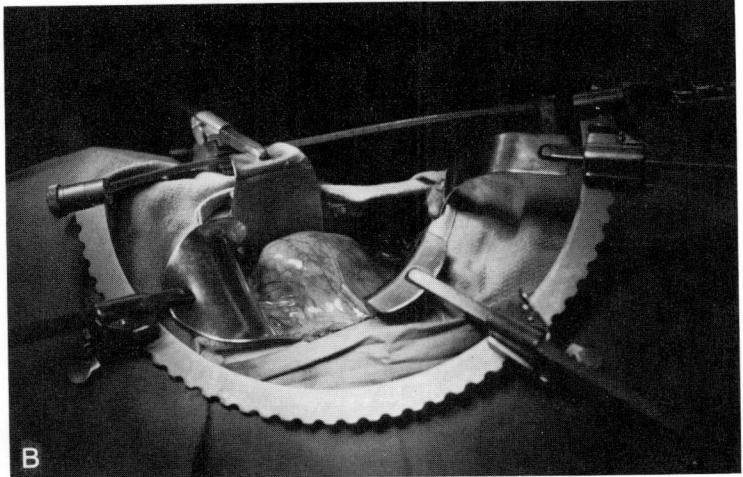

Figure 13–2. *A*, The split ring attachment to the Bookwalter retractor provides superior exposure for flank and thoracoabdominal incisions. *B*, Large transitional cell carcinoma of the renal pelvis invading the renal parenchyma. Note the ability to provide circumferential retracton.

followed by contralateral radical nephrectomy two to three weeks later. The patient should always be apprised preoperatively of the potential need for dialysis. Many patients with bilateral synchronous tumors have evidence of disseminated disease, rarely surviving as long as one year. Some patients, felt to have localized bilateral tumors, must be considered for bilateral nephrectomy followed by chronic hemodialysis or transplantation. The risks of such treatment are considerable, as are the risks of tumor recurrence in an immunosuppressed patient.

Renal cell cancers extending into the vena cava represent a unique surgical challenge. Accurate determination of the distal extent of the thrombus is crucial for preoperative planning. Subdiaphragmatic thrombi can be managed by an abdominal or a thoracoabdominal approach, but those extending into the superior vena cava (SVC) or cardiac chambers are best managed by extracting the tumor thrombus through the SVC or right atrium via a median sternotomy, utilizing circulatory bypass and hypothermic cardioplegia. The reader is referred to several recent studies for further details of operative technique.[4, 8, 9] Basic principles include liver mobilization by division of the coronary and triangular ligaments, ligation of several small hepatic veins as they enter the IVC, and complete proximal and distal control of the IVC, including the opposite renal vein and lumbar branches. We temporarily place a de Weese clip above the tumor thrombus to prevent distal migration of any fragments during removal. We believe that the use of a Foley catheter to extract the thrombus, as described by some authors, is unnecessary and potentially dangerous. When a thoracoabdominal approach is used, we favor an incision on the right side. Either kidney can be removed through this, and wider exposure of the vena cava is possible. For tumor thrombi that extend into the atrium, we use two-dimensional transesophageal cardiac ultrasonography intraoperatively to continuously monitor the tumor thrombus, cardiac wall motion, and right atrial filling.

Much has been written about the fascinating extrarenal manifestations of RCC, which may include neurologic, hematologic, biochemical, or endocrine abnormalities.[10] These paraneoplastic syndromes are felt to be secondary to hormonal substances elaborated by the tumor. It may require two to three months following nephrectomy for these abnormalities to disappear. Persistent symptoms should prompt re-evaluation for potential metastatic disease.

The wide variation in patterns of progression of metastatic lesions (particularly lung metastases) after nephrectomy has led to the popular concept of spontaneous regression. A more critical evaluation of this phenomenon in 10 combined series demonstrated the incidence to be only five of 1,348 patients or 0.4 per cent.[11] We believe that many ill-advised nephrectomies are performed in patients with widely disseminated disease in the hope of inducing such an event. As in all areas of cancer management, one must maintain a realistic appreciation of the limitations of surgery in these situations.

TREATMENT OF ADVANCED DISEASE

Renal cell carcinomas are not radiosensitive, and various chemotherapeutic trials have produced response rates of less than 10 per cent. Hormonal manipulation with progestational agents has not produced objective responses. The most promising form of adjunctive therapy involves various attempts to stimulate an immunologic response to the tumor or metastatic lesions with interferon, autologous tumor preparations, or sensitized lymphocyte preparations. Data from these trials are very preliminary and few statements regarding alteration of survival can be made. In the largest series of patients with metastatic RCC so far reported, 108 patients received lymphokine-activated killer cells plus interleukin 2 with a 33 per cent complete or partial response rate.[12] Interleukin 2 causes considerable transient toxicity (hypotension, fluid retention, oliguria, prerenal azotemia, and hyperbilirubinemia) and intensive in-hospital monitoring is required. We participated in a phase II multicenter trial of recombinant human interleukin 2 and alpha interferon in patients with metastatic RCC in which a 22 per cent partial objective response was seen. Preliminary data from other similar trials suggest that radical nephrectomy, even in the presence of disseminated disease, may increase the response rate to adjuvant immunologic therapy. The reader is referred to several recent studies that discuss various immunotherapeutic modalities.[13, 14]

REFERENCES

1. Zbar, B., Brauch, H., Talmadge, C., et al.: Loss of alleles of loci on the short arm of chromosomes 3 in renal cell carcinoma. Nature *327:*721–727, 1987.
2. Droller, M.F., Stuppler, S.A., Kandzari, S.J., and Milan, D.F.: Hypernephroma and associated ureteral involvement. Urology *8:*575–578, 1976.
3. Holland, J.M.: Proceedings: Cancer of the kidney—natural history and staging. Cancer *32:*1030–1042, 1973.
4. Libertino, J.A., Zinman, L., and Watkins, E.: Long-term results of resection of renal cell cancer with extension into inferior vena cava. J. Urol. *137:*21–24, 1987.
5. Thompson, I.M., and Peek, M.: Improvement in survival of patients with renal cell carcinoma—the role of the serendipitously detected tumor. J. Urol. *140:*487–490, 1988.
6. Novick, A.C., Zincke, H., Neves, R.J., et al.: Surgical enucleation for renal cell carcinoma. J. Urol. *135:*235–238, 1986.
7. Robey, E.L., and Schellhammer P.F.: The adrenal gland and renal cell carcinoma: Is the ipsilateral adrenalectomy a necessary component of radical nephrectomy? J. Urol. *135:*453, 1986.
8. Kearney, G.P., Waters, W.B., Klein, L.A., et al.: Results of inferior vena cava resection for renal cell carcinoma. J. Urol. *125:*769, 1981.
9. Shabian, D.M., Libertino, J.A., Zinman, L.N., et al.: Resection of cavoatrial renal cell carcinoma employing total circulatory arrest. Arch. Surg. *125:*727–732, 1990.
10. Marshall, F.F., and Walsh, P.C.: Extrarenal manifestations of renal cell carcinoma. J. Urol. *117:*439–440, 1977.
11. Freed, S.Z., Halperin, J.P., and Gordon, M.: Idiopathic regression of metastases from renal cell carcinoma. J. Urol. *118:*538–542, 1977.
12. Rosenberg, S.A., Lotze, M.T., Muul, L.M., et al.: A progress report on the treatment of 157 patients with advanced cancer using lymphokine-activated killer cells and interleukin 2 or high-dose interleukin 2 alone. N. Engl. J. Med. *316:*889–897, 1987.
13. Osband, M.E., Lavin, P.T., Babayan, R.K., et al.: Effect of autolymphocyte therapy on survival and quality of life in patients with metastatic renal cell carcinoma. Lancet *335:*994–998, 1990.
14. Fisher, R.I., Coltman, C.A. Jr., Doroshow, J.H., et al.: Metastatic renal cell cancer treated with interleukin 2 and lymphokine activated killer cells: A phase II clinical trial. Am. Inst. Med. *108:*518–523, 1988.

TESTICULAR CANCER
by Paul A. Church, M.D.

Testicular cancer is a relatively rare neoplasm overall, but represents a significant clinical challenge because it generally occurs in a younger age group at which time otherwise healthy men are in their most productive and fertile years. It is the most common solid tumor in men between 20 and 34 years of age. Fortunately, dramatic progress has been made in the management and treatment of testicular tumors over the past 20 years, so that it is now one of the most curable of all cancers.

ORIGIN AND CLASSIFICATION

Almost all testicular malignancies (90 to 95 per cent) are of germ cell origin. Primitive "totipotential" germ cells undergo malignant transformation, yielding lines of cells known as seminoma or a heterogeneous group of nonseminomatous tumors, which may display various types of differentiation as embryonic or extraembryonic structures. From a clinical and therapeutic standpoint, the classification of germ cell tumors as seminoma or nonseminoma is most relevant. The histologic classification most commonly used in the United States divides these tumors into single histologic types and mixed types (Table 13–2).

Seminoma is the most common histologic type (40 per cent) followed in incidence by mixed tumors. Yolk sac tumors occur primarily in children. Embryonal carcinoma is generally composed of highly malignant, primitive epithelial cells that tend to metastasize early. Teratoma is composed of the tissues normally derived from two or more embryonic germ cell layers (endoderm, mesoderm, and ectoderm) and may be immature or mature, often forming mucus-secreting glands or cartilage. The mixture of teratoma and embryonal carcinoma is often termed "teratocarcinoma." Pure choriocarcinoma is extremely rare but highly malignant. Unlike other cell types, choriocarcinoma tends to spread hematogenously rather than through lymphatic drainage.

Rapid growth rates and the capability of secreting biologic "marker"

TABLE 13–2. CLASSIFICATION OF TESTICULAR CARCINOMA

Single Cell Types	Mixed Cell Types
Seminoma	Seminoma and other types
Embryonal	Embryonal and teratoma
Choriocarcinoma	(teratocarcinoma)
Teratoma	Choriocarcinoma/yolk sac and
Yolk sac tumor	other types

substances common to fetal and placental tissue characterize the primitive and multipotential nature of testicular carcinoma. The two most important clinical markers are the beta subunit of human chorionic gonadotropin (HCG), usually the product of syncytiotrophoblasts, and alpha-fetoprotein (AFP), secreted by yolk sac elements.

INCIDENCE

Cryptorchidism is associated with a higher risk of developing testicular cancer. Orchiopexy does not eliminate the risk of cancer, but does make the testis more accessible for physical examination. It has also been observed that there is an elevated risk of malignancy in the contralateral, normally descended testis.[1]

Atrophic testes, particularly resulting from mumps, may also be somewhat more susceptible to developing testicular neoplasms.[2] A history of trauma is often present in patients with testicular cancer, but this is more likely a mechanism for its discovery rather than a causative factor in its development.

PRESENTATION AND DIAGNOSIS

Any mass arising from the testicle itself is suspect for malignancy until proved otherwise. Typically, a testis tumor presents as a painless scrotal mass that does not transilluminate on examination. The mass may be noticed while bathing or during sexual activity. Some patients seem to harbor feelings of guilt or denial about the development of these lesions within their genitalia. Such feelings, coupled with considerable public ignorance regarding testicular cancer, often contribute to delays in seeking medical attention. Some patients will have local symptoms caused by inflammation, hemorrhage within the tumor, hydrocele formation, or even concomitant infection. This may result in misdiagnosis and delay in proper treatment in up to 50 per cent of patients with testicular cancer.[3] Occasionally, men will have symptoms resulting from metastatic disease, since as many as one-third of patients will have metastases at the time of diagnosis. Gynecomastia may also be present from HCG secretion by tumor cells.

Examination of the scrotal mass by a trained urologist should help differentiate between epididymitis, spermatocele, varicocele, hydrocele, and testicular cancer. Transillumination is a useful technique to evaluate solid versus fluid-containing masses. Ultrasonography may be helpful in evaluating scrotal masses especially if there is a surrounding tense hydrocele that impairs palpation of the testis. A good quality ultrasound study should be able to distinguish lesions arising within the testicle from those that are extratesticular. However, the ultrasound study should not be a substitute for a careful physical examination and exercise of clinical judgment.

When a testicular neoplasm is suspected or considered, exploration through an inguinal approach is mandatory. A scrotal incision is contraindicated, as this may create problems with inadequate surgical margins during orchiectomy, local tumor recurrence, and atypical metastatic patterns due to violations of local lymphatic drainage. If a testicular mass is confirmed at surgical exploration, a radical orchiectomy is performed removing the testis and spermatic cord to the level of the internal ring.

Serum markers (beta HCG and AFP) should be drawn before surgery, since this may provide useful information about the cell type and serve as a monitor for subsequent therapy. Since most seminomas and some nonseminomatous tumors do not produce beta HCG or AFP, negative markers should not deter or delay surgery if a tumor is suspected.

STAGING

Testicular cancer has a very predictable pattern of spread to regional lymphatics accompanying the venous drainage (Fig. 13–3). The lymphatics from the right side terminate mainly in interaortocaval lymph nodes around the entrance of the right spermatic vein into the inferior vena cava. On the left side, lymph nodes lateral to the aorta and near the renal hilum, where the left spermatic vein joins the renal vein, are usually involved first. Other retroperitoneal lymph nodes become involved following initial spread along the primary venous drainage. Subsequently, further dissemination may occur, usually to mediastinal lymph nodes or lung parenchyma.

Following inguinal orchiectomy, staging studies are performed to determine further treatment. Stage I disease is limited to the testis. When retroperitoneal lymph nodes are involved (stage II), an effort is made to quantify the volume of disease into subgroups (see Table 13–3). Stage III disease refers to visceral involvement or lymphatic involvement above the diaphragm.

Abdominal CT scanning has proved to be the most useful imaging modality for evaluation of the retroperitoneum. However, there is a 20 to 30 per cent false-negative staging error with CT scans, primarily resulting

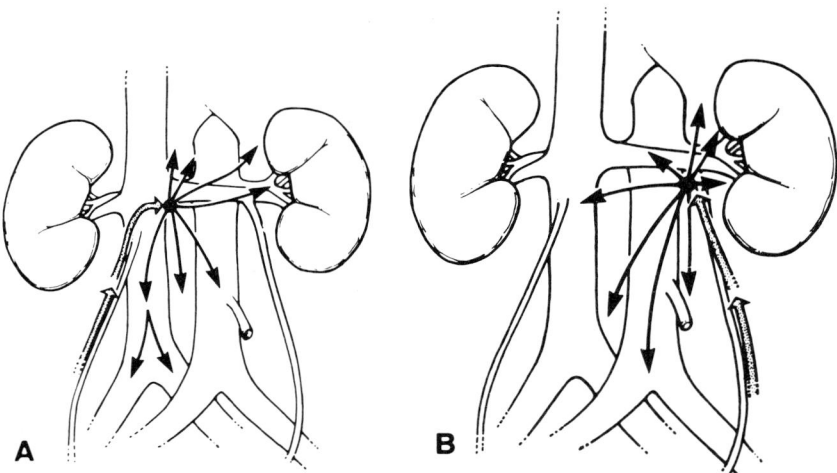

Figure 13–3. The usual sites for right- *(A)* and left-sided *(B)* metastases from testicular neoplasms. After involvement of the primary zone, metastases may spread to surrounding nodal areas (arrows). (From Gillenwater, J.Y., Grayhack, J.T., Howards, S.S., and Duckett, J.W.: Adult & Pediatric Urology. Year Book Medical Publishers, Vol. 2, p. 1387, 1987.)

TABLE 13–3. STAGING SYSTEM FOR TESTICULAR CANCER

Stage I	Tumor confined to testis and epididymis
Stage II	Retroperitoneal metastases
IIA	Microscopic LN involvement (<2 cm)
IIB	Macroscopic LN involvement (2–5 cm)
IIC	Bulky retroperitoneal disease (2–5 cm, may be palpable)
Stage III	Supradiaphragmatic LN metastases or extralymphatic disease (liver, bone, lung)

from microscopic involvement, which does not produce nodal enlargement. The addition of lymphangiogram (LAG) may reduce the staging error somewhat, but the study is time-consuming and requires considerable experience for accurate interpretation. MRI may also be useful in the retroperitoneal staging of testicular cancers. The chest is generally evaluated by tomography or CT scan.

Serum markers are also helpful in staging, since elevation of beta HCG or AFP after orchiectomy indicates the presence of active neoplasm. Overall, more than 70 per cent of nonseminomatous testis tumors elaborate one or both serum markers. AFP is produced only by nonseminomatous tumors, while 5 to 10 per cent of pure seminomas are known to secrete beta HCG. The risk of metastatic disease is greater in patients with vascular or lymphatic invasion within the primary tumor. Local extension of the testicular neoplasm into the epididymis or spermatic cord also is a poor prognostic sign. There is conflicting evidence linking the histology of the primary tumor to risk of relapse or metastatic disease. Most studies have found that tumors with an embryonal cell component are at greater risk.[4] The stage and histologic type are the most important factors determining treatment recommendations for men with testicular tumors. The prognostic features outlined above may also have important implications in clinical decision-making for nonseminomatous tumors.[5]

TREATMENT

The mainstay of treatment for low-stage seminoma continues to be radiation therapy. Only 20 to 30 per cent of patients with seminomas have metastatic disease at the time of diagnosis. This fact, together with the known radiosensitivity of pure seminoma, has made orchiectomy followed by radiation therapy highly effective treatment for stage I and some stage II tumors. Radiotherapy is directed to the retroperitoneal node-bearing areas and ipsilateral groin and iliac fossa. For bulkier retroperitoneal involvement or stage III disease, chemotherapy is presently considered the treatment of choice. Advanced stage pure seminomas are unusual, and every effort must be made to exclude other cell types that would result in reclassification as a nonseminomatous tumor.

In contrast to seminoma, two-thirds of the patients with nonseminomatous tumor have metastatic disease when first diagnosed. In the United States surgical excision of the retroperitoneal lymph nodes has been performed for its value both as an accurate staging tool and as a therapeutic procedure in some patients with early metastatic disease. Older studies have shown that over 50 per cent of patients with metastatic disease in the retroperitoneum can be cured by surgical excision alone.[6]

In the United States, retroperitoneal lymph node dissection (RPLND) is still the standard treatment for low-stage (I, IIA, and IIB) nonseminomatous germ cell tumors (NSGCT). In a full RPLND, excision of lymphatics surrounding the aorta and vena cava is performed from the renal hilum to the bifurcation of the iliacs. Resection of the lumbar sympathetic chains and the presacral branches of the hypogastric plexus almost always results in loss of ejaculatory function. Although patients maintain their erectile potency, the loss of ejaculation may create disturbing infertility issues in this younger population of cancer patients. In an effort to reduce the incidence of this unfortunate complication of surgery, a modified dissection is now often performed in patients who appear to have no metastatic disease at the time of operation. The modified dissection spares the contralateral nodal packages and presacral areas, thereby reducing the incidence of ejaculatory disturbances to 20 to 25 per cent.[7,8]

RPLND is performed on patients with a clinical stage I and early stage II disease. Because of inherent staging errors, some patients with clinical stage I disease will prove to have pathologic stage II disease at surgery. Although some of these patients with stage II disease will be cured by surgery, others will relapse with active malignancy again, almost always outside of the retroperitoneum. In patients with less bulky retroperitoneal disease, this risk of relapse is generally in the range of 30 or 40 per cent. Stage II patients who have undergone surgery may be managed by close observation and full treatment (four cycles) of chemotherapy if relapse occurs. Alternatively, patients in this group may be offered adjuvant chemotherapy (two cycles) rather than observation alone. Both approaches offer cure rates approaching 100 per cent,[9] and management decisions are basically determined by patient/physician preference. Close, reliable follow-up is imperative, especially in patients being managed by observation postoperatively.

Presently there is nearly uniform agreement that patients with more advanced disease (bulky stage II and stage III) should be treated initially with chemotherapy. Surgery is reserved for those patients who continue to have residual retroperitoneal masses after combination chemotherapy. In patients undergoing RPLND for residual mass, approximately 40 per cent will have only necrosis and fibrosis, 40 per cent will have residual malignant elements, and the remaining 20 per cent will have mature teratoma. This residual teratoma probably represents the transformation of the malignant elements into their benign counterparts. Resection of teratoma is therapeutic since local growth can continue causing organ damage and even death. Resection of residual neoplasms serves mainly to re-stage this group of patients for additional chemotherapy. The prognosis, even with additional cycles of therapy, is particularly poor in this group of incomplete responders who continue to harbor residual disease.

Perhaps the most significant advance in the treatment of testicular cancer came from the advent of effective chemotherapeutic regimens capable of inducing remissions in patients with metastatic disease. Multi-drug regimens containing cisplatin, which is the single most active agent against testicular cancer, are now commonly used for treatment of advanced stage disease and as an adjuvant to surgery in some patients with less bulky retroperitoneal involvement. Vinblastine, bleomycin, and platinum (PVB) regimens originated out of work at Indiana University (Einhorn). Somewhat more complicated protocols of cyclophosphamide, vinblastine, actinomycin, bleomycin, and platinum (VAB) were developed simultaneously at Memorial Sloan-Kettering with roughly comparable results. Drug toxicities are considerable, but are generally well tolerated in this young age group with close monitoring. More recently, another chemotherapeutic agent, etoposide, is proving to be very effective in multi-drug regimens. Initially used with cisplatin for salvage therapy in refractory patients, etoposide may now be replacing more toxic agents, like vinblastine, in first line treatment of metastatic testicular cancer. Chemotherapy may aggravate or contribute to the infertility problems faced by testicular cancer patients. Overall, chemotherapy and integrated treatment programs with surgery and multi-drug regimens can now cure 70 to 80 per cent of patients with stage III disease.[10]

One aspect of management now receiving considerable clinical attention, as well as provoking some degree of controversy, is the "observational protocol" for clinical stage I NSGCT. This surveillance approach is based on the rationale that although 10 to 20 per cent of clinical stage I nonseminoma patients proved to have more disease at the time of RPLND, salvage chemotherapy is highly effective for curing patients who relapse when their lesions are identified early. The surveillance protocols are an effort to spare the other 80 to 90 per cent of the patients, who do not have additional disease, from being subjected to surgery. These admirable attempts to eliminate "over-treatment" of patients at low risk for relapse must be proved not to jeopardize the high cure rate presently achieved by standard management techniques. Patients must be highly selected with negative staging studies, normal markers after orchiectomy, and often undergo LAG in addition to CT scans. Men with poor prognostic parameters (see section on staging) are often rejected from surveillance protocols. The ability and motivation to comply with close follow-up that would result in early detection of relapse is also important. Until the long-term survival statistics are available for surveillance protocols and can be compared with the excellent results obtained by lymphatic surgery, these programs must still be regarded as investigational.

In those patients who develop recurrent disease during follow-up, over 90 per cent will relapse within one year. Only rarely do relapses occur after two years. It is presently recommended that patients have very close follow-up during the initial two-year period after diagnosis. Modern treatment programs have yielded cure rates greater than 95 per cent in low-stage disease for both seminoma and nonseminomatous testicular cancer. Advances in chemotherapy and the effectiveness of integrated surgery/chemotherapy protocols are responsible for dramatic improvement in the prognosis for high-stage disease, such that cure rate between 80 and 90 per cent can now be expected.

REFERENCES

1. Hogan, J.M., and Johnson, D.E.: Etiology of testicular tumors. *In* Johnson, D.E. (Ed.): Testicular Tumors, ed 2. Flushing, NY, Medical Examination Publishing Co., Inc., 1976, p. 31.

2. Gilbert, J.B.: Tumors of the testis following mumps orchitis: Case report and review of 24 cases. J. Urol. *51:*296, 1944.
3. Donahue, J.P.: Tumors of the testis. *In* Kendall, A.R. and Karafin, L. (Eds.): Urology, vol. 2. Philadelphia, Harper & Row, 1982.
4. Freedman, L.S., Parkinson, M.C., Jones, W.G., et al.: Histopathology in the prediction of relapse of patients with stage I testicular teritoma treated with orchidectomy alone. Lancet *2:*294, 1987.
5. Heslath, P.J., and Krane, R.J.: Prognostic assessment in nonseminomatous testicular cancer: Implications for therapy. J. Urol. *144:*1–9, 1990.
6. Whitmore, W.F., Jr.: Germinal testis tumors in adults. Seventh National Cancer Conference Proceedings. 1983, p. 795.
7. Richie, J.P., and Garnick, M.B.: Limited retroperitoneal lymphadenectomy for patients with clinical stage I testicular tumor, abstract 179: Proceedings of the 20th Congress of the International Society of Urology, Vienna, 1985, p. 113.
8. Weissbach, L., and Aboderin-Boedefeld, B.: Modified RPLND as a means to preserve fertility, abstract 160. Proceedings of the 20th Congress of the International Society of Urology, Vienna, 1985, p. 113.
9. Williams, S.D., Stablein, D.M., Einhorn, L.H., et al.: Immediate adjuvant chemotherapy versus observation with treatment at relapse in pathological stage II testicular cancer. N. Engl. J. Med. *317:*23, 1433–1438, 1987.
10. Loehrer, P.J., Sr., Williams, S.D., and Einhorn, L.H.: Testicular cancer: The quest continues. J. Natl. Cancer Inst. *80:*1373, 1988.

TRANSITIONAL CELL CARCINOMA OF THE BLADDER
by Robert Eyre, M.D.

INCIDENCE AND EPIDEMIOLOGY

Transitional cell carcinoma of the bladder is the third most prevalent malignant disease among males and the tenth among females in the United States. Over 45,000 new cases are diagnosed annually, and about 11,000 patients per year will die from their disease. The incidence of bladder cancer increases with age; the mean age for diagnosis for both sexes is 68 years. In the United States, the age-adjusted bladder cancer rate in white men is nearly twice that in blacks, and the overall male:female sex ratio of affected individuals is 4:1. Bladder cancer is more prevalent among the higher social classes, particularly among those individuals in "white-collar" occupations.

Cigarette smoking and occupational exposure to arylamines are well-established risk factors. A recent National Bladder Cancer Study suggested that about half of the cases of bladder cancer in men and about one-third of those in women are attributable to cigarette smoking. It appears that bladder cancer risk is reduced in former smokers and those who use filtered cigarettes.[4] Occupational exposure to arylamines can occur in workers handling aniline dyes, leather tanning products, or in the production of rubber and paint products. A weak association between coffee consumption and

CHAPTER 13 / UROLOGIC CARCINOMA: Transitional Cell Carcinoma of The Bladder—299

increased risk of bladder cancer has been found. There appears to be no increased risk associated with the use of artificial sweeteners.

CLINICAL EVALUATION

Macroscopic or microscopic hematuria is the presenting symptom of bladder cancer in approximately 80 per cent of patients. In the outpatient population, however, hematuria is most commonly caused by prostatic obstruction or urinary tract infection. In addition to a thorough physical examination, initial evaluation should include a microscopic urinalysis, urine culture, and urine cytology. Cystographic films from an intravenous urogram (IVP) cannot diagnose bladder tumors with sufficient sensitivity; therefore, complete evaluation for hematuria must include a cystoscopic evaluation of the bladder mucosa. Bladder tumors can assume two general configurations (Fig. 13–4). Papillary or pedunculated tumors are more common, can grow to a considerable size, and tend to be noninfiltrating. Nonpapillary solid tumors produce flat, ill-defined defects with little or no intraluminal projection on cystography. These lesions tend to be of higher grade, and often invade the bladder wall. Because of this, they can produce fixation and rigidity of the bladder wall, which can be detected on the later cystogram films of an intravenous urogram. Other important information to be obtained from an IVP includes the status of the upper tracts, as a urothelial tumor involving the renal pelvis or ureter may produce satellite tumors in the bladder. Ureteral obstruction associated with bladder carcinoma is an ominous prognostic sign, and usually indicates deep infiltration of the muscle wall by tumor in the area of the trigone or intravesical ureter.

Once the clinical diagnosis is made, the patient must have careful clinical and pathologic staging. A cystoscopy under anaesthesia should be done that

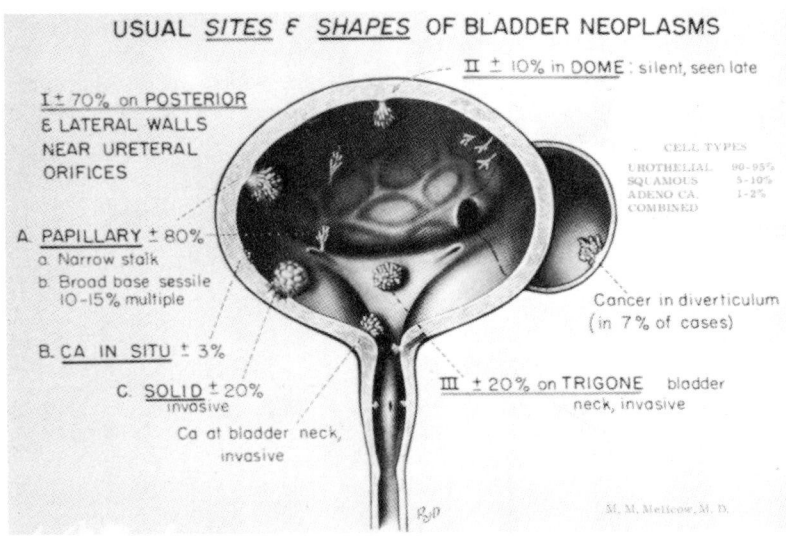

Figure 13–4. Usual sites and shapes of bladder neoplasms. (From Melicow, M.M.: Tumors of the bladder: A multifaceted problem. J. Urol. *112*:467, 1974.)

allows cold-cup biopsy of any visible tumor as well as any area of mucosal abnormality suspicious for carcinoma in situ (CIS). These may appear as raised, roughened, or reddish areas of the bladder mucosa. In addition to any suspicious areas of the bladder, selected mucosal biopsies of the bladder urothelium should be done. In patients with superficial bladder tumors, adjacent mucosal atypia or in situ carcinoma is associated with a higher probability of tumor recurrence.[5] It is important to initially biopsy bladder tumors without the use of cauterization so that an accurate assessment of tumor depth may be done without introducing coagulation artifact. Following biopsy of small papillary tumors, one may completely resect the areas transurethrally. An important adjunct to this initial evaluation and treatment under anaesthesia is a bimanual examination to assess the presence of any masses within the bladder wall. A palpable mass strongly suggests a muscle-invasive tumor.

A number of different staging systems have been proposed for bladder carcinoma. The Jewett and Strong system, as modified by Marshall, describes the depth of bladder wall invasion by tumor as well as the extent of metastatic disease. Although clinical understaging is common relative to pathologic staging at the time of cystectomy, this system continues to provide useful information regarding the management of patients with bladder carcinoma. A more sophisticated TNM system for pathologic staging of tumors has gained increasing acceptance over the last few years, as urologists attempt to categorize subsets of patients who may benefit from several newer treatment modalities currently under investigation for bladder cancer (Fig. 13–5).

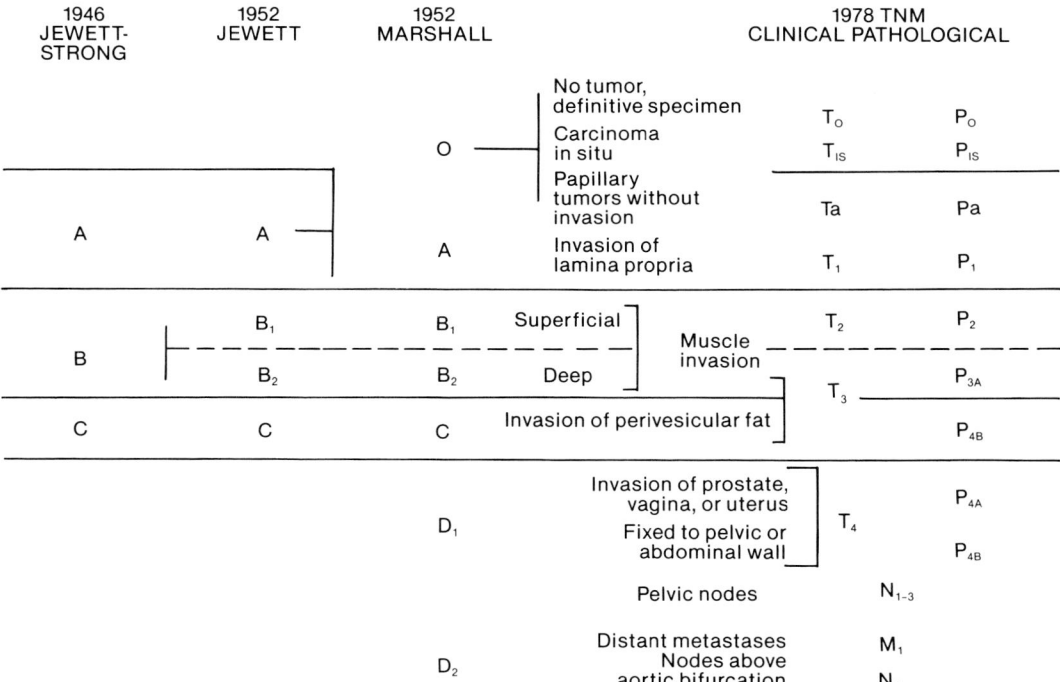

Figure 13–5. Comparisons of American and TNM staging systems for bladder cancer. (Fom Skinner, D.G.: Current state of classification and staging of bladder cancer. Cancer Res. 37:2838–2842, 1977.)

SUPERFICIAL BLADDER CARCINOMA

Superficial bladder tumors include noninvasive papillary transitional cell tumors confined to the bladder mucosa, CIS, and papillary tumors that have invaded through the lamina propria into the submucosa but not into the bladder muscle. These account for 75 to 85 per cent of all newly diagnosed lesions. Approximately 70 per cent of patients with lesions in this category develop tumor recurrences. About one in four patients will have progression to a higher histologic grade, and 10 to 15 per cent of patients who initially had superficial cancer will develop invasive lesions. Initial treatment for superficial bladder tumors should be complete transurethral resection after the tumor has been carefully biopsied without use of electrocautery. Patient follow-up should include interval cystoscopy and urine cytology. Because of the processing demands and interpretive difficulties with cytologies, flow cytometric analysis of urine from patients with bladder cancer has been proposed as a clinically useful alternative. An adequate number of cells for cytologic analysis can usually be obtained on a voided urine specimen; however, a catheterized urine or bladder washing is often necessary to produce enough cells for flow cytometry. A recent study comparing the two techniques showed that flow cytometry was significantly more sensitive than cytology in detecting low-grade papillary superficial bladder tumors.[6]

One of the most difficult jobs for the clinical urologist treating patients with bladder cancer is to select a therapeutic modality and follow-up program that takes into account an individual's risk for tumor recurrence and tumor progression. Several factors that significantly increase the risk for both recurrence and progression include higher tumor grades, lamina propria invasion, invasion of vascular or lymphatic spaces within the tumor, nonpapillary tumor configurations, tumor multiplicity, or associated CIS.[7] It is estimated that between 30 and 70 per cent of bladder cancers may have associated CIS in adjacent urothelium. The frequency of this finding increases with higher tumor grade. It is seen in less than 5 per cent of patients in the absence of other visible tumors. It is an aggressive lesion, as a recent report by Prout et al showed that only one of 12 patients with CIS treated by transurethral resection alone reached five years without a cystectomy or disease progression.[8]

Several experimental techniques have been used to more accurately predict which tumors have a higher potential for recurrence or progression. In 1981 Catalona published a study evaluating the natural history of bladder tumors that had been retrospectively characterized by the presence or absence of red blood cell antigens on the tumor surface epithelium. In patients whose tumors lacked cell surface antigen, recurrence was noted in about 90 per cent; those who were antigen-positive recurred half as often. Two-thirds of antigen-negative patients developed tumor invasion compared with 4 per cent of antigen-positive patients.[9]

Other experimental techniques have included detection of abnormal marker chromosomes in certain tumors, and tumor aneuploidy as demonstrated by flow cytometry. These methods are not available to most clinicians, and no single method has proved so accurate that it has gained widespread clinical usefulness.

Intravesical chemotherapy plays an important role in the management of patients with superficial bladder cancers. Available agents include thiotepa, mitomycin C, and doxorubicin (Adriamycin). All of these agents have about the same success rate in eradicating recurrent tumors, and all of them have been largely supplanted by the intravesical use of bacille Calmette-Guerin (BCG). Many experimental studies have been done on BCG since it was introduced by Morales in 1976, and this agent appears to be clearly superior to the other intravesical therapies.[10] Its mechanism of action is not completely understood, and probably results from a combination of a local inflammatory response of the bladder mucosa and nonspecific stimulation of the host immune system. Complete and durable response rates of 60 per cent or higher in treating residual tumor and 70 to 75 per cent in treating CIS are seen. In our practice, patients receive weekly installations for six weeks, with a few requiring an additional six-week course. Treatment failure after two or more courses is associated with progression to invasive tumor in 30% and metastases in 50 per cent of patients.[11] We recommend BCG for management of any patient who has residual superficial tumors, recurrent tumors, multiple tumors, tumors associated with CIS, or who has positive urine cytologies following transurethral resection of the tumor. In addition, any patient who has a high-grade superficial lesion (grade II to III) with lamina propria invasion receives BCG to decrease the likelihood of tumor recurrence or progression.

INVASIVE BLADDER CANCER

When tumors have invaded the muscular wall of the bladder, aggressive surgical therapy is indicated. A metastatic evaluation including chest x-ray, abdominal and pelvic CT scan, and bone scan should be carried out. Lymphangiography has not been widely advocated for preoperative metastatic evaluation because of its limitations in demonstrating the internal iliac and obturator node chains, which are the first to be involved in metastatic bladder tumors.

Pathologic examination of pelvic lymph nodes removed at the time of radical cystectomy demonstrates that a significant percentage of patients are understaged by clinical evaluation. Skinner et al found that 30 per cent of their patients with clinical stage B lesions and over 50 per cent of patients with stage C lesions (perivesical fat involvement) had positive lymph nodes at the time of pelvic lymphadenectomy. Their data suggest a clear survival advantage for patients with microscopic nodal involvement who have an en bloc pelvic lymphadenectomy at the time of radical cystectomy.[12] A more recent study found that 14 per cent of patients who had grossly normal pelvic lymph nodes at the time of cystectomy had unsuspected micrometastases in one or more nodes upon examination of pelvic lymphadenectomy specimens.[13]

Several clinical trials over the past decade have evaluated the efficacy of neo-adjuvant pelvic radiation therapy in an attempt to sterilize nodal metastases and downstage tumors prior to radical cystectomy. Although downstaging of the bladder lesion was seen in some patients, a survival advantage has not been demonstrated and preoperative radiation has largely been eliminated from contemporary treatment protocols.

Radiation therapy as the sole treatment modality for bladder cancer is used rarely today. It is now generally accepted that bladder cancers exhibit a wide variability in radioresponsiveness. Papillary lesions tend to be much more radiosensitive than flat, spreading, or infiltrating lesions. Conventional external beam therapy, using modern megavoltage techniques, will permanently eradicate local bladder cancer in 30 to 50 per cent of patients. Experimental studies using open cystotomy plus intraoperative radiation therapy delivered to the tumor by electron beam or radioactive seed implants followed by additional external beam irradiation to the bladder have shown impressive preliminary results in terms of low recurrence rates, preservation of bladder function, and five-year survival.[14] Clearly, this treatment needs further investigation.

The mainstay of therapy for invasive bladder cancer remains radical cystectomy with urinary diversion. Control of local disease is achieved in 70 to 90 per cent of patients. Although this tumor commonly affects patients in their seventh and eighth decades of life, age alone should rarely preclude this treatment option. To minimize morbidity, several points should be considered when performing this surgery on elderly patients. These considerations include a preoperative nutritional assessment with more detailed study and correction of abnormalities as needed, preoperative and postoperative enterostomal therapy evaluation and teaching, meticulous anesthetic monitoring with a pulmonary artery catheter, and use of an epidural catheter for intraoperative and postoperative pain management. The epidural catheter (which may remain in place for 24 to 48 hours postoperatively) dramatically reduces the parenteral narcotic requirement, facilitates quicker ventilatory weaning and promotes improved pulmonary function in the immediate postoperative period. After inspecting the pelvis for gross nodal metastases, the ileal conduit should be constructed up to the point of stomal maturation before proceeding with cystectomy. If any hemodynamic or cardiac instability has been encountered, the stoma is matured and cystectomy is deferred for 10 to 14 days. In the author's experience, staged procedures in elderly patients are very rarely necessary, and combined radical cystectomy and urinary diversion are accomplished with very low morbidity and no mortality.

An important recent contribution by Walsh has been the description of a nerve-sparing technique for performing radical cystectomy.[15] The success rate in preserving sexual potency postoperatively using this technique directly correlates with patient age. In Walsh's series fewer than 50 per cent of patients over age 60 maintained their erectile function. Nevertheless, this concept is a major contribution to the field for it offers the younger male patient with invasive bladder cancer optimum therapy without a guaranteed loss of sexual function. Other advantages offered by Walsh's technical modifications include improved hemostasis and better definition of anatomic planes, resulting in a safer, technically easier and quicker operation.

When sexual dysfunction does occur following radical pelvic surgery, potency can usually be restored by the use of small doses of vasoactive agents (e.g. papaverine, prostaglandin E_1) injected directly into the corpora cavernosa. This medication bypasses the normal neurologically mediated initiation of corporal vasodilatation leading to tumescence. Some patients prefer to have a penile prosthetic implant placed.

Although the ileal conduit as described by Bricker remains the diversion of choice for most patients with bladder carcinoma, several different procedures have recently been described for creating continent urinary reservoirs in carefully selected patients with a longer life expectancy. The Kock pouch and the cecoileal reservoir ("Indiana pouch") have been most widely used. All of these procedures use small or large intestinal segments that are reconfigured in such a way that peristaltic contractions become disorganized, thus increasing reservoir compliance. Nonrefluxing ureterointestinal anastomoses are created by tunnelling or intestinal intussusception ("Hendren nipple"), and outflow resistance through a catheterizable segment is increased by plicating or intussuscepting the bowel. For an overview of these procedures, the reader is referred to several recent excellent monographs.[16, 17] Patients who choose this option are not required to wear a cutaneous appliance, but must catheterize a stoma placed on the lower abdominal wall four to five times per day to empty their urinary reservoirs. The type of continent diversion favored by the authors (Indiana pouch) also allows the possibility for direct anastomosis of the urinary reservoir to the urethra or vaginal wall so that catheterization can be done through the penis or female "neo-urethra."

Slight modifications to the continent diversion technique allow the surgeon to create a highly compliant internal reservoir that can be directly anastomosed to the male urethra in such a way that normal voiding may be accomplished. This is not a reconstructive option for females because of short urethral length, and the success of current procedures is still limited by a high percentage of patients having nocturnal incontinence. This can be corrected in most patients by placement of an artificial urinary sphincter at the level of the bulbous urethra.

Continent diversions or functional internal reservoirs are more technically demanding and take longer to perform than ileal conduit urinary diversion. They are also associated with higher potential postoperative morbidity. However, for the carefully selected patient, they may offer significant advantages in terms of self-image, interpersonal relations, and sexuality over more traditional forms of urinary diversion requiring an external collection device. Although our short-term results are excellent, there is insufficient length of follow-up with continent diversions or internal reservoirs to predict the long-term risks of renal deterioration or electrolyte disturbances.

THERAPY FOR ADVANCED DISEASE

The prognosis for patients with muscle-invasive bladder cancer treated by cystectomy or radiation therapy (either alone or in combination) is poor, with five-year survival ranging from 25 to 50 per cent. In two-thirds of patients, the cause of death is metastatic disease. Laboratory and clinical studies looking at various chemotherapeutic agents active against transitional tumors have, until recently, had disappointing results. Clinical responses were typically seen in a minority of patients, most of which were partial, and lasted less than six months.

In 1986, Sternberg et al reported their preliminary results in 25 patients with advanced stage bladder cancer (N + MO and NOM+) using a combination of cisplatin, methotrexate, Adriamycin, and vinblastine (M-VAC) as neo-adjuvant (up-front) chemotherapy. A recent update of 83 patients followed until death or for a minimum of 22 months showed complete remission in 37 per cent of the patients clinically, pathologically, and after surgical resection of residual disease. Partial remissions occurred in 31 per cent, while 32 per cent had either a minor response or progressed.[18]

Our experience using neo-adjuvant M-VAC parallels that of Sternberg at Memorial-Sloan Kettering (M-SK). While the early results are encouraging, several points must be stressed: (1) partial responders appear to do as poorly as nonresponders; (2) in the M-SK patients, brain metastases occurred within 6 to 42 months in 18 per cent of the responders, half of whom never had systemic relapse; (3) M-VAC appears to be active only against transitional cell tumor elements. Many high-grade tumors (grade III to IV) exhibit areas of squamous and adenocarcinomatous dedifferentiation that are not affected by therapy; and (4) drug toxicity is significant. No survival advantage has been demonstrated if M-VAC therapy is given when metastatic disease is discovered at cystectomy or subsequently. Controlled studies are needed to assess its role in an adjuvant setting.

Despite these issues, M-VAC or other platinum-based drug regimens appear to offer a major therapeutic tool in the treatment of advanced bladder cancer. A multi-institutional prospective trial of cisplatin and full-dosage radiation therapy in patients with invasive bladder tumors who were not suitable for cystectomy yielded an overall 70 per cent complete response rate and 51 per cent survival at four years.[19] A randomized prospective trial of neo-adjuvant M-VAC plus cystectomy versus cystectomy alone in patients with muscle-invasive tumors has begun.

Major issues to be resolved include (1) the optimum number of drug cycles prior to cystectomy (should it be based on tumor response as evaluated by cystoscopy, biopsy, and CT, knowing that clinical staging errors may approach 38 per cent?) and (2) the number of cycles of chemotherapy that should be given following cystectomy, both for patients who are complete responders pathologically, and for those who were felt to have a good clinical response but at cystectomy are found to have residual disease in the bladder or lymph nodes. It will likely be several years before statistically valid conclusions can be drawn from the various protocols utilizing platinum-based chemotherapy. It seems clear, however, that multimodality therapy will be required to improve the survival of this challenging group of patients.

In conclusion, one can appreciate the tremendous clinical and research efforts which have redefined the way we treat bladder cancer over the past few years: more sensitive methods of surveillance, more effective intravesical agents, potential predictors of tumor progression, surgical innovations that may allow potency and urinary continence, newer radiation therapy methods, and combinations of radiation and surgery with more effective chemotherapy.

TRANSITIONAL CELL CARCINOMA OF THE RENAL PELVIS AND URETER

Transitional cell cancers arising in the renal pelvis account for about 15 per cent of all primary renal tumors. Gross or microscopic hematuria should prompt a careful evaluation of the urinary tract. An IVP may show delayed or absent renal function. Retrograde ureteropyelography will usually demonstrate a radiolucent filling defect in the ureter or renal pelvis, which must be differentiated from a stone or blood clot. Calyceal distortion may be present. The radiographic finding of pyelolymphatic or pyelovenous retrograde filling on a properly performed, low-pressure retrograde pyelogram should alert the clinician to a possible lesion. Urine cytologies may be very helpful in diagnosing upper tract lesions, and the yield may be further improved by retrograde barbotage of the ureter and renal pelvis (forceful saline irrigation with 5 to 10 ml of fluid). Lesions of the ureter or renal pelvis can be biopsied and fulgerated endoscopically using a rigid or flexible ureteroscope.

Further diagnostic evaluation may include abdominal CT, bone scan, and chest x-ray. Whenever a urothelial cancer is diagnosed, a full evaluation of the urinary tract must be undertaken initially and at regular intervals subsequently as 2 to 3 per cent of patients with bladder cancer will have or will later develop an upper tract lesion,[1] and 30 to 50 per cent of patients with upper tract tumors will have synchronous or subsequent bladder tumors.[2] Because upper tract tumors tend to be multifocal or are associated with other areas of in situ cancer, surgical therapy should include en bloc radical excision of the kidney and entire ureter including a cuff of bladder surrounding the ureteral orifice to minimize the risk of tumor recurrence. The prognosis for aggressively treated superficial tumors is excellent. Ureteral cancers may penetrate through the thin muscular wall to involve regional lymphatics early in the natural history of the disease, hence invasive lesions are associated with a relatively poor prognosis.[3]

With improved endourologic techniques and instrumentation over the past five years, it has become possible to perform percutaneous endoscopic resection of upper tract tumors. However, recurrence rates are very high (probably because of the multifocal nature of many renal pelvic tumors, and the frequent finding of diffuse carcinoma in situ), and this technique should only be considered when conventional surgical therapy is impossible. Intravesical chemotherapeutic agents, such as thiotepa and BCG, have been used as primary or adjuvant therapy in small numbers of patients with reported successes.

Segmental ureterectomy has been proposed by some as a reasonable treatment option for solitary low-grade tumors. Although we have occasionally performed this in patients with compromised renal function or in those with a solitary kidney with good success, we have found that final pathologic analysis frequently showed other areas of epithelial dysplasia, or the tumor was of higher grade than was suggested by urine cytology or ureteral biopsy. These factors all increase the risk of tumor recurrence, thus the most prudent surgical management is to perform radical nephroureterectomy in all appropriate circumstances. We have one elderly patient with recurrent grade II to III tumors in the renal pelvis of a solitary kidney whose lesions have been managed for several years by partial nephrectomy, YAG laser fulgeration via a rigid ureteroscope and interval thiotepa, and BCG delivered through a ureteral catheter as an outpatient who has been clinically tumor-free with negative urine cytologies for five years. Obviously, one cannot be dogmatic in managing individual patients.

Single or multiple agent chemotherapy for regional or disseminated disease may produce some short-lived, partial responses but the overall prognosis remains poor.

REFERENCES

1. Babaian, R.J., and Johnson, D.E.: Primary carcinoma of the ureter. J. Urol. *123:*357, 1980.
2. Kakizoe T., Fujita, J., Tatsuro, M., et al.: Transitional cell carcinoma of the bladder in patients with renal pelvic and ureteral cancer. J. Urol. *124:*17, 1980.
3. Nocks, B.N., Heney, N.M., Daly, J.T., et al.: Transitional cell carcinoma of the renal pelvis. Urology *19:*472–477, 1982.
4. Hartge, P., Silverman, D., Hoover, R., et al.: Changing cigarette habits and bladder cancer risk: A case-control study. J. Natl. Cancer Inst. *78:*1119–1125, 1987.
5. Smith, G., Elton, R.A., and Beynon, L.L.: Prognostic significance of biopsy results of normal-looking mucosa in cases of superficial bladder cancer. Br. J. Urol. *55:*665–669, 1983.
6. Badalaurent, R.A., et al.: The sensitivity of flow cytometry compared with conventional cytology in the detection of superficial bladder carcinoma. Cancer *59:*2078–2085, 1987.
7. Skinner, D.G., and Lieskovsky, G.: Diagnosis and management of genitourinary cancer. Philadelphia, W.B. Saunders, 1988, p. 284.
8. Prout, G.R., Griffin, P.P., and Daly, J.J.: The outcome of conservative treatment of carcinoma in situ of the bladder. J. Urol. *138:*776–770, 1987.
9. Catalona, W.J.: Practical utility of specific red cell adherence test in bladder cancer. Urology *18:*113–117, 1981.
10. Herr, H.W., Laudone, V.P., and Whitmore, W.F.: Overview of intravesical therapy for superficial bladder tumors. J. Urol. *138:*1363–1368, 1987.
11. Catalona, W.J., Hudson, M.A., Gillen, D.P., et al.: Risks and benefits of repeated courses of intravesical Bacillus Calmette-Guerin therapy for superficial bladder cancer. J. Urol. *137:*220–224, 1987.
12. Skinner, D.G.: Management of invasive bladder cancer: A meticulous pelvic node dissection can make a difference. J. Urol. *128:*34–36, 1982.
13. Wishnow, K.I., Johnson, D.E., Ro, J.V., et al.: Incidence extent and location of unsuspected pelvic lymph node metastasis in patients undergoing radical cystectomy for bladder cancer. J. Urol. *137:*408–410, 1987.
14. Shipley, W.U., Kaufman, S.D., and Prout, G.R.: Intraoperative radiation therapy in patients with bladder cancer: A review of techniques allowing improved tumor doses and providing high cure rates without loss of bladder function. Cancer *60:*1485–1488, 1987.
15. Schlegel, P.N., and Walsh, P.C.: Neuroanatomical approach to radical cystoprostatectomy with preservation of sexual function. J. Urol. *138:*1402–1406, 1987.
16. Skinner, D.G., Lieskovsky, G., Boyd, S. D., et al.: Urinary diversion, *In* Ravitch, M.M. (Ed.): Current Problems in Surgery, Vol. XXIV, No. 7. Chicago, Year Book Medical Publishers, Inc., 1987.
17. Fowler, J.E., Jr.: Continent urinary reservoirs and bladder substitutes in the adult: Parts I & II. Monographs in Urology, Vol. 8, No. 2. Stamey, T.A. (Ed.), Princeton, NJ, Custom Publishing Services, Inc., 1987.
18. Sternberg, C.N., Yagoda, A., Scher, H.I., et al.: M-VAC (methotrexate, vinblastine, doxorubicin and cisplatin) for advanced transitional cell carcinoma of the urothelium. J. Urol. *139:*461–469, 1988.
19. Shipley, W.U., Prout, G.R. Jr., Einstein, A. B., et al.: Treatment of invasive bladder cancer by cisplatin and radiation in patients unsuited for surgery. JAMA *258:*931–935, 1987.

14

GYNECOLOGIC ONCOLOGY

by Jonathan M. Niloff, M.D., F.A.C.S., F.A.C.O.G., F.R.C.S.(C.), and Howard M. Goodman, M.D.

The management of gynecologic tumors has undergone major changes over the last two decades. We now have a better understanding of the natural histories of the reproductive neoplasms. This has resulted in recently published modified staging classifications for carcinomas of the ovary, cervix, and endometrium. This has also led to a greater individualization of therapy and less reliance on clinical stage for treatment decisions. The importance of surgical staging, particularly in endometrial and ovarian cancer, has now been accepted. Although surgery remains the cornerstone of management for the major gynecologic cancers, combined therapy with either radiation therapy or chemotherapy is often employed. Ovarian cancer is one of the few solid tumors commonly responsive to chemotherapy. In the following sections, these advances, as they apply to each of the gynecologic tumors, will be discussed.

OVARIAN CANCER

Ovarian cancer is the fifth most common cause of cancer-related mortality among women. It has a high death to case ratio, most likely attributable to its insidious onset. Most patients present with advanced disease manifested clinically by ascites or epigastric distress. The peak incidence for epithelial ovarian tumors is in the fifth to seventh decades of life. An efficacious screening technique is not currently available.

Three hereditary ovarian cancer syndromes have been described: familial ovarian cancer, familial ovarian and breast cancer, and a multiple cancer syndrome that often includes carcinoma of the colon. Women in such families typically present with their ovarian tumors at an early age. The recognition of these families has led to the suggestion that some women might benefit from prophylactic bilateral oophorectomies[1] if they have two or more first-degree relatives with ovarian cancer, especially if a mother or sister developed ovarian cancer at an early age. This operation should only be considered after these women have completed their desired childbearing. However, bilateral oophorectomies are not completely protective inasmuch as several cases have been reported in which pelvic-abdominal tumors have arisen, histologically indistinguishable from ovarian carcinoma, after prophylactic castration.[2] These are presumed to arise from the pelvic peritoneum, which has an embryologic derivation similar to that of the surface epithelium of the ovary. Prophylactic unilateral oophorectomy does not decrease the subsequent risk for ovarian cancer.

Natural History and Staging

Epithelial ovarian cancer spreads intraperitoneally, producing diffuse intraabdominal metastases on the peritoneal and visceral surfaces. Common sites are the diaphragm, especially in its posterior portion, omentum, lateral colonic gutters, and the mesentery of the small bowel. Ascites is common, resulting from tumor obstruction of diaphragmatic lymphatics. A second route of spread is via lymphatics that accompany the ovarian vessels resulting in para-aortic lymph node metastases. The cancer usually remains confined to the peritoneal cavity until later into its course. Deaths are commonly due to small bowel obstruction and progressive inanition.

Management of Ovarian Cancer

Paramount to the management of ovarian cancer is an accurate assessment of stage. In contrast to some of the other gynecologic tumors, staging for ovarian cancer is always performed surgically. The International Federation of Obstetricians and Gynecologists has recently published a revised staging system, which is presented in Table 14–1. Prognosis is closely related to stage and to the amount of residual tumor remaining after primary surgery. Grade, although not included in the staging system, is also an important prognostic factor.

The importance of a meticulous and organized approach to the surgical staging of ovarian cancer was highlighted by a study reported by the Ovarian Cancer Study Group.[3] Thirty-one per cent of 100 patients with putative stage I or II ovarian cancer who were subjected to a second staging procedure were upstaged. Seventy-seven per cent of these lesions were advanced to stage III. The sites of occult metastases are illustrated in Table 14–2. The most common extrapelvic sites were the para-aortic lymph nodes and the omentum.

Laparotomy for ovarian cancer should be performed through an adequate midline incision that will permit satisfactory exploration of the entire abdominal cavity. Hemostasis should be maintained on opening the abdomen, avoiding contamination of peritoneal washings, which should be obtained on

TABLE 14–1. FIGO STAGING FOR CARCINOMA OF THE OVARY (1985)

Stage I	Growth limited to the ovaries
Stage IA	Growth limited to one ovary; no ascites. No tumor on the external surface; capsule intact.
Stage IB	Growth limited to both ovaries; no ascites. No tumor on the external surface; capsules intact.
Stage IC	Tumor either stage IA or IB but with tumor on the surface of one or both ovaries; or with capsule ruptured; or with ascites present containing malignant cells or with positive peritoneal washings
Stage II	Growth involving one or both ovaries with pelvic extension
Stage IIA	Extension and/or metastases to the uterus and/or tubes
Stage IIB	Extension to other pelvic tissues
Stage IIC	Tumor either stage IIA or IIB but with tumor on the surface of one or both ovaries; or with capsule(s) ruptured; or with ascites present containing malignant cells or with positive peritoneal washings.
Stage III	Tumor involving one or both ovaries with peritoneal implants outside the pelvis and/or positive retroperitoneal or inguinal nodes. Superficial liver metastasis equals stage III. Tumor is limited to the true pelvis but with histologically verified malignant extension to small bowel or omentum.
Stage IIIA	Tumor grossly limited to the true pelvis with negative nodes but with histologically confirmed microscopic seeding of abdominal peritoneal surfaces
Stage IIIB	Tumor of one or both ovaries with histologically confirmed implants of abdominal peritoneal surfaces, none exceeding 2 cm in diameter. Nodes negative
Stage IIIC	Abdominal implants >2 cm in diameter and/or positive retroperitoneal or inguinal nodes
Stage IV	Growth involving one or both ovaries with distant metastasis. If pleural effusion is present there must be positive cytologic test results to allot a case to stage IV. Parenchymal liver metastasis equals stage IV.

Data from: Am. J. Obstet. Gynecol., 1987.

entering the peritoneal cavity. One hundred ml of saline are instilled into the peritoneal cavity and then aspirated and sent for cytologic evaluation. If ascites is present, washings are not necessary and it is sufficient to simply send a sample of the ascitic fluid for cytologic examination. The volume of ascites should be recorded. The pelvis is then inspected. The presence or

TABLE 14–2. SITES OF OCCULT METASTASES AT SECONDARY STAGING IN 61 PATIENTS REFERRED WITH APPARENT STAGES IA–IIB OVARIAN CANCER

Site	Biopsies (Positive/Total)	%
Paraaortic nodes	6/52	12
Omentum	6/57	11
Other abdominal tissue	4/45	9
Diaphragm	2/58	3
Cul-de-sac peritoneum	3/51	6
Other pelvic tissue	4/43	9

From Young, R. C., Decker, D. G., Wharton, J. T., et al.: Staging laparotomy in early ovarian cancer. JAMA 250:3072–3076, 1983.

absence of excrescences on the surface of the ovary or adhesion to the pelvic sidewall or other structures are noted. All sites of adhesion should be biopsied to evaluate tumor extension in these locations. Exploration of the upper abdomen is performed. Special attention is directed to palpation of the diaphragm, the surface of the liver, the lateral colonic gutters, the omentum, the root of the mesentery, and the para-aortic lymph nodes. Suspicious areas should be biopsied. Random biopsy of the diaphragm in the absence of any palpable disease has not been fruitful. An omental biopsy is always performed. In the absence of observing gross tumor in the omentum, it is not necessary to perform a total omentectomy. A specimen consisting of the most dependent 2 cm of the omentum is satisfactory. This is the area most likely to contain metastatic tumor.

We reserve aortic lymph node biopsies for stage I and II patients who are at risk for such metastases and in whom the information gained will alter our therapeutic plan. Studies have demonstrated that patients with well-differentiated tumors are at negligible risk for metastases to the para-aortic nodes.[4] Patients with gross tumor in the upper abdomen have already met the criteria for stage III and their treatment plans will therefore not be altered by the detection of occult tumor in the para-aortic region. We therefore limit para-aortic lymph node dissections to patients with poorly differentiated tumors confined to the ovary. These are the patients in whom our treatment plan will be altered by the knowledge of such metastases. The dissection is performed by incising the peritoneum over the aorta. The duodenum is displaced cephalically with a retractor. The nodal tissue is then removed from the renal vein caudally, care being taken not to injure the inferior mesenteric artery. Inasmuch as this is a staging procedure, only a lymph node sampling is necessary.

Management of a Pelvic Mass

The management of a presumed ovarian mass is dependent on the patient's age and menopausal status. In the reproductive age group, most palpable ovarian masses will be physiologic in nature. Such masses, of limited size, may be followed for a period of four to eight weeks. Suppressive therapy with oral contraceptives is often prescribed. Most physiologic cysts will resolve over this period of observation. If the mass persists, surgery is indicated to rule out a neoplasm. If a mass is greater than 8 cm at presentation, it is unlikely to resolve and surgery may be undertaken without delay. An ultrasound evaluation may be helpful in distinguishing ovarian masses from other pelvic pathology. This modality is superior to computed tomography (CT) for this purpose. The presence of an ovarian tumor must always be ruled out in a postmenopausal woman with a pelvic mass. Indeed, any palpable ovary in a postmenopausal woman should raise the suspicion for ovarian cancer, and laparotomy is indicated. In cases of uncertainty, a laparoscopy may be considered to clarify the diagnosis.

Surgical Management of Early-Stage Ovarian Cancer

The standard surgical procedure for ovarian cancer is total abdominal hysterectomy, bilateral salpingo-oophorectomy, and meticulous surgical staging as previously described, including peritoneal washings, omental biopsy, and aortic lymph node biopsies in selected circumstances. However, a more conservative procedure may be considered for young women with a strong desire to maintain their reproductive capability. Surgery for such patients should consist of unilateral salpingo-oophorectomy, biopsy of the contralateral ovary, and the usual staging procedures, including peritoneal washings and omental biopsy. Candidates for such a procedure should have stage I encapsulated borderline or well-differentiated epithelial ovarian tumors. Young women with stage I germ cell or stromal tumors are also candidates for this conservative approach. In patients with dysgerminomas, an ipsilateral pelvic and para-aortic lymph node dissection should also be included in the staging procedure. This issue of fertility conservation should be discussed with young patients prior to laparotomy and they should understand the potential for needing a second operation if more advanced occult disease is detected after histologic evaluation of the staging specimens.

Surgical Management of Advanced Ovarian Cancer

The prognosis among patients with advanced ovarian cancer is strongly related to the volume of tumor remaining after the primary surgical procedure.[5–7,9] It is thus now common practice to perform aggressive cytoreductive procedures in an attempt to excise most, if not all, of both the primary tumor and abdominal metastases. The beneficial effect of this surgery is presumed to result from an increase in the growth fraction in the remaining tumor, rendering it more sensitive to chemotherapy. The literature concerning cytoreductive surgery is difficult to evaluate in that randomized studies have not been performed. However, as illustrated in Table 14–3, there are many studies that report an increase in survival following such procedures. This improved survival, as presented in Table 14–4, appears to be mediated by an improvement in the objective response rate to chemotherapy. The most dramatic effect is observed in the complete response rate, as determined by second-look laparotomy. Complete responses to chemotherapy are essentially limited to those patients having undergone successful cytoreductive operations.

Before beginning an aggressive cytoreductive operation, the surgeon must make a careful assessment of the tumor and its metastases for resectability. If the anatomic location of any tumor dictates that a large tumor mass (greater than 1.5 to 3 cm) will have to be left behind, then the procedure

TABLE 14–3. SURVIVAL AND MAXIMUM RESIDUAL MASS SIZE FOLLOWING PRIMARY CYTOREDUCTIVE SURGERY

Author (reference)	Mass Size (cm)	Number of patients	Median Survival (months)
Griffiths (4)	<1.5	41	22
	>1.5	26	11
Hacker et al (5)	<0.5	7	40
	0.5–1.5	24	18
	>1.5	16	6
Wharton et al (6)	<2.0	29	28
	>2.0	53	15
Vogel et al (8)	<2.0	12	>40
	>2.0	26	15

TABLE 14–4. RESPONSE RATES TO CHEMOTHERAPY BY LARGEST RESIDUAL MASS SIZE FOLLOWING PRIMARY CYTOREDUCTIVE SURGERY

Drug (s)	Mass Size (cm)	Number of patients	Objective response rate (%)	Complete response rate (%)	Reference rate (%)
Melphalan	≤2	11	73	18	7
	>2	26	46	15	
Melphalan	≤2	45	29	18	6
	>2	59	24	5	
Cisplatin	≤2	6	50	0	8
	>2	15	60	7	
HEXACAF	≤2	8	100	100	7
	>2	32	69	16	
H (C/F) AP	≤3	16	100	87	9
	>3	43	95	7	

HEXACAF = hexamethylmelamine, cyclophosphamide, methotrexate, 5-fluorouracil.
H (C/F) AP = hexamethylmelamine, cyclophosphamide or 5-fluorouracil, doxorubicin, cis-platinum.

should be abandoned as survival will not be improved. Thus, deep parenchymal liver metastases exceeding the designated size limit or retroperitoneal disease above the renal vein and involving the celiac or superior mesenteric artery would render a lesion unresectable. Similarly, patients with bulky tumor involving the portal vein are not candidates for an aggressive cytoreductive procedure.

The goal should be to render the patient free of tumor or, if not technically possible, attempt to leave no single mass greater than 0.5 cm in maximum diameter. Dissection commences in the upper abdomen with an omentectomy. When a large "omental cake" is present, the dissection is facilitated by entering the lesser sac. The gastroepiploic vessels may then be isolated and ligated to decrease the blood loss during dissection. Despite the initial appearance of the tumor intimately involving the transverse colon, it is usually possible to develop a plane between the omentum and transverse colon and thus remove the omentum without resecting the transverse colon.

Tumor sometimes extends across the transverse colon to involve the spleen and its hilum. In such cases splenectomy is performed. This is facilitated by first controlling the blood supply to the spleen by ligating the splenic artery as it courses along the superior border of the pancreas. One should not hesitate to perform a bowel resection if this will permit completion of a satisfactory cytoreductive procedure. The pelvic dissection is performed retroperitoneally entering the pararectal and paravesicle spaces. The ovarian vessels are ligated as they cross the pelvic brim with the ureter under direct vision. The uterine arteries may be ligated at their origin from the hypogastric artery. If there is extensive tumor in the anterior cul-de-sac, an anterior cystotomy may facilitate the dissection of this tumor from the bladder. If bulky tumor is present in the posterior cul-de-sac, the vagina may be divided first and a retrograde hysterectomy performed.[13] In this manner, the cul-de-sac tumor may be dissected from the rectum and the tumor-bearing peritoneum is resected en bloc with the specimen. If this is not possible, an anterior resection may be performed.

A frequent problem is how best to manage a woman who, due to anatomic limitations, cannot undergo a satisfactory primary cytoreductive operation. Published data have consistently demonstrated that survival is better the earlier in the course of a patient's disease the operation is performed.[14–16] This is likely explained by the fact that the rationale for cytoreductive surgery requires that it be followed by effective chemotherapy. The likelihood of the emergence of resistant tumor populations increases with the longevity of prior chemotherapy. It is thus important that every effort be made to perform a good cytoreductive operation at the time of the patient's first presentation. If this has not been possible, it has been our practice to proceed with a second attempt after two cycles of chemotherapy if the patient has demonstrated a good response. Cytoreductive surgery can be successfully performed (< 2 cm residual mass size) in over 75 per cent of cases.[17–19] This success rate is also achievable among lesions referred to as "inoperable."[17]

Chemotherapy and Radiation Therapy

Patients with stage I well-differentiated ovarian cancers do not require additional therapy. All other patients must be considered for either chemotherapy or radiation therapy. The single most active agent for ovarian cancer is cisplatin. Response rates and survival with combination chemotherapy are superior to that of single agents alone. However, the superiority of combination chemotherapy appears to be limited to those patients with small residual disease after surgery.[10] The commonly employed regimen was the combination of cisplatin, cyclophosphamide, and Adriamycin.

Recent studies have suggested that the combination of cisplatin and cyclophosphamide is equally efficacious as the three-drug combination with respect to both response rates and survival.[9] We have therefore been using the latter two drug combination avoiding the cardiotoxicity of Adriamycin. The optimal number of cycles of chemotherapy is not established. It has been our practice to administer four cycles of cisplatin and cyclophosphamide to patients with early stage disease and no residual tumor. Among patients with advanced stage disease and/or residual tumor, we have been administering six to eight courses of this regimen. However, it is not clear that the survival among patients with bulky residual disease, who have received multiple agent chemotherapy, is superior to those receiving a single alkylating agent. Therefore, one may consider treating patients with bulky residual disease with a single oral alkylating agent such as melphalan. This will significantly decrease the toxicity of the therapy, thus permitting an improved quality of life. However, given the improved response rates with combination chemotherapy, this therapy is appropriate for patients with bulky disease who have symptoms requiring palliation.

The propensity for upper abdominal spread in ovarian cancer requires that radiation therapy for this disease treat the whole abdomen. The literature is in agreement that patients with residual gross tumor after surgery are poor candidates for this modality. Similarly, patients with grade 3 tumors respond poorly. Therefore, appropriate candidates to be considered for whole abdomen radiation therapy are those patients with grade 1 or grade 2 tumors who have undergone complete cytoreductive operations.[20, 21]

Second-look Surgery

It has become common practice over the last two decades to perform a second-look operation on patients clinically free of disease after the completion of chemotherapy. This has been invaluable in the evaluation of chemotherapy regimens. However, one must question the benefit it accrues to the individual patient. It would be useful if it identified patients with persistent tumor who were then to receive an efficacious second-line therapy. We must therefore answer two questions: (1) Is the procedure predictive of survival, and (2) Is an effective second-line treatment available?

First, are there any alternatives to second-look laparotomy? Computed tomography has been evaluated in this clinical setting. It has a high specificity, ranging from 77 to 100 per cent, but a limited sensitivity of only 32 per cent.[22, 23] If one combines a CT scan with percutaneous biopsy, one can demonstrate persistent tumor in 20 per cent of patients. It is therefore worthwhile to perform a CT scan prior to second-look surgery as it may obviate the need for a laparotomy in one of five patients.[22] The serum tumor marker, CA125, has also been evaluated prior to second-look surgery. Although a normal CA125 level may be encountered in up to one half of patients with occult intraperitoneal tumor, an elevated CA125 level uniformly indicates the presence of intraperitoneal tumor and places a patient at high risk for a subsequent clinical recurrence.[24, 25] Thus, unless further cytoreductive surgery is contemplated, a laparotomy to determine the need for additional therapy is not necessary among patients with elevated CA125 levels.

Among patients undergoing second-look laparotomy, approximately 40 per cent will be free of tumor and 60 per cent will be positive. This ratio is dependent on the initial stage, initial grade, and the amount of residual disease after primary surgery. Reported survivals based on surgical findings vary greatly, but in general survival is diminished among patients with macroscopic tumor. One recent study highlights the limitations of this operation. One hundred and thirty-five patients with no macroscopic tumor at second-look surgery were followed for a minimum of four and one-half years.[26] No grade 1 tumors recurred, whether microscopically positive or negative. Among patients with grades 2 and 3 tumors, whether microscopically positive or negative, approximately one half of the tumors recurred. In another study looking at patients who survived over four years after second-look surgery, more than one-half of these patients had positive second-look procedures.[27] Of note, deaths were observed due to marrow toxicity resulting from second-line therapies.

Our armamentarium for patients, in whom primary cisplatin-based combination chemotherapy has failed, is limited. Although new cytotoxic agents, intraperitoneal therapy, and immunotherapy are under intense investigation and may hold promise, such second-line therapies have not yet been demonstrated to provide survival advantage. Whole abdomen radiation therapy after the completion of multiple courses of chemotherapy is poorly tolerated and is associated with significant gastrointestinal toxicity.[28] It similarly has not been demonstrated to provide a survival advantage. For these considerations, we do not routinely perform second-look surgery. We limit this procedure to patients enrolled in protocols evaluating chemotherapy and for patients who are under consideration for second-line treatment protocols.

Epithelial Tumors of Low Malignant Potential

Epithelial tumors of low malignant potential or "borderline tumors" are a distinct class of ovarian neoplasms. They have a unique natural history and good survivals. Five-year survival rates for stage I tumors are reported at 95 per cent with 10-year survivals of 73 to 95 per cent.[29, 30] Five-year survival rates for stage III and IV disease are reported at 87 per cent.[30] The recurrences of these tumors are very late. Young women with borderline tumors are appropriate candidates for conservative surgery, as previously described, if they wish to maintain reproductive function.[31] A complete unilateral salpingo-oophorectomy should be performed. In patients with more advanced tumors, every attempt should be made to perform a complete cytoreductive procedure. There is no evidence that these tumors respond to either chemotherapy or radiation therapy. We therefore do not administer adjuvant therapy. Patients are followed closely and re-explored should they manifest clinical recurrence. This occurs typically many years after the initial diagnosis.

Tumor Markers

Alpha fetoprotein and human chorionic gonadotropin have been used to monitor the course of endodermal sinus tumor, embryonal carcinoma, and choriocarcinomas of the ovary. Several monoclonal antibodies have been produced that identify cell membrane antigens on epithelial ovarian cancers. An assay has been developed using one of these monoclonal reagents (OC125) that measures CA125 in serum. This assay is elevated in over 80 per cent of patients with epithelial ovarian cancers.[32] It is also elevated among patients with other müllerian-derived adenocarcinomas as well as among some patients with nongynecologic tumors such as pancreatic, lung, breast, and colorectal carcinomas. It may be elevated in patients with cirrhosis and hepatomas as well as in patients with endometriosis and inflammatory processes involving the ceolomic epithelia. An elevated level, however, is encountered in not greater than 1 per cent of healthy individuals. Given the presence of elevated serum levels in patients with nonovarian malignancies, the CA125 assay is of limited value in the determination of the primary site of an unknown metastatic tumor.

Serial CA125 assays correlate with tumor burden reflecting tumor regression or progression.[32] It is interesting to examine the predictive value of an assay performed after three months of chemotherapy. An elevated serum CA125 at this time is inconsistent with a complete response to chemotherapy.[33] Prior to second-look surgery, a normal CA125 level does not confirm the absence of intraperitoneal tumor, and indeed occult tumor will be found in up to one half of cases.[24, 25] However, the tumor encountered in patients with normal CA125 levels will be of limited size. On the other hand, an elevated CA125 level at this time is always indicative of the presence of intraperitoneal tumor. This correlates well with the likelihood for clinical recurrence. A patient with an elevated CA125 level at the time of second-look surgery has a 60 per cent chance of manifesting a clinical recurrence within four months, whereas patients with normal CA125 levels have only a 5 per cent chance of clinical recurrence within the same four-month period.[34]

The CA125 assay is also a strong predictor of clinical recurrence among patients who are clinically free of tumor later in follow-up. In one study, clinical recurrences were preceded by an elevated serum CA125 level in 94 per cent of cases.[34] The median lead time was three months. Serum CA125 levels performed during the follow-up of ovarian cancer are also predictive of survival.[35]

The last two decades have witnessed major advances in the management of ovarian cancer, particularly in the fields of surgery, chemotherapy, and tumor markers. However, although survival has improved, it appears that the same proportion of patients are succumbing to their tumors. Further significant progress in this cancer will require the emergence of new chemotherapeutic agents.

CARCINOMA OF THE ENDOMETRIUM

Carcinoma of the endometrium is the most common of the gynecologic malignancies. Its incidence peaks in the latter half of the sixth decade. It is rare before the age of 40. The constitutional risk factor most strongly associated with endometrial cancer is obesity. Weaker associations are also present with diabetes, hypertension, and late menopause. Endometrial carcinoma is also more common in women who are anovulatory. This is attributable to chronic estrogenic stimulation of the endometrium unopposed by progesterone. Through a similar mechanism, endometrial carcinomas are also observed in women with estrogen-secreting neoplasms and in women receiving exogenous estrogen, unopposed by progestin, as menopausal replacement therapy. The risk associated with estrogen is negated if progesterone is also administered. Combination oral contraceptives decrease the risk for endometrial cancer.

A satisfactory screening technique for endometrial cancer is not available. Cytologic endometrial specimens are difficult to interpret and precursor lesions (hyperplasia) are not detected. Women with appropriate risk factors should be considered for histologic sampling of the endometrium. A cervical pap smear is similarly inadequate for screening or diagnosis. However, postmenopausal women with normal endometrial cells in their cervical cytologic samples have a 6 per cent risk of an occult endometrial neoplasm and should undergo histologic evaluation of the endometrium.[36]

The most common presenting symptom is vaginal bleeding. Every woman with postmenopausal bleeding should undergo histologic evaluation of the endometrium.

Pathology and Patterns of Spread

Endometrial cancer spreads locally by direct extension to the cervix and adjacent pelvic organs via lymphatics to pelvic, aortic, and, less commonly, inguinal lymph nodes, and hematogenously, most commonly to the lung. During the last decade, intraperitoneal spread in a manner similar to ovarian cancer has been recognized. This latter mode of dissemination is commonly encountered with, although not limited to, the uterine papillary serous variant of endometrial cancer. These aggressive tumors have a complex architecture and are cytologically highly anaplastic. Psammoma bodies may be observed. Uterine papillary serous carcinomas have a five-year relapse-free survival rate of only 50 per cent and a high rate of recurrence in the peritoneal cavity.[37]

The risk for lymph node metastases is most strongly related to tumor grade. Depth of myometrial invasion is also correlated with histologic grade, but, independent of grade, depth of myometrial invasion is an independent risk factor for nodal metastases. These relationships are in turn related to survival. The best estimation of prognosis is obtained by combining tumor grade and depth of myometrial invasion as illustrated in Table 14–5.

Staging

FIGO recently introduced a surgical staging classification for endometrial cancer (Table 14–6). Fractional dilation and curettage is no longer required. The new staging system incorporates the important prognostic factors: grade, depth of myometrial invasion, and lymph node metastases. The revised grading classification includes cytologic atypia as well as tumor architecture. The factor of size of the uterus, which was an unreliable variable, has been omitted.[38] This new FIGO staging classification is a major improvement.

Treatment

Endometrial Hyperplasia

Hyperplasias are noninvasive lesions of the endometrium. They are related to either exogenous or endogenous estrogenic stimulation. Cystic hyperplasias have a low neoplastic potential. In contrast, adenomatous hyperplasias may be precursors of endometrial carcinoma. The risk appears to be most related to the degree of cytologic atypia.[39]

The treatment of adenomatous hyperplasia is guided by the patient's menopausal status and desire for reproduction. Premenopausal women are managed with hormonal manipulation, including combination oral contraceptives or, if pregnancy is desired, ovulation induction. Perimenopausal women are treated with progestational agents. Prior to treatment with hormones, a coexisting invasive endometrial carcinoma must be excluded and consideration given to the etiology of the hyperplasia. All patients

TABLE 14–5. PROGNOSIS IN RELATION TO HISTOLOGIC GRADE AND DEPTH OF INVASION

Depth of Myometrial Invasion	5-Year Survival (%)			
	Grade 1	*Grade 2*	*Grade 3*	*Grade 4*
None	95	93	64	62
Less than half	92	73	50	50
More than half	33	37	27	14

Modified from Ng, A. B. P., and Reagan, J. W.: Incidence and prognosis of endometrial carcinoma by histologic grade and extent. Obstet. Gynecol. 35:437–452, 1970.

TABLE 14–6. INTERNATIONAL FEDERATION OF GYNECOLOGY AND OBSTETRICS (FIGO) STAGING SYSTEM FOR ENDOMETRIAL CANCER

Stages

IA G123	Tumor limited to endometrium.
IB G123	Invasion to <1/2 myometrium.
IC G123	Invasion to >1/2 myometrium.
IIA G123	Endocervical glandular involvement only.
IIB G123	Cervical stromal invasion.
IIIA G123	Tumor invades serosa and/or adnexae and/or positive peritoneal cytology.
IIIB G123	Vaginal metastases.
IIIC G123	Metastases to pelvic and/or paraaortic lymph nodes.
IVA G123	Tumor invasion bladder and/or bowel mucosa.
IVB	Distant metastases including intraabdominal and/or inguinal lymph node.

Histopathology-Degree of Differentiation

Cases of carcinoma of the corpus should be grouped with regard to the degree of differentiation of the adenocarcinoma as follows:

G1 = 5% or less of a nonsquamous or nonmorular solid growth pattern.
G2 = 6–50% of a nonsquamous or nonmorular solid growth pattern.
G3 = more than 50% of a nonsquamous or nonmorular solid growth pattern.

Notes on Pathologic Grading

(1) Notable nuclear atypia, inappropriate for the architectural grade, raises the grade of a grade I or grade II tumor by 1.
(2) In serous adenocarcinomas, clear cell adenocarcinomas, and squamous cell carcinomas, nuclear grading takes precedence.
(3) Adenocarcinomas with squamous differentiation are graded according to the nuclear grade of the glandular component.

From FIGO. Int. J. Gynecol. Obstet. 28:189–190, 1989.

managed with hormonal regimens must have follow-up histologic evaluation of the endometrium to ensure complete resolution of the lesion. Hysterectomy is recommended for women with severely atypical hyperplasias and postmenopausal patients.

Invasive Cancer

The cornerstone of therapy for endometrial carcinoma is hysterectomy. An extrafascial hysterectomy should be performed and bilateral salpingo-oophorectomy always included. It has been common practice in the past to administer preoperative radiation therapy. We prefer to surgically explore all patients first and then select those individuals appropriate for adjuvant radiation therapy based on the surgical and pathologic findings. The literature demonstrates that surgical evaluation will increase the stage in 15 to 33 per cent of cases.[41–43] Primary exploration permits accurate assessment of the depth of myometrial invasion, the status of the peritoneal surfaces, and the presence of lymph node metastases. It results in fewer irradiated patients primarily by eliminating those at low risk for recurrence as well as those with disseminated disease outside the treatment field. Equivalent survivals have been reported with this approach. The number of patients receiving radiation therapy will depend on the nature of the referral population to a given hospital and the indications employed. Reports have ranged from 8 to 28 per cent.[44, 45]

Aortic lymph node sampling is recommended for patients with tumors that are poorly differentiated, exhibit deep myometrial invasion, or involve the cervix (Table 14–7). The aortic lymph node status aids in the selection of patients for postoperative radiation therapy and guides the treatment fields.[43]

It is difficult to make firm statements concerning the value of adjuvant radiation therapy in endometrial cancer. Because the overall prognosis is so good, sufficiently large randomized studies to demonstrate treatment advantages have not been performed. It is well-established that radiation therapy decreases vaginal vault recurrences.[46] In terms of prognosis, the patients that appear to benefit from postoperative pelvic radiation are those with poorly differentiated tumors invading more than one-half the myometrial thickness.[47]

Our general treatment plan among early-stage patients has been to proceed with primary surgery consisting of a total (extrafascial) abdominal hysterectomy, bilateral salpingo-oophorectomy, omental biopsy, and peritoneal washings. Aortic lymph node sampling is performed on selected high-risk patients.

Patients with moderately invasive well-differentiated tumors are given postoperative vaginal intracavitary radiation therapy. Patients with poorly differentiated or deeply invasive tumors are selected for pelvic external beam radiation therapy. With modern radiation therapy techniques, it is not necessary to also use brachytherapy in this population.[48] Patients with aortic lymph node metastases are either spared the morbidity of pelvic radiation therapy or, if appropriate candidates, considered for extended field radiation therapy. Preliminary experience with para-aortic irradiation therapy in endometrial cancer has been encouraging, but the risk of significant enteric morbidity must be considered.[49, 50]

The significance of positive peritoneal cytology remains unsettled with conflicting data in the literature.[51, 52] We are not currently administering adjuvant therapy to patients with peritoneal washings as their only high-risk

TABLE 14–7. PELVIC AND AORTIC LYMPH NODE METASTASES IN CLINICAL STAGE I ENDOMETRIAL CARCINOMA CORRELATED WITH GRADE AND DEPTH OF MYOMETRIAL INVASION

Depth of Invasion	Grade	Pelvic Nodes (%)	Aortic Nodes (%)
Endometrium only	1 2 3	2	1
Superficial	1 2	1	0
Superficial	3	23	39–46
Intermediate	1	0	0
Intermediate	2 3	23	8–14
Deep	1	25	0
Deep	2 3	45	35–44

Modified from Boronow, R.C., Morrow, C.P., Creasman, W.T., et al.: Surgical staging in endometrial cancer: Clinical-pathologic findings of a prospective study. Obstet. Gynecol. 63:825–832, 1984.

factor. Consideration has been given to whole abdomen irradiation therapy for patients with positive peritoneal washings combined with other risk factors or for patients with the high-risk uterine papillary serous variant of endometrial carcinoma. The value of this potentially morbid therapy remains unproven.

Patients with stage I endometrial carcinomas and morbid obesity or other major medical problems that place them at high risk from an abdominal operation may be treated with vaginal hysterectomy and bilateral salpingo-oophorectomy with comparable survival rates.[53]

Progestational therapy used in an adjuvant manner for stage I tumors has not been demonstrated to improve survival.[54, 55] Survival rates for patients with stage I endometrial cancer are illustrated in Table 14–8. Patients with stage II disease are treated with extrafascial hysterectomy and radiation therapy. The disease-free survival rate exceeds 80 per cent at 10 years. Survival is significantly superior among patients with microscopic cervical involvement compared with those with gross tumor visible on the cervix.[56]

The evaluation of data concerning the management of stage III endometrial cancer is clouded by confusion between clinical and surgical stage. Hysterectomy should be performed in all instances when it is technically feasible. Furthermore, data suggest that survival is improved when a cytoreductive procedure removing all gross tumor is performed.[57] This is followed by radiation therapy. Overall survival with stage III disease is 54 per cent.[58] Survival is far superior with metastases limited to the tubes and ovaries compared with metastases to other pelvic sites.

Nonsurgical candidates are managed with radiation therapy, with the uterus as the most common site of recurrence when hysterectomy has not been performed.[40] Five-year survival rates for stages I, II, and III are 51, 50, and 37 per cent, respectively.[59] There is rarely a role for surgery in patients with recurrent endometrial cancer. Only about one-third will have tumor limited to the pelvis. One-third of patients with central pelvic recurrences can be salvaged with radiation therapy. Surgery should be considered for previously irradiated patients if the tumor is central in location with anticipated three-year disease-free survival rates of 20 per cent.[60] A metastatic evaluation must first be performed. Patients with tumor extension to the pelvic sidewall or with lymph node or distant metastases are not surgical candidates.

Systemic therapy is disappointing for this tumor. One-third of patients

TABLE 14–8. SURVIVAL FOR STAGE I ENDOMETRIAL ADENOCARCINOMA BY FIGO SUBSTAGES

Stage	5-Year Absolute Survival (%)
IaG1	93
IaG2	87
IaG3	68
IbG1	90
IbG2	76
IbG3	63

Data from Malkasian, G.D., Jr., Annegers, J.F., and Fountain, K.S.: Carcinoma of the endometrium: Stage 1. Am. J. Obstet. Gynecol. *136*:872–888, 1980.

will respond to progestational agents. Progesterone receptor studies are helpful in selecting appropriate candidates.[61] The cytotoxic regimens employed usually include cisplatin and Adriamycin. Response is typically of short duration.

Uterine Sarcomas

Uterine sarcomas are managed with total abdominal hysterectomy and bilateral salpingo-oophorectomy. Adjuvant radiation therapy decreases the pelvic recurrence rate but does not alter survival due to the high rate of distant metastases.

CARCINOMA OF THE CERVIX

Properly planned cervical cytology screening programs have significantly reduced the incidence of and mortality from cervical cancer.[62] We recommend annual screening. To maximize the potential benefit of screening programs, proper evaluation of women with abnormal cytology is imperative. In the past, women with abnormal cytology were managed with either hysterectomy or cervical conization. With the increasing incidence of cervical intraepithelial neoplasia in younger women of reproductive age and with the realization that these surgical procedures are "radical" treatment of localized noninvasive disease, simpler locally destructive techniques such as cryocautery and laser ablation have been developed. Selection of patients appropriate for management by these techniques requires accurate assessment of the cervix possible only with the magnification provided by the colposcope.

The colposcope was developed in 1925 by Hinselman in Germany. This instrument is an operating microscope capable of illuminating and magnifying the surface of the cervix specifically enabling the clinician to identify the so-called transformation zone. The transformation zone is that area of the cervix that has undergone squamous metaplasia, a process by which the columnar epithelium present on the exocervix in virtually all women entering menarche is converted to stratified squamous epithelium. This dynamic process, when acted upon by potentially carcinogenic agents (i.e., herpes simplex virus, human papillomavirus), may give rise to cervical neoplasia. The vast majority of cervical lesions arise in the transformation zone.

All women with abnormal pap smears should undergo colposcopic examination as their initial evaluation. An endocervical curettage is performed to rule out the presence of high endocervical disease, which, if present, is a contraindication to a locally destructive procedure and demands an excisional cone. The patient may be treated conservatively with either laser ablation or cryocautery if the following criteria are fulfilled:

1. The entire lesion must be visualized without extension up the endocervical canal.

2. The entire transformation zone (area at risk) must be visualized.

3. The endocervical curettage must be negative.

4. There must be agreement amongst colposcopic, cytologic, and histologic diagnoses.

5. Patient compliance must be expected.

6. No evidence of invasive disease, either histologically, cytologically, or colposcopically, may be present.

If any of these criteria are not fulfilled, a diagnostic conization is performed.

Eighty to 85 per cent of women may be adequately and completely evaluated and treated on an outpatient basis with either cryocautery or laser ablation, obviating the need for anesthesia and a surgical procedure. In general, most patients who are candidates for local procedures may be adequately treated with cryocautery. Laser is usually reserved for women with cervical intraepithelial neoplasia III, large or multifocal lesions, involvement of the endocervical glands, or following cryocautery failure. The subsequent evaluation of patients who have been lasered is easier than that following cryotherapy as the transformation zone is usually more easily visualized. The overall cure rates for these modalities approaches 95 per cent.

Cervical conization is both a diagnostic and therapeutic procedure. It may be considered total treatment for those women whose lesions are not amenable to local procedures, and it is diagnostic in that it provides tissue for the pathologist to rule out the presence of invasive disease. A cervical conization is performed under general or regional anesthesia. A cone-shaped piece of tissue encompassing the transformation zone and endocervical canal is excised. The colposcopic examination and the status of the endocervical curettage permit the clinician to tailor the cone specimen to the specific anatomic location of disease so that an adequate specimen with a minimal amount of cervical stroma is removed. Curettage of the residual endocervical canal is then performed. An endometrial sampling is left to the discretion of the surgeon.

The cure rate for cone biopsy as treatment for cervical intraepithelial neoplasia is 98 per cent with negative surgical margins and 70 per cent with disease extending to the histologic margin.[63] In this latter circumstance, residual disease is likely to be destroyed during the inflammatory response of healing. Patients having undergone cone biopsy for cervical intraepithelial neoplasia with negative surgical margins are therefore fully treated. Hysterectomy is reserved for women with positive margins, if reproductive capacity is not desired, or for those women with coexisting pelvic pathology.

Technique for Cervical Conization

Cervical conization is performed in the operating room with either regional or general anesthesia. With the patient in lithotomy position, the bladder is catheterized and an examination under anesthesia performed to confirm the absence of coexistent pelvic pathology. Using a weighted speculum, the cervix is visualized and stained with an iodine solution, Lugol's or Schiller's, to localize the lesion and guide the excision. The descending cervical branches of the uterine artery are ligated with deep Polyglactin sutures placed in the cervix at 3 and 9 o'clock. A dilute solution of vasopressin,

20 units in 20 ml normal saline (only in women without a history of either hypertension or cardiac disease), or plain saline is injected in the cervical stroma. A circular incision is then made maintaining a margin beyond the lesion as identified by iodine staining or colposcopy. The cone specimen is then removed with either knife or scissor dissection, taking care to avoid early entry into the cervical canal. A typical cone ranges in height from 1.5 to 2 cm. The specimen is marked with a suture in the stroma at the 12 o'clock position for pathologic orientation. An endocervical curettage is then performed followed by a D&C if indicated. The cone bed is electrocoagulated to achieve hemostasis, and sutures, if needed, are placed. Bleeding is minimal with this technique and most patients are discharged within six hours of surgery. Patients are instructed to abstain from douching, insertion of tampons, and intercourse for several weeks.

Excisional cone biopsy is also easily performed with the carbon-dioxide laser. Using this technique, the procedure may be done under local anesthesia in an ambulatory setting. Local infiltration of vasopressin is essential and no sutures are required. A small spot size should be selected and the cone biopsy performed with colposcopic guidance. The colposcopic magnification permits tailoring of the excision to suit the lesion.

Invasive Carcinoma of the Cervix

Microinvasive Carcinoma

The concept of a minimally invasive cervical carcinoma, so-called microinvasive carcinoma of the cervix, was first proposed by Mestwerdt in 1947 and is now generally accepted.[64] The criteria for diagnosis, however, remain controversial. The diagnosis of microinvasive carcinoma of the cervix suggests that disease is confined to the cervix with a very low probability of lymph node metastases or parametrial spread, enabling these patients to be treated with simple hysterectomy, thereby obviating the need for radical surgery or radiation therapy. Lesions that breach the basement membrane and involve the cervical stroma to a depth of 3 mm or less with no involvement of capillary-like spaces are associated with a risk of occult nodal spread of 1 per cent or less. Lesions fulfilling these criteria may therefore be treated with simple hysterectomy performed either abdominally or vaginally. The excess mortality of radical pelvic surgery or radiation therapy versus simple hysterectomy is approximately equal to this 1 per cent chance of nodal metastases.

Staging

The staging of cervical cancer is clinical. It consists of a complete physical examination, pelvic examination, preferably performed under anesthesia, chest radiograph, intravenous pyelography, cystoscopy, and proctoscopy. Barium enema and skeletal x-rays are permitted but are not usually performed unless the history or physical examination suggests metastases to these locations. The updated FIGO staging system is presented in Table 14–9.

TABLE 14–9. FIGO CLINICAL STAGING OF INVASIVE CERVICAL CANCER

Stage 0   CIS, intraepithelial carcinoma.

Stage I   Carcinoma is confined to the cervix.
    Ia Preclinical carcinoma, those diagnosed only by microscopy.
        Ia1 Minimal microscopically evident stromal invasion.
        Ia2 Lesions detected microscopically that can be measured. Depth of invasion from the base of epithelium not more than 5 mm, horizontal spread not greater than 7 mm.
    Ib All other stage I lesions. Occult cancer should be marked "occ."

Stage II   Carcinoma extends beyond the cervix but has not extended to the pelvic wall. It involves the vagina, but not the lower third.
    IIa No obvious parametrial involvement.
    IIb Obvious parametrial involvement.

Stage III   Carcinoma has extended to the pelvic wall. On rectal examination, there is no cancer-free space between the tumor and the pelvic wall. The tumor involves the lower third of the vagina. All cases with hydronephrosis or nonfunctioning kidney.
    IIIa No extension to the pelvic wall.
    IIIb Extension to the pelvic wall and/or hydronephrosis or nonfunctioning kidney.

Stage IV   Carcinoma has extended beyond the true pelvis or has clinically involved the mucosa of the bladder or rectum. A bullous edema is not classified as Stage IV.
    IVa Spread of the growth to adjacent organs.
    IVb Spread to distant organs.

Management of Invasive Carcinoma of the Cervix

Surgical treatment of frankly invasive cervical carcinoma originated over 100 years ago when Freund described a total hysterectomy with removal of lymph node metastases.[65] Although he reported an operative mortality of 50 per cent, there was no other treatment modality available at that time. In 1895, Clark, while a surgical resident at the Johns Hopkins Hospital, performed two radical hysterectomies.[66] Finally, in 1899 Wertheim of Vienna performed what we recognize today as a radical hysterectomy and pelvic lymphadenectomy.[67] By 1907, he reported 500 cases with an operative mortality approaching 20 per cent.[68]

The discovery of x-rays by Roentgen in 1895 was followed, shortly thereafter, by the purification of radium by the Curries. The recognition that radiation was capable of curing cancer led to the widespread acceptance of radiation therapy for treatment of carcinoma of the cervix to avoid the prohibitive operative mortality associated with radical surgery. In several centers worldwide, however, surgeons (Bonney in the United Kingdom, Schauta in Germany, and Okabayashi in Japan) continued the work of Wertheim in an attempt to refine the radical surgical approach. In 1939 Meigs reintroduced the radical abdominal hysterectomy to the United States, reporting a 1.7 per cent mortality rate and a 9 per cent fistula rate in 500 cases performed by 1955.[69, 70] He advised total pelvic lymphadenectomy rather than the removal of just the enlarged lymph nodes as originally described by Wertheim.

The clinician now has the luxury in early invasive cervical carcinoma, stages IB or IIA, of choosing between two very effective treatment modalities—radical hysterectomy and radiation therapy. Survival with either modality or by combining these modalities is 85 per cent. Radical pelvic surgery is usually selected for women with small lesions and for younger patients in whom preservation of ovarian function is desirable. Additionally, vaginal function is superior following radical hysterectomy than with radiation therapy. This must also be taken into consideration when treating the elderly sexually active woman whose vaginal canal may already be somewhat compromised as a result of the aging process.

The major complication following radical hysterectomy is urinary fistula, usually ureteral in origin. With meticulous technique, retroperitoneal suction drainage and postoperative bladder catheterization, the incidence should be reduced to 2 per cent or less.

Lesion size appears to be of prognostic importance in stage I disease, especially when surgery is selected.[72, 73] This may be a manifestation of the increased difficulty in achieving adequate surgical margins around large lesions, but may also reflect a high incidence of lymph node involvement, which, when extensive, may be better treated with radiation therapy. Lesions greater than 4 cm in size, therefore, are usually treated with radiation therapy.

In an extensive review, Delgado reported a five-year survival for clinical stage IB tumors of 80 to 85 per cent regardless of treatment modality.[71] The most important prognostic factor following stage is the presence or absence of pelvic lymph node metastases. Five-year survival falls to 50 per cent when these nodes are involved. Although external beam radiation therapy is usually added, there is little evidence that survival may be improved. There are some preliminary studies suggesting that survival may be enhanced when platinum-based chemotherapy is added to postoperative radiation therapy in these high-risk cases. Postoperative radiation therapy is beneficial in the presence of positive surgical margins.

Patients with barrel-shaped cervices pose a special problem. High central failure rates are observed with radiation therapy, as the large tumor volume presents poor geometry for intracavitary therapy. The radical surgical approach is compromised as a result of the technical difficulty in achieving adequate margins about the enlarged cervix. These patients are therefore best treated with a combined approach consisting of external beam radiation therapy to the whole pelvis, followed by one intracavitary radium application, followed by an extrafascial hysterectomy. Meticulous technique is required, as the risk of fistula formation following radiation to the pelvis is significant.

Patients with greater than stage IIA lesions are treated with radiation therapy. External beam radiation therapy in conjunction with intracavitary or interstitial techniques is prescribed depending on the clinical circumstance.

Technique of Radical Hysterectomy

The abdomen is entered through a midline or transverse muscle-splitting incision. A complete upper abdominal examination is performed with special attention to the retroperitoneal lymph nodes. Any enlarged nodes along the common iliac or aortic vessels are biopsied and sent for frozen section. Metastases to these nodes are associated with a poor outcome and contradict radical surgery. The abdomen is closed and the patient is treated with radiation therapy.

Attention is then turned to the pelvis in which the size of the cervix and uterus is noted. The parametria and paracolpos are now assessed for tumor extension and, if found, the operation is aborted and radiation therapy employed. Isolated pelvic lymph node metastases in the absence of higher disease is not a contraindication to performance of the radical hysterectomy.

The retroperitoneal spaces are entered by dividing the round ligaments. The pararectal and paravesical spaces are developed isolating the parametria and allowing the ureters to be identified (Fig. 14–1). The ovarian vessels or utero-ovarian pedicles are ligated and divided with the ureter in view. The ovaries may be removed or conserved depending on the patient's age. The peritoneum overlying the lower uterine segment is divided, allowing the bladder to be dissected from the cervix, the upper vagina, and the parametria. The hypogastric arteries are then dissected, and the uterine arteries and adjacent veins are ligated and divided at their origins. Attention is then turned posteriorly where the cul-de-sac peritoneum is divided. Entering the rectovaginal septum, the rectum is dissected from the posterior vagina for approximately one-half of its length. This allows the uterosacral ligaments to be isolated after separating the ureter from the medial leaf of the broad ligament. The uterosacral ligaments are then divided adjacent to the sacrum. This provides maximum mobility and exposure prior to the ureteral dissection. The ureter is dissected from the paracervical tunnel within the parametrium and retracted laterally (Fig. 14–2). The remainder of the uterosacral ligaments and cardinal ligaments may then be divided at the pelvic sidewall (Fig. 14–3). The uterus and parametria are finally removed along with the upper third of the vagina. The vaginal cuff is closed after which a pelvic lymphadenectomy is performed from the level of the common iliac vessels to the inguinal ligament. Metallic clips are used liberally to prevent lymphocele formation. Suction catheters are placed in the retroperitoneal spaces bilaterally after which the abdomen is closed.

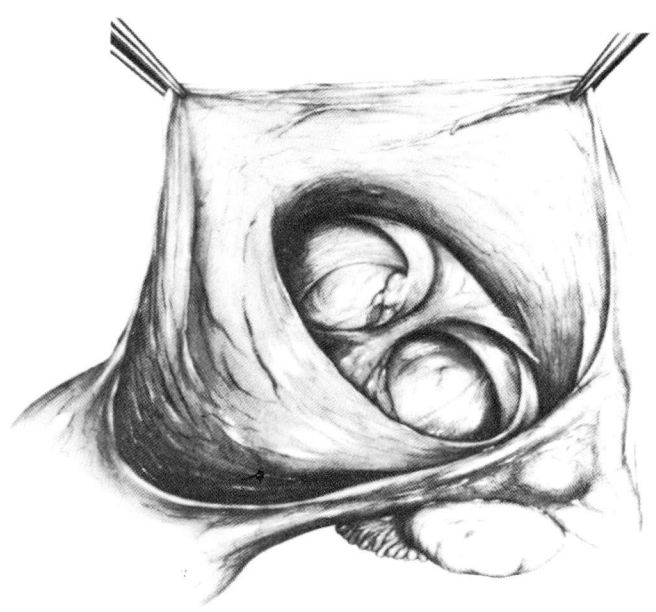

Figure 14–1. Radical Hysterectomy. The pelvic sidewall has been opened, with the paravesical and pararectal spaces developed. (From Mattingly, R.F.: TeLinde's Operative Gynecology, 5th Ed. Philadelphia, J.B. Lippincott, 1977, p. 723.)

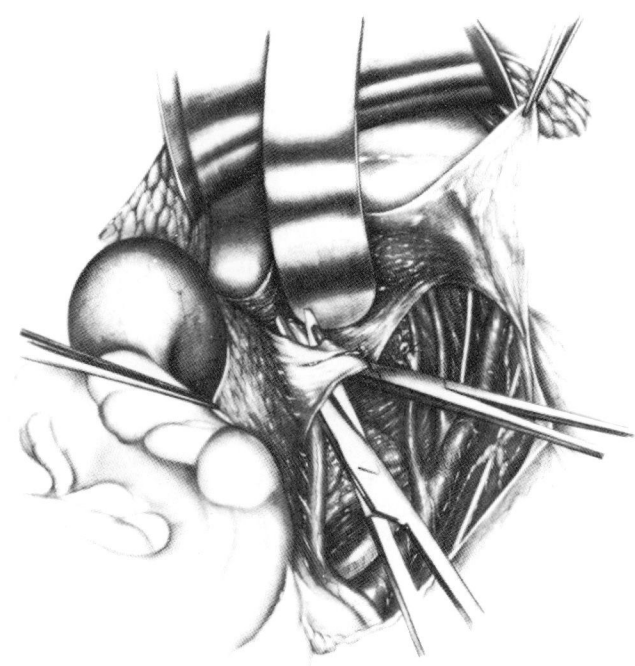

Figure 14-2. Radical Hysterectomy. The parametrial tunnel has been opened and clamped with the ureter in view. (From Mattingly, R.F.: TeLinde's Operative Gynecology, 5th Ed. Philadelphia, J.B. Lippincott, 1977, p. 727.)

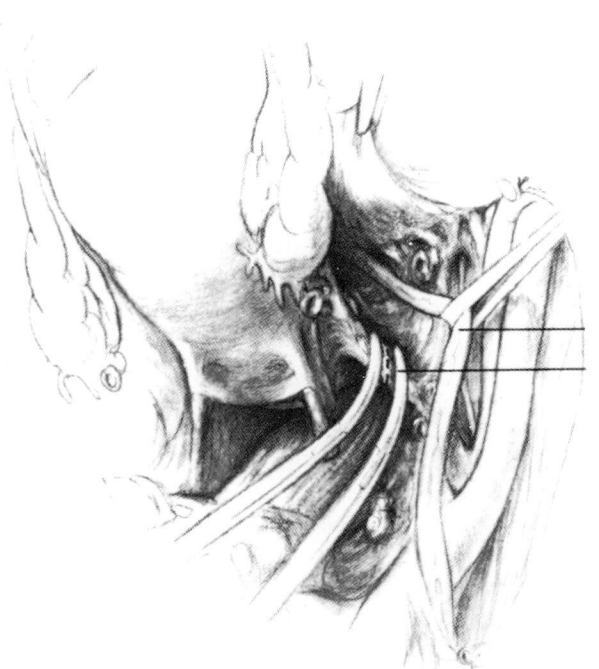

Figure 14-3. Radical Hysterectomy. The uterosacral ligament has been divided. The ureter is retracted laterally with clamps applied to the cardinal ligaments. (From Nelson, J.H.: Atlas of Radical Pelvic Surgery, 2nd Ed. New York, Appleton-Century-Crofts, 1976, p. 157.)

Management of Recurrent Cervical Cancer

Surgery again plays a role in women with pelvic recurrence following radiation therapy. There is currently no effective systemic treatment for recurrent cervical cancer. Pelvic exenteration, originally described by Brunschweig in 1948, may be considered for recurrent disease confined to the central pelvis.[74] Patients with distant metastases, sidewall involvement, or positive nodes should be considered inoperable, as long-term survival in these women is routinely poor and does not justify the morbidity and mortality associated with this procedure.

Depending on the anatomic location of tumor, either the bladder or rectum may be spared. However, in general, a total pelvic exenteration and full lymphadenectomy is performed with creation of a urinary conduit and permanent colostomy.

Brunschweig's original report described 22 patients with an operative mortality of 23 per cent. Urinary diversion consisted of a wet colostomy. This was associated with a prohibitive incidence of pyelonephritis and renal failure. Later, Bricker described separating the excretory streams by creating an isolated ileal conduit.[75] The risk of urinary leaks at the uretero-ileal anastomoses secondary to radiation induced changes in both the ureters and intestinal segments lead Nelson to suggest the use of nonirradiated bowel such as transverse colon for the urinary conduit.[76] Indwelling ureteral stents are used to minimize the risk of an anastomotic leak.

Preoperative assessment should include a complete physical examination, CT scan of the abdomen and pelvis, chest x-ray, and routine blood studies to rule out the presence of metastatic disease and to assess the patient's general medical condition prior to such radical surgery.

The patient must have a good understanding of the planned procedure, and consultation with a psychiatric social worker, psychiatrist, or psychologist may be considered. Preoperative teaching and stoma site marking by an enterostomal therapist is very useful. The question of sexual function and vaginal reconstruction should be discussed with each patient and, if desired, should be performed at the completion of the primary procedure. Mechanical and antibiotic bowel preparation should be performed prior to surgery and consideration given to preoperative total parenteral nutrition if the patient's preoperative nutritional status is compromised.

A description of the exenterative procedure may be found in gynecologic or general surgical atlases. Patients with disease localized high in the vagina or uterus may be spared the perineal phase of the operation. Intestinal continuity may be restored with a low anastomosis and the anus preserved without sacrificing curability in some patients. In such cases with radiated patients, a temporary protective colostomy is recommended. A transverse colon conduit is used in conjunction with indwelling ureteral Silastic stents.

Pelvic reconstruction is performed to minimize the complications associated with the denuded pelvic cavity such as sepsis, adhesion formation, bowel obstruction, and fistula formation. Myocutaneous gracili or posterior thigh flaps may be mobilized to close the pelvic defect. This brings an additional blood supply to the pelvis and allows the construction of a neovagina. The pelvic roof is created with omentum, if it is present, or vicryl mesh to minimize the incidence of postoperative small bowel complications.

With proper patient selection (excluding patients with sidewall involvement, positive nodes, or peritoneal metastases), five-year disease-free survivals ranging from 30 to 50 per cent may be anticipated.[78] Operative mortality is minimized by optimal preoperative and postoperative care, modern anesthesia techniques, and, as described above, improved surgical techniques. Operative mortality ranges from 1 to 5 per cent.

CARCINOMA OF THE VULVA

Carcinoma of the vulva accounts for approximately 4 per cent of gynecologic malignancies in the United States, the vast majority of which are squamous in histology. Over 90 per cent of women with vulvar carcinoma are postmenopausal at presentation with the peak incidence occurring in the seventh decade. In contrast, in situ vulvar neoplasia appears to be a disease of the reproductive age group with a peak age now in the late fourth decade.

In contrast to cervical neoplasia, in which in situ disease appears to be a definite precursor of invasive cancer, vulvar carcinoma in situ has only rarely been observed to progress to invasive disease. The 30-year difference in median age at diagnosis similarly argues against the premise that in situ vulvar disease progresses to frank invasion. However, in situ and invasive vulvar neoplasms are often seen together.

Often vulvar malignancies are associated with some other vulvar abnormality. In areas in which granulomatous diseases of the vulva such as lymphogranuloma venereum and granuloma inguinale are endemic, virtually all cases of vulvar carcinoma are associated with these conditions. Similarly, condylomatous lesions appear to predispose to the development of vulvar neoplasia.

The chronic vulvar dystrophies, a generic term referring to lichen sclerosus and hyperplastic dystrophy, also appear to play a role in the etiology of vulvar malignancy. Morley estimated that 50 per cent of vulvar carcinomas arise in areas of chronic vulvar dystrophy; however, only 2 to 4 per cent of patients with these conditions will ultimately go on to develop cancer.[78]

In situ vulvar neoplasia has been divided into several categories including Bowen's disease, erythroplasia of Queyrat, carcinoma simplex, and Paget's disease. The former three are biologically and histologically so similar that they have been lumped together under the general term carcinoma in situ. Paget's disease will be discussed separately.

The incidence of vulvar carcinoma in situ is increasing with the majority now found in premenopausal women. The peak age is in the mid to late fourth decade. A strong association with sexually transmitted diseases, especially human papillomavirus infection and synchronous or metachronous cervical neoplasia, has also been noted and should always be suspected in women with preinvasive vulvar neoplasia.[79] Grossly, these lesions are elevated and may appear either hyperpigmented or hypopigmented; occasionally they are erythematous. Although pruritus is occasionally noted, this symptom is usually suggestive of invasive disease.

The treatment for vulvar carcinoma in situ has classically been simple vulvectomy. With a better understanding of the natural history of this disease, less extensive procedures such as wide local excision, skinning vulvectomy with or without grafting, or laser vaporization have been successfully employed.

Paget's Disease

Paget's disease of the vulva is observed in older women with a median age of 65 years. Grossly, these lesions appear velvety red and may involve the entire vulva. Pruritus is a frequent presenting complaint. Although Paget's disease is most commonly described on the breast, involvement of areas richly invested with apocrine glands such as genital, perianal, and axillary skin has been well described.

Histologically, Paget's disease exhibits nests of large pale oval cells infiltrating the dermis or epidermis. These cells contain neutral and acid mucopolysaccharides that stain positive with PAS, mucicarmine, and Alcian blue. These staining characteristics aid in differentiating this lesion from the occasional amelanotic melanoma involving the vulva, which, of course, carries a very different prognosis.

The major significance of extramammary Paget's disease is its frequent association with synchronous invasive carcinoma either of the underlying skin appendages or distal sites such as the breast, rectum, and Bartholin's gland. Treatment of Paget's disease requires excision of the lesion with sufficient subcutaneous tissue to rule out an underlying adnexal carcinoma. This usually mandates a simple vulvectomy. As nests of Paget's cells may be noted several centimeters from the evident margin, a wide rim of normal tissue must be removed. Intraoperative frozen sections may be helpful. Even so, a high incidence of recurrent disease is noted. Identification of an underlying adenocarcinoma mandates radical vulvectomy and groin dissections. Barium enema and mammography may be considered in these women to rule out tumors in these locations.

Invasive Cancer of the Vulva

Histologic evaluation is the cornerstone of management of vulvar lesions. The dystrophies, intraepithelial lesions, and invasive carcinomas are often grossly indistinguishable. Biopsy is easily performed in the office under local anesthesia with a disposable (4 to 5 mm) dermatologic biopsy punch. The biopsy site may be cauterized with silver nitrate or Monsel's solution, although a fine suture may occasionally be required. The need for histologic evaluation of vulvar lesions cannot be over-emphasized. Diagnostic delays of a year or more are common while multiple creams, ointments, and salves are prescribed for what would be readily identified histologically as a neoplastic process.

The current staging system for vulvar carcinoma was adopted in 1971 by FIGO and is illustrated in Table 14–10. It suffers from the usual limitation of a clinical staging system with an error rate of 40 per cent when compared with the final surgical-pathologic stage.

The treatment of choice for invasive vulvar carcinoma remains radical surgery, consisting of radical vulvectomy with bilateral femoral and inguinal lymphadenectomies. This procedure removes the vulvar tissue to the level

TABLE 14–10. FIGO CLINICAL STAGING OF INVASIVE VULVAR CANCER

Stage I	Tumor confined to the vulva, 2 cm or less in greatest diameter, without suspicious groin nodes.
Stage II	Tumor confined to the vulva, greater than 2 cm in diameter, without suspicious groin nodes.
Stage III	Tumor of any size with extension beyond the vulva (vagina, urethra, perineum, anus) and/or suspicious groin nodes.
Stage IV	Tumor of any size with involvement of bladder or rectal mucosa and/or grossly positive groin nodes, and/or fixed to bone and/or distant metastases.

of the deep perineal fascia and the draining lymphatics in the inguinal area. This operation classically has entailed an en bloc resection with extensive mobilization and undermining of skin flaps (Fig. 14–4). The groin dissection removes the regional draining lymph nodes from both the superficial and deep inguinal and femoral compartments. The superficial nodes and adjacent adipose tissue lying above the fascia lata, external oblique aponeurosis, femoral sheath, and inguinal ligament, and below the integument and Camper's fascia are removed (Fig. 14–5). Access to the femoral vessels and deep nodal compartment is made by incising the femoral sheath at its lateral aspect and reflecting this medially, thereby unroofing the femoral artery, femoral vein, and "empty space" overlying the pectineus fascia. The saphenous vein is usually ligated and divided at its juncture with the femoral vein, although some authors suggest retaining this vessel to diminish the incidence of postoperative edema.

In the past, when inguinal or femoral lymph node metastases were found, an extraperitoneal deep pelvic lymphadenectomy was performed. The procedure is now omitted and patients with groin node metastases are treated with postoperative radiation therapy.

With an en bloc resection, the vulvectomy incisions are made from the

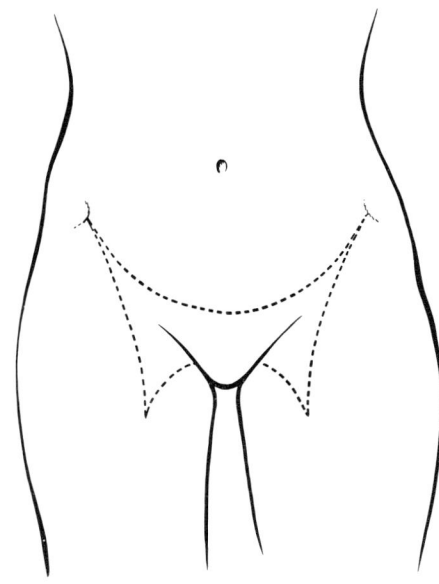

Figure 14–4. En bloc, butterfly-shaped incision for radical vulvectomy with inguinal and femoral lymphadenectomy. (From Mattingly, R.F.: TeLinde's Operative Gynecology, 5th Ed. Philadelphia, J.B. Lippincott, 1977, p. 657.)

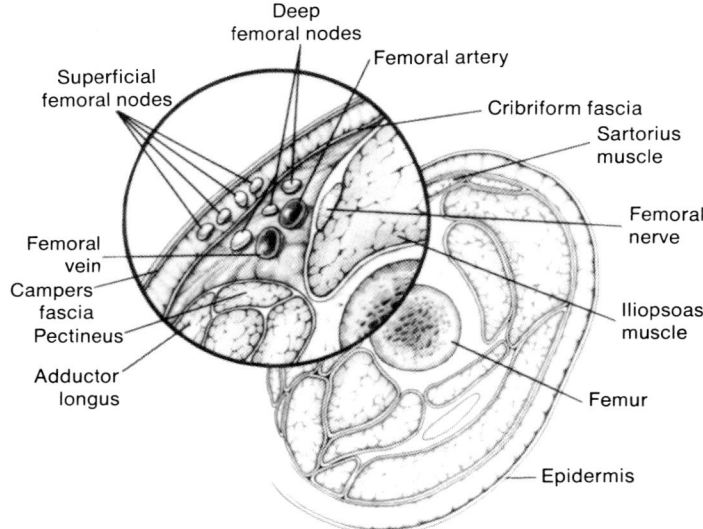

Figure 14–5. The location of the superficial inguinal and femoral lymph nodes between Camper's fascia and the deeper layers is displayed. (From DiSaia, P.L., Creasman, W.T., and Rich, W.M.: An alternative approach to early cancer of the vulva. Am. J. Obstet. Gynecol. *133:* 828, 1979.)

groin through the labial-crural folds and across the top of the anus. With involvement of either the distal urethra or vagina, an extended radical vulvectomy encompassing these areas may be performed. The distal one half of the urethra may be removed without compromising continence. All tissues above the deep perineal fascia are resected. Primary closure is usually possible although random skin flaps, gracilis, or posterior thigh myocutaneous flaps or skin grafting may occasionally be required.

Wound breakdown and infection occur in as many as 50 per cent of cases when large en bloc dissections are performed.[80] Deep vein thrombosis, bleeding, and lymphocyst formation are also encountered. Later complications include urinary incontinence, urinary spraying, pelvic relaxation symptoms with cystocele or rectocele, introital stenosis with dyspareunia, and chronic leg edema.

To minimize the risk of wound breakdown, the large butterfly-shaped (en bloc) incision has been replaced in many centers by a triple incision technique[81] (Fig. 14–6). The groin dissections are performed through bilateral incisions parallel to and just below the inguinal ligament. The vulva is removed with an elliptical incision commencing in the mons and extending to and along the labial-crural fold and across the perineum just above the anus. This incision minimizes wound complications and provides an excellent cosmetic result without compromising survival.

Overall survival for vulvar carcinoma treated with radical vulvectomy approaches 80 per cent.[78] Of major prognostic significance is the presence or absence of inguinal lymph node metastases. With negative nodes, the overall survival is greater than 80 per cent. In women with positive nodes, the survival falls to approximately 40 per cent.

With extensive tumor involvement of the urethra, bladder, vagina, or rectum, primary exenteration is indicated. In small series, survivals approaching 70 per cent have been reported.[83] With bulky tumors, preoperative radiation therapy, chemotherapy, or the two modalities combined have been used. This has been reported to be successful in improving operability and permitting more limited resections with the avoidance of some stomas.[82]

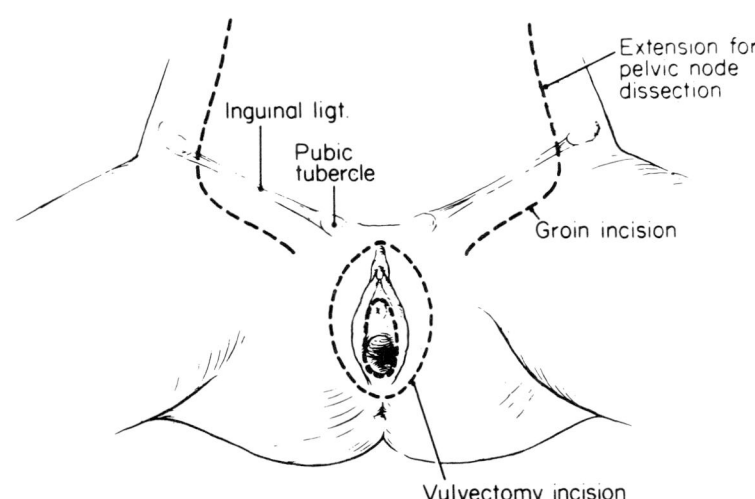

Figure 14–6. Three-in-one incision for radical vulvectomy and inguinal and femoral lymphadenectomy. Cephalad extension for an extra-peritoneal pelvic lymph node dissection is also indicated. (From Hacker, N.F. et al., Obstet Gynecol. 58:575, 1981. Reprinted with permission from The American College of Obstetricians and Gynecologists.)

Treatment of early invasive carcinoma of the vulva remains controversial. Although the definition and treatment of microinvasive carcinoma of the cervix is fairly well accepted, no such definition has been developed for carcinoma of the vulva. It appears that well-differentiated tumors invasive to 1 mm or less, 1 cm or less in diameter, and without capillary or lymphatic-like space involvement may be treated with wide local excision only. The risk of lymph node metastases in these patients is less than 1 per cent. With lesions up to 2 cm in diameter and invasion limited to 3 mm, wide excision with ipsilateral superficial groin dissections may be performed. As suggested by DiSaia, the superficial inguinal nodes may be considered "sentinel nodes."[84] Absence of metastases in these sentinel nodes obviates the need for further treatment. More extensive disease, however, mandates radical vulvectomy and bilateral groin dissections.

Carcinoma of the Bartholin's Gland

Carcinoma of Bartholin's gland accounts for 2 to 3 per cent of all vulvar carcinomas. Bartholin's gland cysts or abscesses are usually seen in the reproductive age group. Any bleeding or enlargement in this region in postmenopausal women must be considered suspicious for neoplasia, and excision or marsupialization with biopsy is mandatory. Late diagnosis probably accounts for the somewhat inferior prognosis in these patients compared with other women with carcinoma of the vulva. The recommended treatment is radical vulvectomy and bilateral groin dissection. Although routine pelvic lymphadenectomy has been recommended in the past, in the absence of documented metastases in the groin, the incidence of pelvic node involvement approaches zero. The location of Bartholin's gland in close proximity to the anterolateral rectal wall may on occasion require abdominoperineal resection to obtain adequate surgical margins.

Melanoma

Melanoma accounts for approximately 3 per cent of all vulvar cancers with an overall five-year survival of 30 per cent.[85] In contrast to squamous carcinoma of the vulva, which is rather indolent and slow growing, melanoma is an aggressive tumor with a propensity for both lymphatic and hematogenous spread. It is best classified based on depth of invasion as opposed to the standard FIGO staging system. Tumor corresponding to Clarke's levels I and II or with invasion to less than 1 mm from the skin surface may be treated with a generous wide local excision.[86] More extensive tumors are classically managed with radical vulvectomy and groin dissection. In anatomically suitable candidates, a radical hemivulvectomy and ipsilateral groin dissection may be considered. Although prognosis is poor in the presence of lymph node metastases, some women are cured with this procedure.

REFERENCES

1. Lynch, H.T., Albano, W.A., Lynch, J.F., et al.: Surveillance and management of patients at high genetic risk for ovarian carcinoma. Obstet. Gynecol. *59:*589–596, 1982.
2. Topacman, J.K., Greene, M.H., Tucker, M.A., et al.: Intraabdominal carcinomatosis after prophylactic oophorectomy in ovarian cancer-prone families. Lancet *2:*795, 1982.
3. Young, R.C., Decker, D.G., Wharton, J.T., et al.: Staging laparotomy in early ovarian cancer. JAMA *250:*3072–3076, 1983.
4. Knapp, R.C., and Friedman, E.A.: Aortic lymph node metastases in early ovarian cancer. Am. J. Obstet. Gynecol. *119:*1013–1017, 1974.
5. Griffiths, C.T.: Surgical resection of tumor bulk in the primary treatment of ovarian carcinoma. Natl. Cancer Inst. Monogr. *42:*101–104, 1975.
6. Hacker, N.F., Berek, J.S., Lagasse, L.D., et al.: Primary cytoreductive surgery for epithelial ovarian cancer. Obstet. Gynecol. *61:*413–420, 1983.
7. Wharton, J.T., Herson, J.: Surgery for common epithelial tumors of the ovary. Cancer *48:*582–589, 1981.
8. Vogel, S.E., Pagano, M., Kaplan, B.H., et al.: Cis-Platin based combination chemotherapy for advanced ovarian cancer. Cancer *51:*2024–2030, 1983.
9. Bertelsen, K., Jakobsen, A., Andersen, J.E., et al.: A randomized study of cyclophosphamide and cis-platinum with or without doxorubicin in advanced ovarian carcinoma. Gynecol. Oncol. *28:*161–169, 1987.
10. Young, R.C., Chabner, B.A., Hubbard, S.P., et al.: Advanced ovarian adenocarcinoma. A prospective clinical trial of melphalan (L-PAM) versus combination chemotherapy. N. Engl. J. Med. *299:*1261–1266, 1978.
11. Gershenson, D.M., Wharton, J.T., Herson, T., et al.: Single agent cis-platinum therapy for advanced ovarian cancer. Obstet. Gynecol. *58:*487–496, 1981.
12. Greco, F.A., Julian, C.G., Richardson, R.C., et al.: Advanced ovarian cancer. Brief intensive combination chemotherapy and second-look operation. Obstet. Gynecol. *58:*199–206, 1981.
13. Hudson, C.N.: Surgical treatment of ovarian cancer. Gynecol. Oncol. *1:*370–378, 1973.
14. Vogel, S.E., Seltzer, V., Calanog, A., et al.: "Second-effort" surgical resection for bulky ovarian cancer. Cancer *54:*2220–2225, 1984.
15. Joyeux, H., Szawlowski, A.W., Saint-Aubert, B., et al.: Aggressive regional surgery for advanced ovarian carcinoma. Cancer *57:*142–147, 1986.
16. Wils, J., Blijham, G., Naus, A., et al.: Primary or delayed debulking surgery and chemotherapy consisting of cis-platin, doxorubicin, and cyclophosphomide in Stage III–IV epithelial ovarian carcinoma. J. Clin. Oncol. *4:*1068–1073, 1986.
17. Piver, M.S., and Baker, T.: The potential for optimal ($\leq$ 2cm) cytoreductive surgery in advanced ovarian carcinoma at a tertiary medical center: A prospective study. Gynecol. Oncol. *24:*1–8, 1986.
18. Heintz, A.P.M., Hacker, N.F., Berek, J.S., et al.: Cytoreductive surgery in ovarian carcinoma: Feasability and morbidity. Obstet. Gynecol. *67:*783–788, 1986.
19. Chen, S.S., and Bochner, R.: Assessment of morbidity and mortality in primary cytoreductive surgery for advanced ovarian carcinoma. Gynecol. Oncol. *20:*190–195, 1985.
20. Dembo, A.J., and Bush, R.S.: Current concepts in Cancer: Ovary—Treatment for stages

III and IV. Choice of postoperative therapy based on prognostic factors. Int. J. Radiat. Oncol. Biol. Phys. *8:*893–897, 1982.
21. Schray, M., Martinez, A., Cox, R., and Ballon, S.: Radiotherapy in epithelial ovarian cancer: Analysis of prognostic factors based on long-term experience. Obstet. Gynecol. *62:*373–382, 1983.
22. Clarke-Pearson, D.L., Bandy, L.C., Dudzenski, M., et al.: Computed tomography in evaluation of patients with ovarian carcinoma in complete clinical remission: Correlation with surgical-pathologic findings. JAMA *255:*627–630, 1986.
23. Brenner, D.E., Shaff, M.I., Jones, H.W., et al.: Abdominopelvic computed tomography: Evaluation in patients undergoing second-look laparotomy for ovarian carcinoma. Obstet. Gynecol. *65:*715–719, 1985.
24. Niloff, J.M., Bast, R.C., Jr., Schaetzl, E.M., and Knapp, R.C.: Predictive value of CA125 antigen levels in second-look procedures in ovarian cancer. Am. J. Obstet. Gynecol. *151:*981–986, 1985.
25. Berek, J.S., Knapp, R.C., Malkasian, G.D., et al.: CA125 serum levels correlated with second-look operations among ovarian cancer patients. Obstet. Gynecol. *67:*685–689, 1986.
26. Copeland, L.J., and Gershenson, D.M.: Ovarian cancer recurrences in patients with no macroscopic tumor at second-look laparotomy. Obstet. Gynecol. *68:*873–874, 1986.
27. Wharton, J.T., Edwards, C.L., and Rutledge, F.N.: Long-term survival after chemotherapy for advanced epithelial ovarian carcinoma. Am. J. Obstet. Gynecol. *148:*997–1004, 1984.
28. Hoskins, W.J., Lichter, A.S., Whittington, R., et al.: Whole abdominal pelvic irradiation in patients with minimal disease at second-look surgical reassessment for ovarian carcinoma. Gynecol. Oncol. *20:*271–280, 1985.
29. Colgan, T.J., and Norris, H.J.: Ovarian epithelial tumors of low malignant potential: A review. Int. J. Gynecol. Pathol. *1:*367–382, 1983.
30. Barnhill, D., Heller, P., Bnzozowski, P., et al.: Epithelial ovarian cancer of low malignant potential. Obstet. Gynecol. *65:*53–59, 1985.
31. Tazelaar, H.D., Bostwick, D.G., Ballon, S.C., et al.: Conservative treatment of borderline ovarian tumors. Obstet. Gynecol. *66:*417–422, 1985.
32. Bast, R.C., Jr., Klug, T.L., St. John, E., et al.: A radioimmunoassay using a monoclonal antibody to monitor the course of epithelial ovarian cancer. N. Engl. J. Med. *309:*883–887, 1983.
33. Lavin, P.T., Knapp, R.C., Malkasian, G., et al.: CA125 for the monitoring of ovarian carcinoma during primary therapy. Obstet. Gynecol. *69:*223–227, 1987.
34. Niloff, J.M., Knapp, R.C., Lavin, P.T., et al.: The CA125 assay as a predictor of clinical recurrence in epithelial ovarian cancer. Am. J. Obstet. Gynecol. *155:*56–60, 1986.
35. Niloff, J.M., Dubeshter, B., Zurawski, V.R., Jr., et al.: Serum CA125 levels correlated with survival in epithelial ovarian cancer. Surg. Forum *38:*470–472, 1987.
36. Ng, A.B.P., Reagan, J.W., Hawliczek, C.T., and Wentz, B.W.: Significance of endometrial cells in the detection of endometrial carcinoma and its precursors. Acta Cytol. *18:*356–361, 1974.
37. Hendrickson, M.R., Ross, J.C., Eifel, P.J., et al.: Uterine papillary serous carcinoma. A highly malignant form of endometrial adenocarcinoma. Am. J. Surg. Pathol. *6:*93–108, 1982.
38. Javert, C.T., and Douglas, R.G.: Treatment of endometrial adenocarcinoma. Am. J. Roentgenol. *75:*508–514, 1956.
39. Welch, W.R., and Scully, R.E.: Precancerous lesions of the endometrium. Hum. Pathol. *8:*503–512, 1977.
40. Yoonessi, M., Anderson, D.G., and Morley, G.W.: Endometrial carcinoma: Causes of death and sites of treatment failure. Cancer *43:*1944–1950, 1979.
41. Cowles, T.A., Magrina, J.F., Masterson, B.J., and Capen, C.V.: Comparison of clinical and surgical staging in patients with endometrial carcinoma. Obstet. Gynecol. *66:*413, 1985.
42. Macasaet, M., Brigati, D., Boyce, J., et al.: The significance of residual disease after radiotherapy in endometrial carcinoma: Clinicopathologic correlation. Am. J. Obstet. Gynecol. *138:*557, 1980.
43. Boronow, R.C., Morrow, C.P., Creasman, W.T., et al.: Surgical staging in endometrial cancer: Clinical-pathologic findings of a prospective study. Obstet. Gynecol. *63:*825, 1984.
44. Bean, H.A., Bryant, A.J.S., Carmichael, J.A., and Mallik, A.: Carcinoma of the endometrium in Saskatchewan. Gynecol. Oncol. *6:*503–514, 1978.
45. Eifel, P.J., Ross, J.C., Hendrickson, M.R., et al.: Adenocarcinoma of the endometrium: Analysis of 256 cases with disease limited to the uterine corpus: Treatment comparisons. Cancer *52:*1026–1031, 1983.
46. Jones, H.W.: Treatment of adenocarcinoma of the endometrium. Obstet. Gynecol. Surv. *30:*147–169, 1975.
47. Aalders, J., Abeler, V., Kolstad, P., and Onsrud, M.: Postoperative external irradiation and prognostic parameters in stage I endometrial carcinoma. Obstet. Gynecol. *56:*419–427, 1980.

48. Kuipers, T.: The role of radiation therapy in conjunction with surgery in the treatment of endometrial carcinoma. *In* Heintz, A.P.M., Griffiths, C.T., and Trimbos, J.B. (Eds.): Surgery in Gynecologic Oncology. The Hague, Matinus Nijhoff Pub., 1983, pp. 236–247.
49. Potish, R.A., Twiggs, L.B., Adcock, L.L., et al.: Paraaortic lymph node radiotherapy in cancer of the uterine corpus. Obstet. Gynecol. *65:*251–256, 1985.
50. Feuer, G.A., and Calanog, A.: Endometrial carcinoma, treatment of positive paraaortic nodes. Gynecol. Oncol. *27:*104–109, 1987.
51. Yazigi, R., Piver, M.S., and Blumenson, L.: Malignant peritoneal cytology as prognostic indicator in stage I endometrial cancer. Obstet. Gynecol. *62:*359–362, 1983.
52. Creasman, W.T., DiSaia, P.J., Blessing, J., et al.: Prognostic significance of peritoneal cytology in patients with endometrial cancer and preliminary data concerning therapy with intraperitoneal radiopharmaceuticals. Am. J. Obstet. Gynecol. *141:*921–927, 1981.
53. Peters, W.A., Anderson, W.A., Thornton, W.N., Jr., and Morley, G.W.: The selective use of vaginal hysterectomy in the management of adenocarcinoma of the endometrium. Am. J. Obstet. Gynecol. *146:*285–291, 1983.
54. Lewis, G.C., Jr., Slack, N.H., Mortel, R., and Bross, I.D.J.: Adjuvant progestogen therapy in the primary definitive treatment of endometrial cancer. Gynecol. Oncol. *2:*368–376, 1974.
55. Malkasian, G.D., Jr., and Decker, D.G.: Adjuvant progesterone therapy for stage I endometrial carcinoma. Int. J. Gynaecol. Obstet. *16:*48–49, 1978.
56. Kinsella, T.J., Bloomer, W.D., Lavin, P.T., and Knapp, R.C.: Stage II endometrial carcinoma: 10-year follow up of combined radiation and surgical treatment. Gynecol. Oncol. *10:*290–297, 1980.
57. Aalders, J.G., Abeler, V., and Kolstad, P.: Clinical (stage III) as compared to subclinical intrapelvic extrauterine tumor spread in endometrial carcinoma: A clinical and histopathological study of 175 patients. Gynecol. Oncol. *17:*64–74, 1984.
58. Bruckman, J.E., Bloomer, W.D., Marck, A., et al.: Stage III adenocarcinoma of the endometrium: Two prognostic groups. Gynecol. Oncol. *9:*12–17, 1980.
59. Rustowski, J., and Kupsc, W.: Factors influencing the results of radiotherapy in cases of inoperable endometrial cancer. Gynecol. Oncol. *14:*185–193, 1982.
60. Aalders, J.G., Abeler, V., and Kolstad, P.: Recurrent adenocarcinoma of the endometrium: A clinical and histopathological study of 379 patients. Gynecol. Oncol. *17:*85–103, 1984.
61. Kauppila, A., Janne, O., Kujansuu, E., and Vihko, R.: Treatment of advanced endometrial adenocarcinoma with a combined cytotoxic therapy. Cancer *46:*2162–2167, 1980.
62. Johannesson, G., Geinsson, G., and Day, N.: The effect of mass screening in Iceland 1965–1974 on the incidence and mortality of cervical carcinomas. Int. J. Cancer *21:*418, 1978.
63. Ahlgren, M., Ingemarsson, I., Lindberg, L.G., and Nordquist, S.R.B.: Conization as treatment of carcinoma in situ of the uterine cervix. Obstet. Gynecol. *46:*135, 1976.
64. Mestwerdt, G.: Fruhdiagnose des kollumkarzinoms zentralblatt fur Gynakologie *69:*326, 1947.
65. Freund, W.A.: Eine neue methode der exstirpatici des ganzen uterus sammlung klinischer. Vortrage no 133. Gynakologie *41:*911, 1878.
66. Clark, J.G.: A more radical method of performing hysterectomy for cancer of the uterus. Bul. Johns Hopkins Hosp. *6:*120, 1895.
67. Wertheim, E.: Zur frage den radicaloperation beim uteruskrebs. Archiv fur Gynakologie *61:*627, 1900.
68. Wertheim, E.: The radical abdominal operation in carcinoma of the cervix uteri. Surg. Gynecol. Obstet. *4:*1, 1907.
69. Meigs, J.V.: Carcinoma of the cervix. The Wertheim operation. Surg. Gynecol. Obstet. *78:*195, 1944.
70. Liu, W., and Meigs, J.V.: Radical hysterectomy and pelvic lymphadenectomy. Am. J. Obstet. Gynecol. *69:*1, 1955.
71. Delgado, G.: Stage Ib squamous carcinoma of the cervix: The choice of treatment. Obstet. Gynecol. Surv. *33:*174–183, 1978.
72. Van Nagell, J.R., Donaldson, E.S., Parker, J.C., et al.: The prognostic significance of cell type and lesion size in patients with cervical cancer treated by radical surgery. Gynecol. Oncol. *5:*142, 1977.
73. Piver, M.S., and Chung, W.S.: Prognostic significance of cervical lesion size and pelvic node metastases in cervical carcinoma. Obstet. Gynecol. *46:*507, 1975.
74. Brunschweig, A.: Complete excision of the pelvic viscera for advanced carcinoma. Cancer *1:*177, 1948.
75. Bricker, E.M.: Bladder substitution after pelvic evisceration. Surg. Clin. North Am. *30:*1511, 1950.
76. Nelson, J.H.: Atlas of radical pelvic surgery. New York, Appleton-Century-Crofts, 1977.
77. Curry, S.L.: Pelvic exenteration. *In* Buschsbaum, H.J., and Sciarra, J.J. (Eds.): Gynecology and Obstetrics. Vol 4. Philadelphia, Harper & Row, 1984, p. 5.

78. Morley, G.W.: Cancer of the vulva. *In* Knapp, R.C., and Berkowitz, R.S. (Eds.): Gynecologic Oncology. New York, Macmillan Publishing Company, 1986.
79. Friedrich, E.G., Wilkinson, E.J., and Fu, Y.S.: Carcinoma in situ of the vulva: A continuing challenge. Am. J. Obstet. Gynecol. *136:*830, 1980.
80. Morley, G.W.: Infiltrative carcinoma of the vulva. Results of surgical treatment. Am. J. Obstet. Gynecol. *124:*874, 1976.
81. Hacker, N.F., Leuchter, R.S., Berek, J.S., et al.: Radical vulvectomy and bilateral groin lymphadenectomy through separate groin incisions. Obstet. Gynecol. *58:*574, 1981.
82. Boronow, R.C.: Combined therapy as an alternative to exenteration for locally advanced vulvo-vaginal cancer. Cancer *46:*6, 1982.
83. Cavanaugh, D., and Shepherd, J.H.: The place of pelvic exenterations in the primary management of advanced carcinoma of the vulva. Gynecol. Oncol. *13:*318–322, 1982.
84. DiSaia, P.J., Creasman, W.T., and Rich, W.M.: An alternative approach to early cancer of the vulva. Am. J. Obstet. Gynecol. *133:*825, 1979.
85. Morrow, C.P., and Rutledge, F.N.: Melanoma of the vulva. Obstet. Gynecol. *39:*745, 1972.
86. Chung, A.F., Woodruff, J.M., and Lewis, J.L.: Malignant melanoma of the vulva. Obstet. Gynecol. *45:*638, 1975.

15

MANAGEMENT OF REGIONAL AND LOCAL TUMOR RECURRENCE

by Peter N. Benotti, M.D., Mohammed Karbassi, M.D., Thanjavur S. Ravikumar, M.D., Albert Bothe, M.D., and Glenn Steele, Jr., M.D.

Local or regional tumor recurrence refers to a tumor recurrence in a previous operative field at an interval after a presumed curative resection. The surgical field includes the tumor bed, gastrointestinal anastomosis, regional lymph drainage area, drain tracts, and surgical scars.

The management of regional recurrence is a difficult problem for surgeons and oncologists. Differences in surgical expertise, experience, and courage will result in variability of the adequacy of initial curative cancer surgery. Many "local recurrences" are not really recurrences but simply a progression of disease left behind at the original resection. The tumor surveillance protocols for a variety of tumors are not well established. Rarely are tumor surveillance protocols rigorously followed in asymptomatic patients. Current imaging techniques are incapable of picking up small asymptomatic recurrences with any degree of certainty. This often results in delays in diagnosis until patients have disabling symptoms, poor performance status, bulky tumor, and narcotic dependence, all of which reflect advanced disease. Nonsurgical therapy for regional tumor recurrence has little to offer beyond short-term palliation of symptoms. Despite this, surgeons have traditionally been reluctant to proceed with major radical resections of recurrent disease because of limited curative potential and a likelihood of substantial morbidity and mortality.

Colorectal carcinoma is the most extensively studied tumor for surgical applications to local and regional recurrence. During the past three decades there has been little improvement in overall survival in patients undergoing curative resection for colorectal carcinoma.[1] Reviews of large series of patients undergoing curative resections suggest that approximately half will develop tumor recurrence. Of these recurrences, 25 per cent will be in the liver and 25 to 30 per cent will be in the abdomen or pelvis.[1,2] Approximately 151,000 new cases of colorectal cancer will be diagnosed in 1991. The annual death rate from colorectal carcinoma is between 50,000 and 60,000. Autopsy studies demonstrate that a significant number of the patients dying of colorectal cancer die from local/regional recurrence-related problems.[3–5]

Clinical and pathologic studies of patients with local recurrence reveal factors both related to the technical aspects of the original resection and to the tumor biology that predispose to local recurrence. The adequacy of the original resection is clearly an important factor contributing to both locally recurrent disease and survival. The significance of surgical expertise is best illustrated in a series of 52 patients reviewed at Memorial Sloan-Kettering referred because of apparent unresectable tumor of the colon. Of this group of patients, 40 actually had resectable disease. Curative resections were performed in 32 patients and palliative procedures in eight patients. Five-year survival in this patient group was 36 per cent with 28 per cent disease-free.[6] Likewise, recurrence data from the Large Bowel Cancer Project in England emphasize the surgeon's technical skill as a risk factor for local recurrence.[7]

Other technical factors important at the original resection include the necessity of obtaining a radial margin for tumors of the mid and lower third of the rectum. This includes resection of the mesorectum below the primary tumor in all cases of low anterior resection with anastomosis.[8,9] The viability of tumor cells at the resection margin is inversely proportional to the distance from the primary tumor. Lesions of the lower third of the rectum tend to recur locally more commonly than tumors of the upper rectum, which is probably related to the technical limitation in the radial margin.[10] The use of stapling techniques to facilitate the performance of low anterior anastomosis does not influence local recurrence rates provided that the previously mentioned technical guidelines are rigorously followed.[11,12]

Regional recurrence for colon carcinoma above the sigmoid is rare. This occurs most commonly at the splenic flexura and in the rectosigmoid.[13] Perforation of tumor is a major factor influencing the likelihood of regional recurrence. The increase in the incidence of local recurrence after resection of a perforated colonic carcinoma is approximately nine-fold.[14] Penetration through the bowel wall into the surrounding adipose tissue or extension of the tumor to contiguous structures is also an ominous sign predisposing to local recurrence.[14] The presence of positive lymph nodes,[15] mucin production,[16] and the degree of differentiation of the tumor[4] are additional factors related to the incidence of local recurrence. When more than one risk factor is present, local recurrence rate can increase to approximately 40 per cent.[17]

The overall incidence of local or regional recurrence after curative resection for colorectal carcinoma varies from 4 to 30 per cent. Schiessel, in a large series of patients with colorectal carcinoma, reported a local recurrence rate of 14.7 per cent for rectal carcinoma and 4.4 per cent for colon carcinoma.[18] Rich reported a local recurrence rate of 16.9 per cent for rectal carcinoma, and an additional 13.3 per cent local recurrence combined with distant recurrence for a total local recurrence rate of 30.2 per cent.[4] Wilking[19] and Pheils,[15] in smaller series of patients undergoing more radical surgery for rectal lesions, demonstrated local recurrence rates of 6 per cent and 9.8 per cent respectively for patients undergoing radical resectional therapy for cancer of the rectum. The lower rates in this series were attributed to more radical resections incorporating uterus and posterior vaginal wall when indicated. McDermott, in another large series of patients with rectal cancer undergoing resectional therapy, reported a local recurrence rate of 11 per cent with an additional 9 per cent occurring locally in combination with distant recurrence.[5]

Malcolm reported that isolated local recurrence is extremely rare after curative resections of right, transverse, and left colon tumors. However, local failure, either isolated or in combination with distant disease, is much more common for sigmoid carcinoma.[13] Gunderson, in 1974, reviewed the Wangensteen second-look operations performed in patients at high risk for local recurrence (i.e., patients with positive nodes or extension through the bowel wall at their original curative procedure). In this group, 50 per cent had isolated local recurrence. Local failure in combination with distant failure occurred in 92 per cent of patients.[17]

Numerous other clinical series confirm these observations.[14, 20] Autopsy studies suggest that the incidence of single-site regional recurrence in colorectal carcinoma is 27 per cent.[2] The importance of these observations is that a substantial number of patients dying of colorectal carcinoma succumb only to isolated regional recurrence.[2, 3, 21]

METHODS

Since 1982, we have prospectively evaluated and explored 51 consecutive patient cases for regionally recurrent abdominal and pelvic tumors. The diagnoses included 38 patients with colorectal carcinoma, four patients with ovarian carcinoma, three patients with cervical carcinoma, two patients with carcinoma of the anus, and one patient each with sacral chordoma, carcinoma of the bladder, carcinoma of the uterus, and melanoma.

In each of these patients, the recurrence was isolated with no other metastatic lesions noted on preoperative testing. In 84 per cent of the patients, the isolated recurrence involved the pelvis. The remaining 14 per cent had intraperitoneal recurrence.

All of these patients were referred for surgical therapy because of progressive symptomatology that led to the diagnosis of recurrence by CT scanning, endoscopy, and x-ray contrast studies. Many of the cases were referred as treatment failures after courses of external beam radiation and chemotherapy.

Pain was the predominate symptom in this series, occurring in 76 per cent of patients. Palpable recurrent tumor was present in 27 per cent, 14 per cent had genitourinary symptoms, and 3 per cent had intestinal fistulae.[22] This clinical presentation is similar to that reported in other series of abdominal and pelvic tumor recurrence. Nearly all patients in this series had their diagnosis of tumor recurrence established only after the development of severe symptoms and not by routine tumor surveillance studies. This is an extremely important factor, which may influence the ultimate salvage rates after resectional therapy in these patients.[18]

A number of studies have addressed the role of carcinoembryonic antigen (CEA) in the detection of recurrent colon cancer and in prognostication. The rationale behind CEA-directed second-look procedures is that early detection and aggressive resection of recurrence can result in long-term survival in a group of patients. However, the overall survival benefits of such second-look procedures are yet to be well documented.[17, 22, 23] Based on single-institutional and multi-institutional data that did not support a clear-cut survival benefit as a result of CEA-directed or blind second-look surgery, our institution has not embarked on any such second-look protocols.

Despite the fact that the resectional therapy for regionally recurrent abdominal cancers in our series was based on symptomatology, CEA levels were obtained preoperatively in most of the patients and were obtained postoperatively at periodic intervals. Serial estimations of CEA are available in 26 of the 38 patients with regional pelvic recurrence of colorectal cancer. The preoperative CEA levels range from 0.4 to 963 ng/ml with a median level of 3.6 ng/ml. In 50 per cent of our patients, CEA was over 5 ng/ml. In 42 per cent of our patients, CEA was not elevated, and no preoperative CEA levels were available in 8 per cent. While CEA is elevated in most of the patients with recurrent disease in the liver, only 30 to 50 per cent of patients with pelvic recurrent tumors have such elevations in other series.[24] Additionally, when one looks at the sites of the recurrences detected in clinically directed and CEA-directed second-look series, pelvic recurrence is mostly detected clinically and less often diagnosed by monitoring CEA elevations.[25] Thus, CEA is not a sensitive test to detect early pelvic recurrences.

All of the patients reported here underwent exploratory laparotomy. In each case, the assessment of operability was made at the time of laparotomy. The operations performed included nine abdominoperineal resections, 17 radical resections of tumor recurrence with involved viscera, and 18 pelvic exenterations, 13 of which were total exenterations. In seven patients, conservative procedures were carried out because of unresectable tumor. These procedures included biopsy and/or colonic diversion only. Preoperative clinical examinations and noninvasive imaging studies were not reliable in assessing operability in these patients. Preoperative clinical signs of incurability, even by radical resection, included fixation to the pelvic side wall on clinical examination, ipsilateral pain and swelling in the leg, and ureteral obstruction.[26] In the presence of these and other indicators of incurability, the decision to proceed with palliative resections was primarily based on an estimate of technical difficulty, the safety of resection, and the anticipated result in controlling symptoms.

At laparotomy, inoperability was determined by extensive bony invasion by tumor of the sacrum and pelvic side walls. The presence of large bulky lesions fixed in the pelvis precluded en bloc dissection and therefore were also deemed inoperable. Attempts to excise such tumors in a piecemeal manner invariably lead to early recurrence and should be discouraged except in rare instances in which short-term palliation of disabling symptoms seems justified.

In 44 instances (86 per cent), major resection was possible. Tumor was unresectable in seven patients (14 per cent) and only a conservative procedure (i.e., biopsy or colonic diversion) was carried out. In 32 patients (63 per cent), the resection was deemed curative in that all gross tumor was successfully removed. In 12 patients (24 per cent), a major resection was carried out with some residual tumor remaining usually fixed to pelvic side walls. In nine patients, intraoperative radiation therapy (IORT) was used as a boost to a course of external beam radiation. This was usually delivered to areas of tumor adherence in the retroperitoneum and/or pelvic side wall. IORT was given only when frozen section confirmed residual tumor.

The management of the open pelvis following abdominoperineal resection or exenteration after a full course of external beam therapy poses a difficult problem. Healing in the pelvis is often delayed because of previous radiation. Delayed healing and contamination at surgery explain the significant problem with chronic nonhealing pelvic abscess cavities. Recurring small bowel obstruction, both early and late, is also related to the open pelvis. We have followed the recommendations of Kraybill et al and attempted whenever possible to fill the pelvis with well-vascularized tissue in such situations.[26] Use of omental or myocutaneous flaps will significantly reduce both early and late morbidity related to infection and bowel obstruction involving the pelvis and perineum. The combination of exenteration with construction of myocutaneous flaps to fill the pelvis can be a lengthy procedure requiring in excess of 12 hours. For this reason, in selected patients, we have chosen to stage these procedures. In certain instances absorbable mesh is secured in place to prevent migration of small bowel loops into the pelvis.[27] This occasionally allows for successful management of the narrow pelvis after abdominoperineal resection and radiation. However, in most circumstances the use of vascularized tissue to fill the pelvis is preferable.

RESULTS

All patients were followed until death or the present; follow-up is 100 per cent. The median follow-up is 24 months (3 to 91 months). Survival data involve only the 38 patients with recurrent colorectal cancer because of the very limited number of patients with other tumors. Overall survival is 35 per cent with seven patients disease-free at a median follow-up of 39 months.

A major resection was performed in 43 (84 per cent) out of 51 patients. Curative resection of all gross tumor was achieved in 32 patients (66 per cent). In patients undergoing palliative resections, small foci of tumor were left behind if densely adherent to pelvic side walls. When indicated, these areas were treated with IORT. Seven patients with unresectable disease underwent biopsy and colonic diversion only. One patient with unresectable disease received IORT.

There were three operative deaths in this series (Table 15–1). Two elderly patients with colorectal carcinoma developed fatal septic complications and the third fatality followed resection of an infected uterine tumor recurrence in a debilitated patient. Problems related to prolonged ileus and intestinal obstruction are not uncommon when major resections are carried out following substantial external beam radiation to the lower small intestine. There was a single urinary bladder leak in the series. This occurred in a patient who underwent partial cystectomy after full-dosage pelvic radiation. Others have stated that partial cystectomy is contraindicated in the irradiated pelvis.[26] Additional complications are summarized in Table 15–1.

Recent published series of patients undergoing resections of regional tumor recurrence or locally advanced primary disease indicate mortality rates that vary from 2 to 16 per cent.[26, 28–36] Review of the data from multiple

TABLE 15–1. COMPLICATIONS (N = 51 PATIENTS)

	N	%
Mortality	3	6
Prolonged ileus	6	12
Hemorrhage	4	8
Superficial wound infection	4	8
Bowel obstruction	2	4
Deep venous thrombosis	2	4
Renal failure	2	4
Respiratory failure	2	4
Sepsis (perineal/pelvic)	3	6
Miscellaneous	10	20
None	21	41

large series over the past 10 years demonstrates that the mortality and morbidity for these operations has declined significantly. The reason for these improved results is multifactorial. Like other technically demanding procedures, these resections are associated with a substantial learning curve; most of our major complications occurred early in this series. In addition, improved preoperative recognition of nutritional and functional deficits has resulted in delay of surgery for appropriate nutritional rehabilitation. Preoperative nutritional repletion has been shown to reduce major life-threatening and postoperative complications.[37] Preoperative antibiotic therapy for control of active infection within the tumor mass also reduces morbidity.

In those 26 patients with recurrent colorectal cancer undergoing curative resection, nine (35 per cent) are surviving with a median follow-up of 39 months (5 to 91 months). Five of these patients are disease-free and four patients are alive with regional recurrence (Figs. 15–1 and 15–2). Of the 26 patients with colorectal cancer recurrence undergoing curative surgery, 17 have died including two operative deaths with a median survival of 22 months (6 to 91 months). Of these, 15 (83 per cent) had regional recurrence. One died at six months free of tumor and treatment failed in two because of distant disease outside of the abdomen.

There were 12 patients with colorectal cancer recurrence who underwent palliative resection. Eight of these patients (73 per cent) have died with a median survival of nine months. Of the four surviving, the longest survivor underwent colostomy, IORT, and external beam radiation for an unresectable recurrent rectal cancer in the pelvis. This patient is disease-free at 58 months. Overall median survival for patients undergoing palliative resections for recurrent colorectal carcinoma is 12 months (Figs. 15–1 and 15–2).

Analysis of survival after major resection in these patients prompts consideration of the natural history of disease in patients receiving nonsurgical therapy. Survival data after nonsurgical therapy are limited to historic control information of patients who are initially considered for resection and then excluded. No randomized or case-controlled information is available. In Wanebo's series of patients with pelvic recurrence, those not qualifying for resection had a median survival of 15 months with a five-year survival at 3 per cent.[30] Vassilopoulos reported a median survival of eight to 13 months in patients with recurrent colorectal carcinoma undergoing major resection in which gross tumor was left behind.[38] Polk and Spratt reported a median

CHAPTER 15 / MANAGEMENT OF REGIONAL AND LOCAL TUMOR RECURRENCE—347

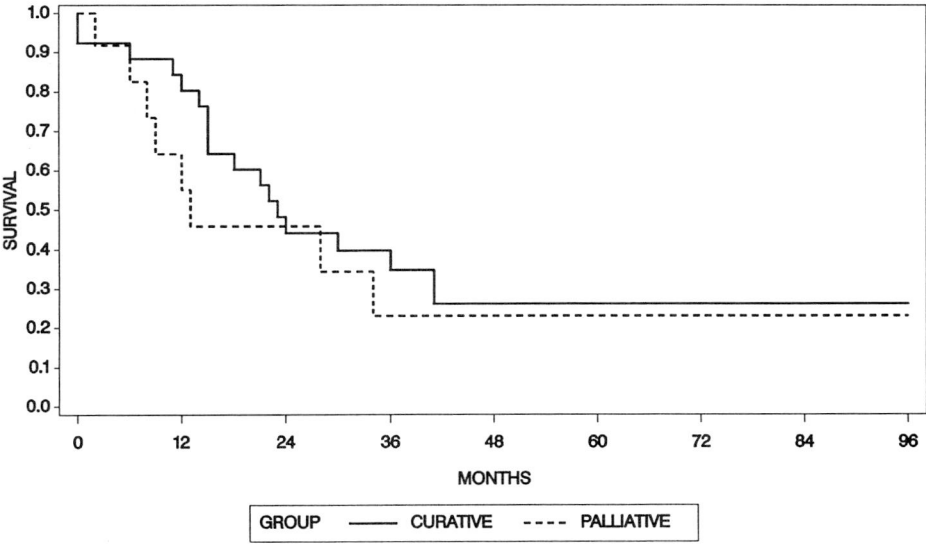

Figure 15–1. Kaplan-Meier survival curves for patients undergoing resection for regional recurrence of colorectal cancer broken down into two groups, as determined by the completeness of the resection.

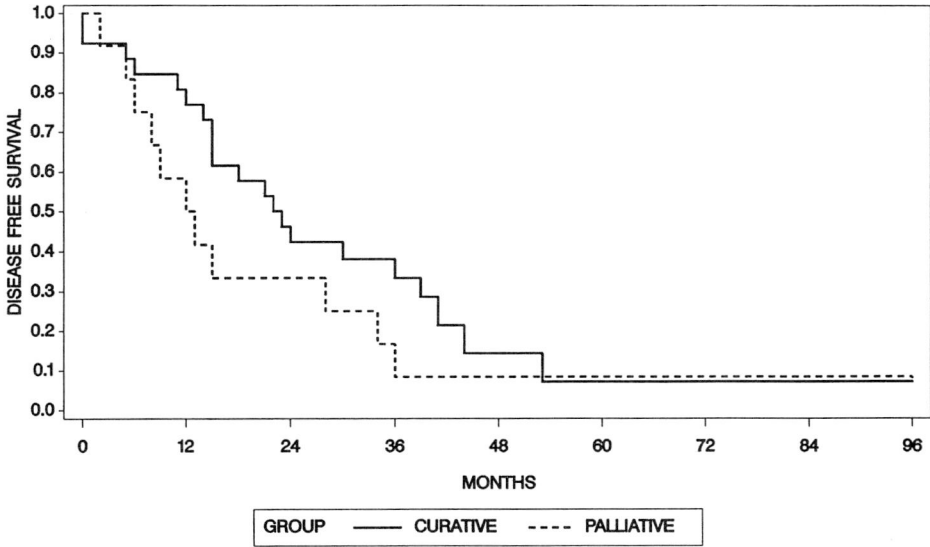

Figure 15–2. Kaplan-Meier disease-free survival curves for patients undergoing resection for regional recurrence of colorectal cancer broken down into two groups, as determined by the completeness of the resection.

TABLE 15–2. SURVIVAL WITH NONOPERATIVE THERAPY FOR REGIONAL TUMOR RECURRENCE

Author	Median Survival	5-Year Survival
Wanebo et al, 1987[30]	15 months	3%
Polk and Spratt, 1971[39]	7 months	
Gunderson et al, 1988[48]		5–10%
Pearlman et al, 1987[29]	12 months	
Schiessel et al, 1986[18]	8 months	

survival of seven months in their patients who did not undergo resection.[39] Schiessel reported a median survival of eight months in patients with recurrent colorectal carcinoma who did not undergo resection.[18] Review of the literature concerning the natural history of nonoperative therapy for pelvic tumor recurrence reveals an overall median survival between eight to 12 months[5, 15, 17, 21] (Table 15–2).

The survival after resection of regional tumor recurrence in the current major series is summarized in Table 15–3. Our own series of patient cases includes a variety of tumor types. In addition, our cases all occurred with disabling symptoms and as failures of other therapies. No patients in our series were asymptomatic or were diagnosed on the basis of tumor surveillance alone. This is in contrast to results that indicate earlier diagnosis of regional recurrence by routine screening before the development of disabling symptoms appears to increase the potential for long-term survival with re-resection.[18]

There was no statistically significant difference in the overall or disease-free survival between patients with normal CEA levels compared with those who had elevated CEA levels on admission. Furthermore, the level of CEA at presentation did not correlate with survival. The median survival of patients with CEA levels over 20 ng/ml was 15 months. This is in contrast to the reported prognostic value of CEA at the time of primary colorectal cancer diagnosis. Single-institutional and multicenter trials have shown that higher levels of plasma CEA correlate with recurrence.[40, 41]

Twenty-five patients have had serial CEA estimations during the follow-up period. CEA levels were normal in 14 of these 25 patients. Nine patients (64 per cent) remain disease-free at a median of 14 months follow-up; three patients (22 per cent) have died from regional/abdominal recurrence. During the same period of follow-up, 11 of the 25 patients demonstrated either

TABLE 15–3. SURVIVAL AFTER RESECTION OF REGIONAL TUMOR RECURRENCE

Author	Operation	N	Median Survival	5-Year Survival
Wanebo et al, 1987[30]	Abdominosacral resection	28	36 months	20%
Pearlman et al, 1987[29]	Sacropelvic exenteration	15	18 months	60%*
Schiessel et al, 1986[18]	Resections for local recurrence	109	14 months	30%*
Gunderson et al, 1988[48]	Resections and x-ray therapy	36	16 months	27%
Polk and Spratt, 1971[39]	Curative Re-resection	11	21 months	25%
Vassilopoulos et al, 1981[38]	Re-resection of abdominal recurrence	12	41 months	34%

*Projected

elevation or lack of normalization of CEA levels. Significantly, 10 out of 11 patients in this group (91 per cent) have died of recurrence predominantly in the regional distribution. Rarely does one see distant metastases to liver, lung, or bone as the pattern of failure. These data support the use of CEA in postoperative monitoring after resection for pelvic recurrence. Obviously this would be more beneficial to the patient if additional therapy were shown to be effective.

At the present time, surgery is the only therapy that offers patients with regional tumor recurrence the possibility of extended survival. High-dosage external beam radiation as a solitary treatment for these patients does offer the potential for short-term palliation, but overall survival is limited. Evidence is increasing that radiation therapy may play a significant role when combined with resection. The use of preoperative external beam therapy in patients with apparent unresectable colorectal tumors renders a significant portion of these tumors resectable.[42–45] These data have been extrapolated to the management of regional recurrence, and the use of external beam to minimize local disease prior to resection is increasing.

The rationale for preoperative radiation therapy involves enhanced control of the local tumor and the possibility for reduction in the risk of tumor dissemination at the time of surgery. In controlled trials, preoperative radiation therapy has been shown to result in downstaging of the tumor and, occasionally, in tumor sterilization.[42]

During the past five years, in several centers intraoperative radiation therapy has been used in clinical trials.[46] The rationale for using intraoperative therapy is that a single larger radiation fraction will have enhanced tumoricidal efficacy. Additionally, toxicity will be reduced by the direct protection of surrounding structures by focused targeting and by appropriate shielding within the operative field.

The efficacy of intraoperative radiation in combination with external beam therapy has been established in the management of patients with locally advanced colorectal cancer receiving large-dosage external beam therapy followed by curative resection.[46] This therapy has also been shown to be effective in patients with colorectal carcinoma undergoing major resection with limited residual local disease and in those patients undergoing resection for isolated local recurrence.[47, 48] Gunderson reported four-year actuarial survivals of 53 per cent in patients undergoing resection of locally extensive primary rectal carcinomas and survivals of 23 per cent in patients undergoing resection of regional recurrence with preoperative and intraoperative radiation therapy.[48]

Because our experience with IORT in this series is limited to nine patients, the precise impact of therapy is unclear. Overall, six of the nine are surviving at a median of 27 months. Four of the nine are disease-free. The growing consensus is that IORT in combination with resection enhances local control in colorectal carcinoma. Interestingly, our only five-year disease-free survivor received IORT after removal of an adherent recurrent colonic carcinoma in the right iliac fossa.

The decision to use IORT as a boost to a preoperative course of external beam therapy should be a clinical decision made by the operating team. Strict reliance on frozen section biopsy material obtained from radiated tissues may result in significant false-negative interpretations. The decision to proceed with IORT should be made on the basis of clinical suspicion of residual tumor, frozen section interpretation, and clinical assessment of the risks of additional radiation.

More effective chemotherapeutic agents are required for better management of regional tumor recurrence. In colon cancer, controlled trials have only recently demonstrated some survival benefit with adjuvant immunochemotherapy.[49] In rectal cancer, the combination of 5-fluorouracil with or without semustine and postoperative radiation therapy shows promise. This modality has been shown in randomized trials to reduce the incidence of systemic metastasis to increase the disease-free survival as well as overall total survival when compared with preoperative radiation therapy alone followed by surgery or postoperative radiation alone.[45, 50, 51] The use of combinations of 5-fluorouracil, leucovorin, and levamisole is promising in preliminary trials and may offer the potential for greater survival benefit when used with radiotherapy as an adjuvant following surgery for high-risk rectal cancer.[50, 52, 53]

A proposed algorithm for the care of patients suspected of developing regional recurrence of colorectal carcinoma is summarized in Figure 15–3. Close surveillance after primary resection is extremely important. Frequent physical examinations, stool studies for occult blood, and CEA determinations will precede imaging studies. Although CT is capable of identifying regional recurrence in the abdomen or pelvis, poor definition limits its sensitivity in detecting early asymptomatic disease. Improved MRI offers potential for earlier diagnosis. Once regional recurrence is identified, studies should be obtained to exclude distant metastatic disease.

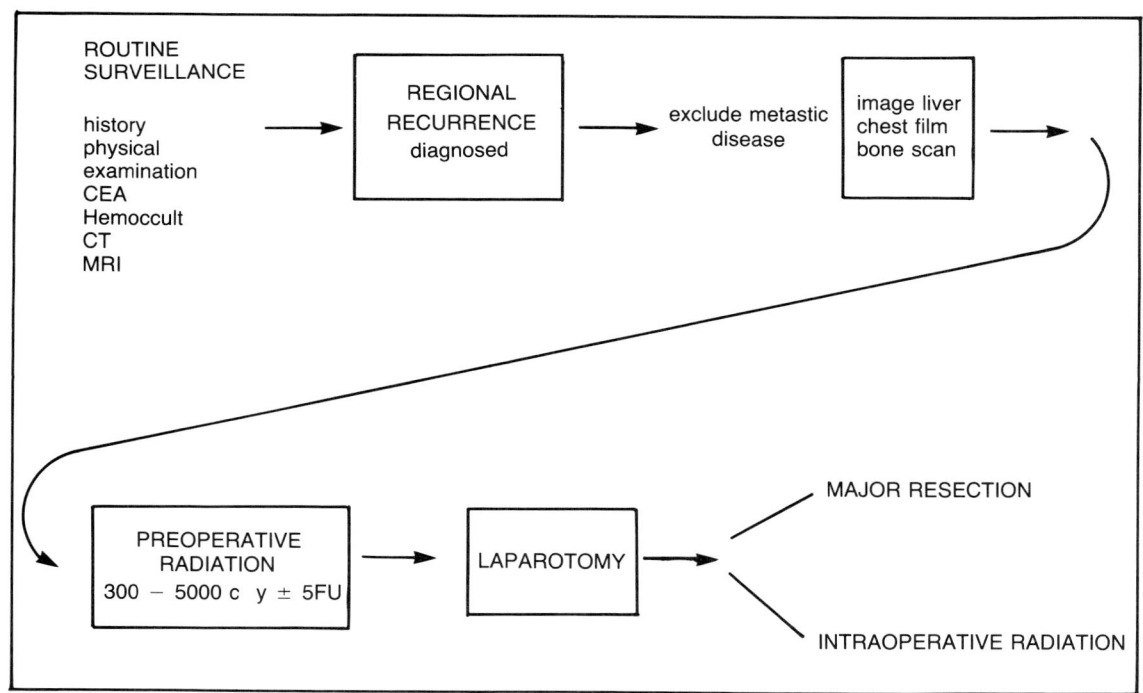

Figure 15–3. Algorithm for management of patients with recurrence of colorectal cancer.

In the patient with a regional recurrence, preoperative radiation of 3000 and 5000 cGy with synchronous 5-fluorouracil infusion should be considered. If extensive small bowel or other radiosensitive vital structures lie in proximity to tumor, radiation may be delayed until after resection.

At exploration, a careful search for occult intraabdominal spread to peritoneum, lymph nodes, and liver parenchyma should be performed. Once an isolated recurrence is confirmed, appropriate resectional therapy is indicated. Intraoperative radiation therapy should be considered for any areas of localized tumor fixation to bony structures within the pelvis or to the musculofascial layers of the posterior retroperitoneum. Areas of dense attachment should be biopsied for frozen section analysis. Suspicious areas, even if frozen-section negative, should be considered for intraoperative radiation on the basis of clinical judgment. When major resections are carried out in irradiated areas, attempts should be made to move well-vascularized tissue into the field to provide better healing. If postoperative radiation therapy is considered, vascularized tissue or synthetic support should be used to keep the small intestine away from the planned radiation field.

The potential for multimodality combinations of more effective systemic adjuvant therapy with external beam intraoperative radiation combined with surgery, either curative or palliative, does offer the potential for significant reduction in mortality of colorectal carcinoma during the next decade.

REFERENCES

1. Welch, J.P., and Donaldson, G.A.: Detection and treatment of recurrent cancer of the colon and rectum. Am. J. Surg. *135*:505–510, 1978.
2. Gilbert, J.M., Jeffrey, I., Evens, M., et al.: Sites of recurrent tumor after curative colorectal surgery: Implications for adjuvant therapy. Br. J. Surg. *71*:203–205, 1984.
3. Rao, A.R., Kagan, A.R., Chan, P.M., et al.: Pattern of recurrence following curative resection alone for adenocarcinoma of the rectum and sigmoid colon. Cancer *48*:1492–1495, 1981.
4. Rich, T., Gunderson, L.L., Lew, R., et al.: Patterns of recurrence of rectal cancer after potentially curative surgery. Cancer *52*:1317–1329, 1983.
5. McDermott, F.T., Hughes, E.S.R., Pihl, E., et al.: Local recurrence after potentially curative resection for rectal cancer in a series of 1008 patients. Br. J. Surg. *72*:34–37, 1985.
6. Newman, H.K., and Stearns, M.W.: Re-exploratory for "unresectable" colonic cancer. Dis. Colon Rectum *18*:576–580, 1975.
7. Phillips, R.K.S., Hittingen, R., Blesovsky, L., et al.: Local recurrence following "curative" surgery for large bowel cancer: 1. The overall picture. Br. J. Surg. *71*:12–16, 1984.
8. Heald, R.J., Husband, E.M., and Ryall, R.D.M.: The mesorectum in rectal cancer surgery— the clue to pelvic recurrence. Br. J. Surg. *69*:613–616, 1982.
9. Phillips, R.K.S., Hittinger, R., and Blesovsky, L.: Local recurrence following "curative" surgery for large bowel cancer II. The rectum and rectosigmoid. Br. J. Surg. *71*:17–20, 1984.
10. Adloff, M., Arnaud, J.P., Schloegel, M., et al.: Factors influencing local recurrence after abdominoperineal resection for cancer of the rectum. Dis. Colon Rectum *28*:413–415, 1985.
11. Rosen, C.B., Beart, R.W., and Ilstrup, D.M.: Local recurrence of rectal carcinoma after hand-sewn and stapled anastomosis. Dis. Colon Rectum *28*:305–309, 1985.
12. Kennedy, H.L., Langevin, J.M., Goldberg, G.M., et al.: Recurrence following stapled coloproctostomy for carcinomas of the mid portion of the rectum. Surg. Gynecol. Obstet. *160*:513–516, 1985.
13. Malcolm, A.W., Perencevich, N.P., Olson, R.M., et al.: Analysis of recurrence patterns following curative resection—for carcinoma of the colon and rectum. Surg. Gynecol. Obstet. *152*:131–136, 1981.
14. Herfarth, C., Schlag, P., and Hohenberger, P.: Surgical strategies in local regional recurrences of gastrointestinal carcinoma. World J. Surg. *11*:504–510, 1987.
15. Phiels, M.T., Chapuis, R.C., and Newland, K.: Local recurrence following curative resection for carcinoma of the rectum. Dis. Colon Rectum *26*:98–102, 1983.

16. Umpleby, H.C., Ranson, D.L., and Williamson, R.E.N.: Peculiarities of mucinous colorectal carcinoma. Br. J. Surg. 72:715–718, 1985.
17. Gunderson, L., and Sosin, H.: Areas of failure found at reoperation (second or symptomatic look) following "curative surgery" for adenocarcinoma of the rectum. Cancer 34:1278–1292, 1974.
18. Schiessel, R., Wunderlich, M., and Herbst, F.: Local recurrence of colorectal cancer: Effect of early detection and aggressive therapy. Br. J. Surg. 73:342–344, 1986.
19. Wilking, N., Herrera, L., Petrelli, N., et al.: Pelvic and perineal recurrences after abdominoperineal resection for adenocarcinoma of the rectum. Am. J. Surg. 150:561–563, 1985.
20. Olson, R.M., Perencevich, N.P., Malcom, A.W., et al.: Patterns of recurrence following curative resection of adenocarcinoma of the colon and rectum. Cancer 45:2969–2974, 1980.
21. Taylor, F.W.: Cancer of the colon and rectum: A study of routes of metastases and death. Surgery 52:305–308, 1962.
22. Benotti, P.N., Bothe, A., Eyre, R.L., et al.: Management of recurrent pelvic tumors. Arch. Surg. 122:457–460, 1987.
23. Attiyeh, F.F., and Stearns, M.W.: Second-look laparotomy based on CEA elevations in colorectal cancer. Cancer 47:2119–2125, 1981.
24. Evans, J.T., Mittleman, A., Chu, M., et al.: Pre and post operative use of CEA. Cancer 42:1419–1424, 1978.
25. Wanebo, H.J.: Re-operative surgery for recurrent colorectal cancer: Role of carcinoembryonic antigen in patient selection. In Levine, J., and Beahrs, O. (Eds.): Colorectal Cancer. New York, Marcel Dekker, 1985, pp. 303–313.
26. Kraybill, W.G., Lopez, M.J., and Bricker, E.M.: Total pelvic exenteration as a therapeutic option in advanced malignant disease of the pelvis. Surg. Gynecol. Obstet. 166:259–263, 1988.
27. Devereux, D.F., Kavanah, M.T., Feldman, M.I., et al.: Small bowel exclusion from the pelvis by a polyglycolic acid mesh sling. J. Surg. Oncol. 26:107–112, 1984.
28. Williams, L., Huddleston, C.B., Sawyers, J., et al.: Is total pelvic exenteration reasonable primary treatment for rectal carcinoma? Ann. Surg. 207:670–678, 1988.
29. Pearlman, N.W., Donohue, R.E., Stiegmann, G.V., et al.: Pelvic and sacropelvic exenteration for locally advanced or recurrent anorectal cancer. Arch. Surg. 122:537–541, 1987.
30. Wanebo, H.J., Gaker, D.L., and Whitehill, R.: Pelvic recurrence of rectal cancer, options for curative resection. Ann. Surg. 205:482–495, 1987.
31. Falk, R.E., Moffat, F.L., Makowa, L., et al.: Pelvic exenteration for advanced primary and recurrent adenocarcinoma. Can. J. Surg. 28:539–541, 1985.
32. Boey, J., Wong, J., and Ong, G.B.: Pelvic exenteration for locally advanced colorectal carcinoma. Ann. Surg. 195:513–518, 1982.
33. Wanebo, H.J., and Marcove, R.C.: Abdominal sacral resections of locally recurrent cancer. Ann. Surg. 194:458–471, 1981.
34. Segall, M.M., Goldberg, S.M., Nevatvongs, S., et al.: Abdominoperineal resection for recurrent cancer following anterior resection. Dis. Colon Rectum 24:80–84, 1981.
35. Ledesma, E.J., Bruno, S., and Mittleman, A.: Total pelvic exenteration in colorectal disease. Ann. Surg. 194:701–703, 1981.
36. Kiselow, M., Butcher, H.R., and Bricker, E.M.: Results of the radical surgical treatment of advanced pelvic cancer. Ann. Surg. 166:428–436, 1967.
37. Muller, J.M., Dienst, C., Brenner, U., et al.: Preoperative parenteral feeding in patients with gastrointestinal carcinoma. Lancet 1:68–71, 1982.
38. Vassilopoulos, P.P., Ledesma, E., Yoon, J.M., et al.: Surgical treatment of metastatic colorectal adenocarcinoma. Dis. Colon Rectum 24:265–271, 1981.
39. Polk, H.C., and Spratt, J.S.: Recurrent colorectal carcinoma: Detection, treatment, and other considerations. Surgery 69:9–23, 1971.
40. Goslin, R., Steele, G., Jr., MacIntyre, J., et al.: The use of preoperative plasma CEA levels for the stratification of patients after the curative resection of colorectal cancers. Ann. Surg. 192:747–751, 1980.
41. Steele, G., Jr., Ellenberg, S., Ramming, K., et al.: CEA monitoring among patients in multi-institutional adjuvant GI therapy protocols. Ann. Surg. 196:162–169, 1982.
42. Duncan, W.: Preoperative radiotherapy in rectal cancer. World J. Surg. 11:429–445, 1987.
43. Pilepich, M.V., Munzenrider, J.E., Tak, W.K., et al.: Preoperative irridation of primarily unresectable colorectal carcinoma. Cancer 42:1077–1081, 1978.
44. Bjerkeset, T., and Dahl, O.: Irradiation and surgery for primarily inoperable rectal adenocarcinoma. Dis. Colon Rectum 23:298–303, 1980.
45. Boulis-Wassif, S., Gerard, A., Loygus, J., et al.: Final results of a randomized trial on the treatment of rectal cancer with preoperative radiotherapy alone or in combination with 5-flourouracil, followed by radical surgery. Cancer 53:1811–1818, 1984.
46. Gunderson, L.L., Shipley, W.U., Suit, H.D., et al.: Intraoperative irradiation. A pilot study combining external beam photons with "boost" dose intraoperative electrons. Cancer 49:2259–2266, 1982.

47. Tepper, J.E., Cohen, A.M., Wood, W.C., et al.: Intraoperative electron beam radiotherapy in the treatment of unresectable cancer. Arch. Surg. *121:*421–423, 1986.
48. Gunderson, L.L., Kirk Martin, J., and Beart, R.W.: Intraoperative and external beam irradiation for locally advanced colorectal cancer. Ann. Surg. *20:*52–59, 1988.
49. Moertel, C.G., Fleming, T.R., MacDonald, J.S., et al.: Levamisole and fluorouracil for adjuvant therapy of resected colon carcinoma. N. Engl. J. Med. *322:*352–358, 1990.
50. Gastrointestinal Tumor Study Group: Prolongation of disease-free interval in surgically treated rectal carcinoma. N. Engl. J. Med. *312:*1465–1472, 1985.
51. Gastrointestinal Tumor Study Group: Survival after postoperative combination treatment of rectal carcinoma. N. Engl. J. Med. *315:*1294–1295, 1986.
52. Laurie, J., Moertel, C., Fleming, T., et al.: Surgical adjuvant therapy of poor prognosis colorectal cancer with levamisole alone or combined levamisole and 5-fluorouracil. Proc. Am. Soc. Clin. Oncol. *5:*81, 1986.
53. Madajewicz, S., Petrelli, N., and Rustum, Y.M.: Phase II trial of high dose calcium leucovorin and 5-fluorouracil in advanced colorectal cancer. Cancer Res. *44:*4667–4669, 1984.

INDEX

Page numbers in *italics* refer to illustrations; page numbers followed by a (t) refer to tables.

Achalasia, 88
Acid phosphatase
  in prostate cancer, 279
Adenocarcinoma
  esophageal, *90*, 90–91
Adenoma
  colon cancer and, 157–158
Adenosquamous carcinoma
  esophageal, 91
Adrenal gland
  cancer of, 230
Adriamycin (doxorubicin)
  in soft tissue sarcoma, 266, 267, 268
Alcohol
  esophageal cancer and, 88
  head and neck cancer and, 24, 24(t)
Alpha-fetoprotein (AFP)
  in ovarian cancer, 317
  in testicular cancer, 293, 294, 295
Aminoglutethimide
  in prostate cancer, 282
Androgen
  antagonists of
    in prostate cancer, 283
  deprivation of
    in prostate cancer, 282
  total blockade of
    in prostate cancer, 283
Angiography
  in liver cancer, 187
Anus
  cancer of, 171, 179–180
    biopsy in, 180
    lymphatic metastases from, 172–173
    prognosis in, 179
Apnea
  sleep
    post-treatment
      in oral cavity cancer, 53
Arteriography
  in head and neck cancer, 32
  in renal cell carcinoma, 286–287
  in soft tissue sarcoma, 254
Arylamines
  bladder cancer and, 298
Aspergillus flavus
  liver cancer and, 185

Bacille Calmette-Guérin (BCG)
  in bladder cancer, 302

Barrett's esophagus
  esophageal cancer in, 88–89, *90*
Bartholin's gland
  cancer of, 335
Bile acids
  in colon cancer, 151
Biopsy
  in anal cancer, 180
  in breast cancer, 205–214, *206–209*, 210(t)
  in gastric cancer, 140–141
  in head and neck cancer, 31
  in lung cancer, 112, 113, 114(t)
  in ovarian cancer, 312
  in prostate cancer, 276
  in soft tissue sarcoma, 251, 255(t), 255–257, *256*, *257*
Bladder
  cancer of, 298–306
    arylamines and, 298
    chemotherapy in, 304–305
    cigarette smoking and, 298
    clinical evaluation of, *299*, 299–300, *300*
    epidemiology of, 298–299
    follow-up for, 301
    hematuria in, 299
    incidence of, 298–299
    invasive, 302–304
    metastases from, 302
    nonpapillary, 299, *299*
    papillary, 299, *299*
    recurrence of, 301
    shapes of, *299*
    sites of, *299*
    staging of, 300, *300*
    superficial, 301–302
    treatment of
      bacille Calmette-Guérin in, 302
      chemotherapy in, 304–305
      continent urinary reservoirs in, 303–304
      intravesical chemotherapy in, 301–302, 304–305
      radiation therapy in, 302–303
      radical cystectomy in, 303
      sexual dysfunction and, 303
      transurethral resection in, 301
Blood transfusion
  in colon cancer, 163

Bone marrow
  monoclonal antibody staining of
    in breast cancer, 196
Bowen's disease, 331. See also *Vulva, cancer of.*
Brachytherapy
  in soft tissue sarcoma, 264–265, *265*
Breast
  cancer of, 195–216
    advanced, 214–215
    axillary dissection in, 202, 212
    biology of, 195–197
    bone marrow monoclonal antibody staining in, 196
    chemotherapy for, 216
    disease-free survival in, 205(t)
    epidemiology of, 198–199
    excisional biopsy of, 205–214, *206–209*, 210(t)
    follow-up for, 16–17, 213
    genetic aspects of, 198, 199
    in situ
      duct, 196, 200–201, 201(t), 202(t)
        microinvasion in, 213
      high-risk, 201, 201(t)
      lobular, 199, 200(t), 201, 202(t)
    inflammatory, 215
    invasive, 202(t)
      nonpalpable, 202–204
      palpable, 204–205, 205(t)
    mammography in, 197–198, 204
    menopausal status and, 198–199
    metastases from
      nodal, 195–196, 204, 212
    microcalcifications in, 200, 201(t)
    micrometastases from, 196, 212
    needle aspiration cytology in, 204
    presentation of, 197–198
    recurrence of
      local, 195, 210, *210*, 213
    treatment of
      chemotherapy in, 13, 197
      lumpectomy for, 202–204
        contraindications to, 210
        follow-up for, 213
        local recurrence after, 213
        margin analysis in, 203
        radiation therapy and, 203, 215–216
      mastectomy for, 213
        reconstruction with, 211
      radiation therapy in, 20, 203, 215–216
      receptors in, 209
      tamoxifen for, 197, 216
    vs. breast cyst, 204–205
    vs. testicular cancer model, 197
  reconstruction of, 20, 211
Bronchoscopy
  in lung cancer, 111, 119

CA125
  in ovarian cancer, 316, 317–318
Calcification
  on mammography, 200, 201(t)
Calcitonin
  in medullary carcinoma, 229
Calcium
  in colon cancer, 151
Carcinoembryonic antigen (CEA)

Carcinoembryonic antigen (CEA) *(Continued)*
  in colon cancer, 11, 12, 15, 16(t), 17(t), 163, 343–344, 348–349
  in hepatic cancer, 186, 191
  in medullary carcinoma, 229
  in thyroid cancer, 299
Carcinoma simplex, 331. See also *Vulva, cancer of.*
Carcinosarcoma
  esophageal, 91
Castration
  in prostate cancer, 282
CEA. See *Carcinoembryonic antigen (CEA).*
Celestin tube
  in esophageal cancer, *94*, 94–95
Cervix
  cancer of, 323–331, 326(t), *328, 329*
    conization for, 324–325
    invasive, 325
      management of, 326–329, *328, 329*
        radical hysterectomy in, 327–328, *328, 329*
      recurrence of
        management of, 330–331
    metastases from, 327
    microinvasive, 325
    size of, 327
    staging of, 325, 326(t)
    treatment of
      conization in, 324–325
      pelvic exenteration in, 330
      radiation therapy in, 326–327
      radical hysterectomy in, 327–328, *328, 329*
      urinary diversion in, 330
  colposcopic examination of, 323–324
  transformation zone of, 323
Chemotherapy
  in anal cancer, 179
  in bladder cancer, 301–302, 304–305
  in breast cancer, 13, 197, 216
  in colon cancer, 165–166, 350
  in endometrial cancer, 322–323
  in esophageal cancer, 94, 99
  in gastric cancer, 146
  in head and neck cancer, 72–76
  in hypopharyngeal cancer, 70
  in laryngeal cancer, 64
  in liver cancer, 192
  in lung cancer, 118, 131–133, *132*, 136
  in malignant melanoma, 242
  in nasopharyngeal cancer, *83*, 83–84
  in ovarian cancer, 313, 314(t), 315
  in prostate cancer, 284
  in rectal cancer, 176–177
  in retroperitoneal sarcoma, 271(t)
  in soft tissue sarcoma, 260, 266–267, 267(t)
  in testicular cancer, 296–297
Cholangiocarcinoma, 187. See also *Liver, cancer of.*
Cholesterol
  serum
    in colon cancer, 151
Cigarette smoking
  bladder cancer and, 298
  renal cell carcinoma and, 286
Cirrhosis
  liver cancer and, 185–186, 188–189, *189*
Clinician/scientist
  characterization of, 5
Colon
  cancer of, 149–167

Colon (Continued)
   age and, 162
   anatomic considerations in, 149–150
   bile acids and, 151
   blood transfusion in, 163
   calcium and, 151
   carcinoembryonic antigen in, 11, 12, 15, 16(t), 17(t), 163, 343–344, 348–349
   chromosomal changes in, 154
   colon diseases and, 153–154
   colonoscopy in, 156
   contiguous organ involvement in, 161
   diagnosis of, 155–157, 158–159
   DNA content in, 163
   double contrast barium enema study in, 156
   etiology of, 150–151
      multistep process in, 154
   familial cancer syndromes and, 152–153, 153(t)
   familial polyposis syndromes and, 152, 153(t), 159–160
   fecapentaenes and, 151
   follow-up of, 15–17, 16(t), 17(t)
      carcinoembryonic antigen in, 11, 12, 15, 16(t), 17(t), 163, 343–344, 348–349
      schedule for, 16(t)
   Gardner's syndrome and, 152–153
   gene products in, 163–164
   genetics of, 151–155, 153(t)
      molecular, 154–155
   hepatic 5-fluorouracil infusion in, 166–167
   inflammatory bowel disease and, 154
   intraoperative considerations in, 158–159
   3-keto steroids and, 151
   Lynch syndrome and, 153, 157
   metastases in
      hepatic, 12, 164
         treatment of, 19, 190, 191
      ovarian, 160–161
      pulmonary, 12
   NIH 1990 Consensus Development Conference on, 166
   obstruction in, 161, 162
   occult blood testing in, 156
   Oldfield syndrome and, 153
   Park's procedure in, 159–160
   pathology of, 162–163
   perforation in, 161
   polypectomy in, 156, 157–158
   polyps and, 157–158
   presentation of, 162
   proctosigmoidoscopy in, 156
   prophylactic oophorectomy in, 160–161
   proto-oncogenes in, 154–155
   pyrolysis and, 151
   recurrence of, 150, 164–165, 341–351
      algorithm for, *350*, 350–351
      carcinoembryonic antigen in, 11, 12, 15, 16(t), 17(t), 343–344, 348–349
      clinical presentation of, 343–345
      evaluation of, 343–345
      incidence of, 342–343
      treatment of, 343–345
         chemotherapy in, 350
         complications of, 346, 346(t)
         pelvic abscess cavity and, 345
         radiation therapy in, 349–350
         results of, 345–351, 346(t), *347*, 348(t)
         survival with, 345, 346, *347*, 348, 348(t)

Colon (Continued)
   risk factors for, 151–155, 153(t)
   screening for, 155–157
   serum cholesterol and, 151
   serum β-lipoprotein and, 151
   sex and, 162
   staging of, 150, 158, 158(t)
   surgical treatment of, 159, *161*
      adjuvant therapy in, 165–167
      chemotherapy and, 165–166
      follow-up in, 164
      liver infusion therapy and, 166–167
      radial margin in, 342
      results of, 161–164
      surgical expertise in, 342
   symptoms of, 155
   tumor DNA content in, 163
   tumor suppressor genes in, 154–155
   Turcot syndrome and, 153
   ulcerative colitis and, 154
Colonoscopy
   in colon cancer, 156
Colorectal cancer. See *Colon, cancer of; Rectum, cancer of.*
Colostomy
   in rectal cancer treatment, 172
Computed tomography
   in esophageal cancer, 92
   in head and neck cancer, 32
   in laryngeal cancer, 61
   in liver cancer, 186
   in lung cancer, 111
   in nasopharyngeal cancer, *79*, 79–80
   in ovarian cancer, 316
   in renal cell carcinoma, 286
   in soft tissue sarcoma, 253, *254*
   in testicular cancer, 294
Conization
   cervical, 324–325
Cryosurgery
   in liver cancer, 192
Cryptorchidism
   testicular cancer and, 293
Cyst
   Bartholin's gland, 335
   breast
      vs. breast cancer, 204–205
   ovarian, 312
   pulmonary
      lung cancer and, 123
Cystadenocarcinoma, 188. See also *Liver, cancer of.*

DCC (deleted in colorectal cancer) gene, 155
Dearterialization
   hepatic
      in liver cancer, 192
Deleted in colorectal cancer (DCC) gene, 155
Deoxyribonucleic acid (DNA)
   in colon cancer, 163
Depression
   post-treatment
      in oral cavity cancer, 53
Diethylstilbestrol (DES)
   in prostate cancer, 282–283
DNA (deoxyribonucleic acid)
   in colon cancer, 163

Doxorubicin (Adriamycin)
   in soft tissue sarcoma, 266, 267, 268
Duke's classification
   in colon cancer, 158, 158(t)
Dysphagia
   in esophageal cancer, 91
Dysplastic nevus syndromes, 234, 237
Dystrophy
   hyperplastic
      vulvar cancer and, 331

EBV (Epstein-Barr virus)
   in nasopharyngeal cancer, 78, 80
Endometrium
   cancer of, 318–323, 319(t), 320(t), 321(t), 322(t)
      invasive
         treatment of, 320–332, 321(t), 322(t)
      metastases from, 319
         nodal, 321, 321(t)
      pathology of, 318–319, 319(t)
      prognosis for, 319
      spread of, 318–319, 319(t)
      stage of, 319, 320(t)
      treatment of, 319–323, 321(t), 322(t)
         chemotherapy in, 322–323
         hysterectomy in, 320
         progestational therapy in, 322
         radiation therapy in, 321, 322
   hyperplasia of
      treatment of, 319–320
Endoprosthesis
   in esophageal cancer, 94, 94–95
Endoscopy
   in esophageal cancer, 93
   in head and neck cancer, 31
   in laryngeal cancer, 61
Epithelium
   gastrointestinal
      premalignant changes in, 12
Epstein-Barr virus (EBV)
   in nasopharyngeal cancer, 78, 80
Erythroplasia of Queyrat, 331. See also *Vulva, cancer of.*
Esophagogastrectomy
   in esophageal cancer, 96–99, *97*, *98*, 99(t)
Esophagogastrostomy
   side-to-side
      in esophageal cancer, 100
Esophagus
   adenocarcinoma of, *90*, 90–91
   adenosquamous carcinoma of, 91
   cancer of, 87–101
      Barrett's esophagus and, 88–89, *90*
      carcinogens in, 24(t)
      demography of, 88
      diagnosis of, 91–93, *92*
         early, 93
         endoscopy in, 93
         roentgenography in, 92, *92*
         screening techniques in, 93
      dysphagia in, 91
      etiology of, 88–89
      location of, 89, *89*
      pathology of, 89–91, *90*
      precancerous lesions of, 88
      prognosis for, 87

Esophagus *(Continued)*
      staging of, 105
      symptoms of, 91–92
      treatment of, 93–101, *94*, 96(t), *97*, *98*, 99(t), *100*, *101*
         bypass in, 100
         chemotherapy in, 94, 99
         combined therapy in, 99–101, *100*, *101*
         endoprosthesis in, *94*, 94–95
         gastrostomy in, 101
         intubation in, 101
         laser coagulation in, 95
         outcome of, 96(t), 99(t), *100*, *101*
         photoirradiation in, 95
         radiation therapy in, 93–94, 99
         stricture dilation in, 95
         surgical, 95–101, 96(t), *97*, *98*, 99(t), *100*, *101*
            discussion of, 105
            outcome of, 99(t)
            technique of, 96–99, *97*, *98*, 99(t)
      types of, 89–91, *90*
   cervical
      cancer of, 68–71
         clinical features of, 69–70
         diagnosis of, 69–70
         treatment of, 70–71
   melanoma of, 91
   oat cell carcinoma of, 91
   pseudosarcoma of, 91
   reconstruction of, 36
   sarcoma of, 91
   squamous cell carcinoma of, 89–90, *90*
Estrogen
   endometrial cancer and, 318
   in prostate cancer, 282
Etoposide
   in testicular cancer, 297

Familial cancer syndromes
   colon cancer and, 152–153, 153(t)
Familial polyposis syndromes
   colon cancer and, 152, 153(t), 159–160
Fasciitis
   proliferative, 249
Fecapentaenes
   in colon cancer, 151
α-Fetoprotein
   in liver cancer, 186
Fibrosis
   radiation
      in head and neck cancer, 37, 38
FIGO staging
   in cervical cancer, 325, 326(t)
   in endometrial cancer, 319, 320(t)
   in ovarian cancer, 310, 311(t)
   in vulvar cancer, 332, 333(t)
Fine needle aspiration
   in prostate cancer, 277
Fistula (fistulae)
   bronchopleural
      in lung cancer treatment, 119, 120, 126–127
5-Fluorouracil (5-FU)
   in colon cancer, 165–166
Flutamide
   in prostate cancer, 283
Follow-up

Follow-up *(Continued)*
  design of, 14–18

Gardner's syndrome, 152–153, 248
Gastric cancer. See *Stomach, cancer of*.
Gastrointestinal tract
  premalignant changes in, 12
Gastrostomy
  in esophageal cancer, 101
Glottis
  cancer of
    clinical features of, 60
    computed tomography in, 61
    diagnosis of, 60–62
    growth of, 57–58
    histology of, 57–58
    metastases from, 26, 57, 58
    staging of, 59(t)
    treatment of, 62–64
      chemotherapy in, 64
      outcome after, 65
      radiation therapy in, 64
Gynecologic cancer, 309–336. See also specific sites, e.g., *Ovary*.

Head and neck
  cancer of, 23–86. See also specific sites, e.g., *Mouth*.
    appearance of, 25
    arteriography in, 32
    biopsy in, 31
    carcinogens in, 24(t), 24–25
    classification of, 27–29
    clinical evaluation of, 29–32
    computed tomography in, 32
    endoscopy in, 31
    etiology of, 24(t), 24–25
    family history in, 29
    laboratory tests in, 31–32
    lung cancer with, 28–29
    magnetic resonance imaging in, 32
    metastases from
      distant, 26–27
      lymphatic, 25–26, 30, 31
      pulmonary, 28–29
    natural history of, 25–27
    neck palpation in, 31
    patient history in, 29–31
    physical examination in, 30–31
    primary site of, 25
    radiologic studies in, 32
    recurrence of
      vs. radiation fibrosis, 38
    staging of, 27–29
    symptoms of, 25, 30
    treatment of
      chemotherapy in, 39–40, 72–76
      combination therapy in, 38
      fundamentals of, 32–40, 34(t)
      hyperbaric oxygen in, 39
      induction chemotherapy in, 72–76
        protocol for, 75
      physical impairment with, 33, 34(t)
      radiation therapy in, 37–38
      surgical, 34–37

Head and neck *(Continued)*
    approach in, 35
    cervical lymphadenectomy in, 36–37
    phases of, 35–37
    radiation therapy and, 38–39
  ultrasound in, 32
Hemangiosarcoma, 188. See also *Liver, cancer of*.
Hemochromatosis
  liver cancer and, 186
Hemorrhoidal artery, 172
Hepatic cancer. See *Liver, cancer of*.
Hepatitis B virus
  liver cancer and, 185
Hepatoblastoma, 187. See also *Liver, cancer of*.
Hepatocellular carcinoma, 187. See also *Liver, cancer of*.
Human chorionic gonadotropin (HCG)
  in ovarian cancer, 317
  in testicular cancer, 293, 294, 295
Hutchinson freckle, 236
Hypernephroma. See *Renal cell carcinoma*.
Hypopharynx
  cancer of, 68–71
    carcinogens in, 24(t)
    clinical features of, 69–70
    diagnosis of, 69–70
    metastases from, 26, 71
    treatment of, 70–71

Immunotherapy
  in malignant melanoma, 242–243
  in nasopharyngeal cancer, 83
  in renal cell carcinoma, 291
Inflammatory bowel disease
  colon cancer and, 154
Interleukin 2
  in malignant melanoma, 242–243
Intravenous pyelography
  in renal cell carcinoma, 286
Intubation
  in esophageal cancer, 101
Iodine
  radioactive
    in thyroid cancer, 227

Keratosis palmaris et plantaris, 88
Ketoconazole
  in prostate cancer, 282
Kidneys
  cancer of, 285–291
    arteriography in, 286–287
    bilateral, 289–290
    computed tomography in, 286
    diagnosis of, 286–288, *288*
    epidemiology of, 286
    extrarenal manifestations of, 290
    incidence of, 286
    intravenous pyelography in, 286
    metastases from, 287, 290
    staging of, 286–288, *288*
    treatment of
      adjunctive therapy in, 290–291
      immunologic, 291
      surgical, 288–290, *289*

Kidneys *(Continued)*
    ultrasound in, 286
    urine cytology in, 287
    vena cava extension of, 290

Langer's lines
  in excisional breast biopsy, *206*
Laryngectomy, 35–36
  subtotal, 35
  vocal rehabilitation after, 35–36
Laryngopharyngectomy
  reconstruction after, 36
Larynx
  cancer of, 56–65
    carcinogens in, 24(t)
    clinical features of, 60
    computed tomography in, 61
    diagnosis of, 60–62
    endoscopy in, 61
    epidemiology of, 59–60
    histology of, 56–59
    metastatic, 57
    nodal metastases from, 26
    staging of, 59(t)
    treatment of, 62–64
      chemotherapy in, 64
      radiation therapy in, 64
  necrosis of
    in head and neck cancer treatment, 39
Laser
  carbon dioxide
    in laryngeal cancer, 63
  ND:YAG
    in esophageal cancer, 95
Levamisole
  in colon cancer, 165–166
Lichen sclerosus
  vulvar cancer and, 331
Linitis plastica. See *Stomach, cancer of.*
β-Lipoprotein
  serum
    in colon cancer, 151
Liver
  cancer of, 185–193
    angiography in, 187
    carcinoembryonic antigen in, 186
    computed tomography in, 186
    epidemiology of, 185–187
    evaluation of, 186–187
    α-fetoprotein in, 186
    magnetic resonance imaging in, 186–187
    metastatic, 190–192
      carcinoembryonic antigen in, 191
      in colon cancer, 164
      surgical therapy of, 190–192
    primary, 187–190, 188(t), *189*
      cirrhosis and, 188–189, *189*
      classification of, 187–188
      fibrolamellar variant of, 189
      pathology of, 187–188
      treatment of, 188–190
        results of, 188(t), 188–190, *189*
    radiology of, 186–187
    treatment of, 188–193
      chemotherapy in, 192
      cryosurgery in, 192

Liver *(Continued)*
      dearterialization in, 192
      orthotopic transplantation in, 192–193
      ultrasound in, 192
    ultrasound in, 187
  5–fluorouracil infusion of
    in colon cancer, 166–167
  transplantation of
    in liver cancer, 192–193
Lungs
  cancer of, 107–133, 135–137
    biopsy in, 112, 113, 114(t)
    bone scan in, 111
    bronchoscopy in, 111, 119
    cell type in, 115(t), 116
    computed tomography in, 111
    diagnosis of, 111–112
      chest films in, 110
    head and neck cancer with, 28–29
    inoperable, 110
    malignant pleural effusion in, 110–111, 130–131, *131*
    mediastinoscopy in, 111–112, 135
    mediastinotomy in, 112
    occult
      case of, *122*, 122–123
    operability in, 110–113, 112(t), 113(t)
    prognosis in, 107–108
    pulmonary cyst and, 123
    pulmonary infection and, 130–131, *131*
    recurrent laryngeal nerve involvement in, 129–130
    screening for, 110
    stage I
      cases of, 121–122, 124, 129–130, *130*
      results in, 108, 110
    stage II
      postoperative chemotherapy in, 118
      surgical therapy of, 115–118, 116(t), 117(t)
        postoperative radiotherapy and, 118
        preoperative radiotherapy and, 117–118
        results of, 116, 116(t), 117(t)
    stage III
      cases of, 121, 123–133, *125–128*, *131*, *1132*
      pleural fluid in, 130–131, *131*
      postoperative chemotherapy in, 118, 131–133, *132*
      surgical therapy of, 115–118, 116(t), 117(t)
        postoperative radiotherapy and, 118, 124–126, *126*
        preoperative radiotherapy and, 117–118
        results of, 116, 116(t), 117(t)
    staging of, 107–108, 108(t), 109(t), 112(t), 113(t), 135–136
    surgical therapy of, 113–121
      anesthesia in, 119
      bronchial closure in, 120
      bronchopleural fistulae and, 119, 120, 126–127
      bronchoscopy in, 119
      case studies of, 121–133, *122*, *125–128*, *130–132*
      chest tubes in, 120–121
      cost of, 118–119
      critique of, 135–137
      for palliation, 119
      limited resection in, 113–115, 114(t), 115(t), 136
        margins in, 114–115

Lungs (Continued)
    results of, 114, 115(t), 116(t)
    morbidity of, 118–119
    mortality of, 118–119
    pneumonectomy and, 121
    position for, 119–120
    postoperative chemotherapy and, 136
    postoperative radiotherapy and, 136
    preoperative radiotherapy and, 136
    stapler in, 120
    technical considerations in, 119–121
  undiagnosed
    risk of, 113, 114(t)
  visceral metastases in, 111, 127–129
  metastases from, 111, 127–129
Lymphocyte activated killer cells
  in malignant melanoma, 242–243
Lymphoepithelioma
  of tongue base, 43
Lymphoma
  hepatic, 188
  oral cavity, 43
Lynch syndrome
  colon cancer and, 153, 157

Magnetic resonance imaging (MRI)
  in head and neck cancer, 32
  in liver cancer, 186–187
  in nasopharyngeal cancer, 80
  in soft tissue sarcoma, 253, *254*
Malignant melanoma. See *Melanoma, malignant.*
Mammography
  in breast cancer, 197–198, 204
Mandible
  osteoradionecrosis of
    in head and neck cancer treatment, 39
Mastectomy, 211, 213
  prophylactic, 199
Mediastinoscopy
  in lung cancer, 111–112, 135
Mediastinotomy
  in lung cancer, 112
Melanin, 234
Melanoma
  malignant, 233–245
    biology of, 238
    clinical presentation of, 235–238
    coloration of, 235–236
    diagnosis of, 238–239
    differential diagnosis of, 237–238
    dysplastic nevi and, 234, 237
    early detection of, 245
    epidemiology of, 233–234
    esophageal, 91
    etiology of, 233–234
    follow-up for, 16, 243
    genetics of, 234
    histologic features of, 235
    laryngeal, 56
    lentiginous
      acral, 237
    lentigo, 234, 236–237
    management of, 239–243
      chemotherapy in, 242
      digit amputation in, 241–242
      excisional closure in, 240

Melanoma (Continued)
      immunotherapy in, 242–243
      limb perfusion in, 242
      local resection in, 239–240
      lymph node dissection in, 240–241
      lymphedema and, 241
    metastases from, 238, 243–245
      dermal, 243–244
      nodal, 244–245
      pulmonary, 244–245
      subcutaneous, 244
      visceral, 244–245
    nodular, 236
    oral cavity, 43
    pathology of, 234–235
    prophylactic lymph node dissection in, 13
    rates of, 233
    recurrence of, 239, 243
    subungual
      amputation for, 241–242
    sun exposure and, 233–234
    superficial, 235–236
    thickness neasurement in, 234–235
    vulvar, 336
Menopause
  breast cancer and, 198–199
Microcalcifications
  on mammography, 200, 201(t)
Mouth
  cancer of, 41–54, 42(t)
    clinical features of, 43–44
    diagnosis of, 44–45
    histology of, 42–43
    metastases from
      nodal, 26
    multifocal, 45
    recurrence of, 53
    staging of, 42(t)
    treatment of
      combined therapy in, 47, 50
      follow-up and, 52–54
      general considerations in, 45–48
      morbidity of, 45–46
      outcome of, 50–51
      primary site excision in, 46, 48–49
      radiation in, 47, 49–50
      sequelae of, 52–53
      surgical, 45–49
        approach for, 48
      survival rates with, 50–52
Mumps
  testicular cancer and, 293
Myositis ossificans, 249

Nasopharynx
  anatomy of, 78
  cancer of, 77–84
    carcinogens in, 24(t)
    computed tomography in, *79*, 79–80
    diagnosis of, *79*, 79–80
    Epstein-Barr virus in, 78, 80
    histology of, 80
    metastases from
      distant, 26
      nodal, 26, 82
    risk factors for, 78
    signs of, 78–79

Nasopharynx *(Continued)*
  staging for, 80–81, 81(t)
  symptoms of, 78–79
  treatment of
    frontiers of, *83*, 83–84
    induction chemotherapy in, *83*, 83–84
    palliative, 82–83
    radiation therapy in, 81–82
    standard, 81–82
Neck. See also *Head and neck, cancer of.*
  dissection of
    in head and neck cancer treatment, 36–37
Neurofibromatosis, 248, 249
Neuropathy
  cranial
    in nasopharyngeal cancer, 79
Nevus (nevi)
  blue, 238
  dysplastic, 237
  junctional, 237
  pigmented, 237
  spindle cell, 237
  Spitz, 237
Nitrates
  gastric cancer and, 140

Oat cell carcinoma
  esophageal, 91
Obesity
  endometrial cancer and, 318
Obstruction
  in colon cancer, 161, 162
Occult blood test
  in colon cancer, 156
Oldfield syndrome
  colon cancer and, 153
Oophorectomy
  in colon cancer, 160–161
  in ovarian cancer, 310
Oral cavity
  cancer of, 41–54, 42(t). See also *Mouth, cancer of; Tongue, cancer of.*
    bony invasion in, 43
    carcinogens in, 24(t)
    clinical features of, 43–44
    diagnosis of, 44–45
    follow-up for, 52–54
    histology of, 42–43
    metastases from
      distant, 26
      nodal, 44
    recurrence of, 53
    second primary in, 44, 45
    treatment of, 45–50
      combined therapy in, 47, 50
      general considerations in, 45–48
      morbidity of, 45–46
      outcome of, 50–52
      primary site excision in, 46, 48–49
      radiation in, 44, 47, 49–50
      sequelae of, 52–53
      surgical, 45–49
        approach for, 48
      survival rates with, 50–52
Oropharynx
  cancer of

Oropharynx *(Continued)*
  bony invasion in, 43
  clinical features of, 43–44
  diagnosis of, 44–45
  histology of, 42–43
  nodal metastases from, 44
  recurrence of, 53
  staging of, 42(t)
  treatment of, 45–50
    combined therapy in, 47, 50
    follow-up and, 52–54
    general considerations in, 45–48
    morbidity of, 45–46
    outcome of, 50–52
    primary site excision in, 46, 48–49
    radiation in, 47, 48, 49–50
    sequelae of, 52–53
    surgical, 45–49
      approach for, 48
    survival rates with, 50–52
Otalgia
  evaluation of, 30
Ovary
  cancer of, 309–318, 311(t), 313(t), 314(t)
    advanced
      treatment of, 313(t), 313–315, 314(t)
    biopsy in, 312
    CA125 in, 316, 317–318
    computed tomography in, 316
    early-stage
      treatment of, 312–313
    epithelial type of, 317
    α-fetoprotein in, 317
    hereditary syndromes of, 309–310
    human chorionic gonadotropin in, 317
    metastases from, 310, 311(t)
    natural history of, 310
    spread of, 310
    staging of, 310, 311(t)
    treatment of, 310–316, 313(t), 314(t)
      chemotherapy in, 313, 314(t), 315
      radiation therapy in, 315
      second-look surgery in, 315–316
    tumor markers in, 317–318
    vs. cyst, 312
  metastatic
    from colon cancer, 160–161
Oxygen
  hyperbaric
    in head and neck cancer, 39

Paget's disease
  vs. duct carcinoma in situ, 196
Paranasal sinuses
  cancer of. See also *Head and neck, cancer of.*
    carcinogens in, 24(t)
Park's procedure
  in colon cancer, 159–160
Paterson-Kelley (Plummer-Vinson) syndrome, 69, 88
Pelvis
  renal
    transitional cell carcinoma of, 305–306
Perforation
  in colon cancer, 161
Pharynx
  reconstruction of, 36

Pheochromocytoma, 230
Photoirradiation
  in esophageal cancer, 95
Pleural effusion
  malignant
    lung cancer and, 110–111, 130–131, *131*, 131
Plummer-Vinson syndrome, 69, 88
Pneumonectomy
  in lung cancer treatment, 121
Polypectomy
  in colon cancer, 156, 157
Polyps
  colon cancer and, 157–158
Polyvinyl chloride, 248
Pregnancy
  breast cancer and, 198
Proctosigmoidoscopy
  in colon cancer, 156
Progestogen
  in endometrial cancer, 322
Prostate
  cancer of, 275–285
    acid phosphatase in, 279
    diagnosis of, 276–277
    digital rectal examination in, 276
    epidemiology of, 275–276
    etiology of, 275
    grade of, 277
    incidence of, 275–276
    metastases from, 278
    needle biopsy in, 276
    nuclear shape in, 277
    ploidy of, 277
    progression of, 276
    prostate specific antigen in, 279
    staging of, 277–278, 278(t)
    transrectal fine needle aspiration in, 277
    transrectal ultrasound in, 276
    treatment of, 279–284
      adrenal ablation in, 283
      aminoglutethimide in, 282
      androgen deprivation in, 282
      anti-androgens in, 283
      castration in, 282
      chemotherapy in, 284
      diethylstilbestrol in, 282–283
      estrogen in, 282–283
      flutamide in, 283
      ketoconazole in, 282
      LH suppression in, 283
      radiation therapy in, 279–281
      radical prostatectomy in, 279–280
      transurethral resection in, 282
Prostate specific antigen
  in prostate cancer, 279
Proteins
  laminin-binding
    in colorectal cancer, 11
Proto-oncogenes
  in colon cancer, 154–155
Pseudosarcoma
  esophageal, 91
  vs. laryngeal carcinoma, 56
Pyrolysis
  in colon cancer, 151

Radiation therapy
  in anal cancer, 179–180
  in bladder cancer, 302–303
  in breast cancer, 20, 203, 215–216
  in cervical cancer, 326–327
  in colon cancer, 165, 349–350
  in endometrial cancer, 321, 322
  in esophageal cancer, 93–94, 99
  in gastric cancer, 146
  in head and neck cancer, 37–38
  in hypopharyngeal cancer, 70
  in laryngeal cancer, 64
  in lung cancer, 117–118, 122–126, 124–126, *126*, 129, 136
  in nasopharyngeal cancer, 81–82
  in oral cavity cancer, 44, 47, 49–50
  in ovarian cancer, 315
  in prostate cancer, 279–281
  in rectal cancer, 175–177
  in retroperitoneal sarcoma, 271(t)
  in soft tissue sarcoma, 260, 263–266, 264(t)
Rectum
  anatomy of, 172–173
  arterial supply of, 172–173
  cancer of, 171–179
    metastases from
      lymphatic, 172–173
      tumor histology and, 174
    prognosis in, 174(t), 174–175, 175(t)
    recurrence of, 173, 175
    surgical therapy of, 177–179, 178(t)
      colostomy after, 172
      local failure of, 175
      node dissection in, 173
      parasacral approach to, 178, 178(t)
      postoperative chemotherapy in, 176–177
      postoperative radiotherapy in, 176–177
      preoperative radiotherapy in, 175–176
      results of, 174(t), 174–175, 175(t)
      trans-sphincteric approach to, 177
      transanal approach to, 177
    ultrasonography in, 179
Recurrent laryngeal nerve
  in lung cancer, 129–130
Renal cell carcinoma, 285–291. See also *Kidneys, cancer of.*
  diagnosis of, 286–288, *288*
  epidemiology of, 286
  incidence of, 286
  management of
    adjunctive therapy in, 290–291
    surgical, 288–290, *289*
  staging of, 286–288, *288*
Renal pelvis
  transitional cell carcinoma of, 305–306
Retroperitoneum
  sarcoma of, 270–271, 271(t)

Salivary glands
  cancer of
    carcinogens in, 24(t)
    histology of, 42–43
    metastases from, 26
Sarcoma
  soft tissue, 247–272
    arteriography in, 254
    aspiration cytology in, 255

Sarcoma *(Continued)*
    biopsy in, 251, 255(t), 255–257, *256, 257*
    bone scan in, 253
    clinical presentation of, 251, 253–259, *254,* 255(t), *256, 257,* 258(t), 259(t)
    computed tomography in, 253, *254*
    core needle biopsy in, 255–256, *256*
    epidemiology of, 247–248
    excisional biopsy in, 256
    follow-up for, 17, *268,* 268–270, 269(t), *270*
    grade of, 249–250, 250(t), *251, 252*
    histologic types of, 248–249, 249(t)
    incisional biopsy in, 256–257, *257*
    magnetic resonance imaging in, 253, *254*
    metastases from, 254
        pathologic examination of, 263
        treatment of, 262–268, 264(t), *265,* 267(t)
            technical considerations in, 262–263
    necrosis in, 250
    pathology of, 248(t), 248–250, 249(t), 250(t), *251, 252*
    prognosis for, 258(t), 259(t)
    punch biopsy in, 256
    radiation and, 247
    radiologic examination in, 253–255, *254*
    recurrence of, *268,* 268–270, 269(t), *270*
        pulmonary, 269–270
        sites of, 269(t)
    retroperitoneal, 270–271, 271(t), *272*
    site of, 248, 248(t)
    staging of, 258(t), 258–259, 259(t)
    survival with, *252, 270*
    treatment of, 250, 259–262
        amputation in, 262
        brachytherapy in, 264–265, *265*
        chemotherapy in, 260, 266–268, 267(t)
        current concepts in, 259–260
        enucleation in, 260
        intraarterial infusion therapy in, 267–268
        local, 260–262
        radiation therapy in, 260, 263–264, 264(t)
            intraoperative, 265–266
        radical resection in, 261–262
        surgical, 260–262, *261, 262*
        wide excision in, 261
    types of, 249(t), *252*
Shoulder
    dysfunction of
        radical neck dissection and, 53
Sleep apnea
    post-treatment
        in oral cavity cancer, 53
Soft tissue sarcoma. See *Sarcoma, soft tissue.*
Speech
    esophageal, 36
Sphincter muscles, 172
Staging
    in bladder cancer, 300, *300*
    in cervical cancer, 325, 326(t)
    in colon cancer, 150, 158, 158(t)
    in endometrial cancer, 319, 320(t)
    in esophageal cancer, 105
    in gastric cancer, 141
    in head and neck cancer, 27–29
    in laryngeal cancer, 59(t)
    in lung cancer, 107–108, 108(t), 109(t), 112(t), 113(t), 135–136
    in nasopharyngeal cancer, 80–81, 81(t)

Staging *(Continued)*
    in oral cavity cancer, 42(t)
    in oropharyngeal cancer, 42(t)
    in ovarian cancer, 310, 311(t)
    in prostate cancer, 277–278, 278(t)
    in renal cell carcinoma, 287–288, *288*
    in soft tissue sarcoma, 258(t), 258–259, 259(t)
    in testicular cancer, *294,* 294–295, 295(t)
    in vulvar cancer, 332, 333(t)
Stapler
    in lung cancer surgery, 120
Steroids
    3-keto
        colon cancer and, 151
Stewart-Treves syndrome, 248
Stomach
    cancer of, 139–147
        benign ulcer disease and, 145
        biopsy in, 140–141
        diagnosis of, 140–141
        dietary factors and, 140
        epidemiology of, 139–140, 140(t)
        lymph node metastases in, 13–14, 144, 146
        nitrates and, 140
        staging in, 141
        superficial, 139, 140(t), 145
        treatment of
            chemotherapy in, 146
            surgical
                follow-up for, 145
                margins in, 146
                omental removal in, 144
                palliative, 143
                radiation therapy and, 146
                subtotal gastrectomy in, 141–145
                total gastrectomy in, 141–145, 142(t)
Stricture
    dilation of
        in esophageal cancer, 95
Stridor
    in subglottic cancer, 60
Subglottis
    cancer of
        clinical features of, 60
        computed tomography in, 61
        diagnosis of, 60–62
        histology of, 58
        nodal metastases from, 58
        staging of, 59(t)
        treatment of, 62–64
            outcome after, 65
Sucrase isomaltase
    in colorectal cancer, 11
Sunlight
    exposure to
        melanoma and, 233–234
Supraglottis
    cancer of
        clinical features of, 60
        computed tomography in, 61
        diagnosis of, 60–62
        histology of, 58
        metastatic, 57
        nodal metastases from, 58, 61
        staging of, 59(t)
        treatment of, 62–64
            chemotherapy in, 64
            outcome after, 65

Supraglottis *(Continued)*
  radiation therapy in, 64
Surgical oncologist
  as patient manager, 18–21
  characterization of, 9
Surgical oncology
  certification in, 9
  training programs for, 1–9, 3(t), *4*, 8(t)
    basic science, 2–7, 3(t), *4*
    clinical, 7–9, 8(t)
    goals of, 6–7

Tamoxifen
  in breast cancer, 197, 216
Testis (testes)
  cancer of, 292–297
    classification of, 292(t), 292–293
    computed tomography in, 294
    cryptorchidism and, 293
    diagnosis of, 293–294
    α-fetoprotein in, 293, 294, 295
    follow-up for, 297
    human chorionic gonadotropin in, 293, 294, 295
    incidence of, 293
    lymphangiogram in, 295
    mumps and, 293
    origin of, 292–293
    presentation of, 293–294
    staging of, *294*, 294–295, 295(t)
    treatment of, 295–297
      chemotherapy in, 296–297
      "observational protocol" for, 297
      retroperitoneal lymph node dissection in, 296
    ultrasound in, 293
    vs. breast cancer, 197
Thorotrast, 248
Thyroid
  cancer of, 219–230
    biology of, 228
    calcitonin in, 299
    carcinoembryonic antigen in, 299
    clinical presentation of, 220–221
    death rate in, 228
    diagnosis of, 221–223
    differentiated, 223–224
      biology of, 228
      risk of, 220
    epidemiology of, 221
    etiology of, 219–220
    follicular, 223–224
    follow-up for, 17
    incidence of, 219–220
    iodine deficiency and, 221
    medullary, 228–229
    needle aspiration cytology in, 221–223, 299
      technique for, 222
    nodal metastases from, 224, 299
    operative approach to, 224–226
      lobectomy in, 225–226
      patient position for, 225
      results of, 227–228
    papillary, 223–224
      microscopic foci of, 220
      nodal metastases from, 224
    pathology of, 223–224
    prognosis in, 13

Thyroid *(Continued)*
    radioactive iodine therapy in, 228
    recurrence of, 228
    risk of, 220
    thyroid function tests in, 222
    thyroid stimulating hormone suppression in, 228
TNM staging
  in bladder cancer, 300, *300*
  in colon cancer, 158, 158(t)
  in head and neck cancer, 27–29
  in laryngeal cancer, 59(t)
  in lung cancer, 107–108, 108(t), 109(t), 112(t), 113(t)
  in nasopharyngeal cancer, 80–81, 81(t)
  in oral cavity cancer, 42(t)
  in oropharyngeal cancer, 42(t)
  in prostate cancer, 277–278, 278(t)
Tobacco
  in esophageal cancer, 88
  in head and neck cancer, 24, 24(t)
  in laryngeal cancer, 59–60
  in oral cavity cancer, 41–42
Tongue
  cancer of, 41–54, 42(t)
    clinical features of, 43–44
    diagnosis of, 44–45
    histology of, 42–43
    recurrence of, 53
    staging of, 42(t)
    treatment of
      combined therapy in, 47, 50
      follow-up and, 52–54
      general considerations in, 45–48
      morbidity of, 45–46
      outcome of, 51–52
      primary site excision in, 46, 48–49
      radiation in, 47, 48, 49–50
      sequelae of, 52–53
      surgical, 45–49
        approach for, 48
      survival rates with, 50–52
Training programs, 1–9, 3(t), *4*, 8(t)
  basic science, 2–7, 3(t), *4*
  clinical, 7–9, 8(t)
  goals of, 6–7
Transplantation
  in liver cancer, 192–193
Turcot syndrome
  colon cancer and, 153
Tylosis, 88

Ulcer disease
  gastric cancer and, 145
Ulcerative colitis
  colon cancer and, 154
Ultrasound
  in head and neck cancer, 32
  in liver cancer, 187, 192
  in prostate cancer, 276
  in rectal cancer, 179
  in renal cell carcinoma, 286
  in testicular cancer, 293
Ureter
  transitional cell carcinoma of, 305–306
Urologic carcinoma, 275–306. See also specific sites, e.g., *Prostate.*

Uterine cervix. See *Cervix*.
Uterus. See also *Endometrium*.
   sarcoma of, 323

Verrucous carcinoma, 43, 56
Vocal cords. See *Glottis*.
Voice
   prosthesis for, 35–36
Von Hippel-Lindau disease, 286
Vulva
   cancer of, 331–336, *333*, 333(t), *334*, *335*
     early treatment of, 335

Vulva *(Continued)*
   invasive, 332–335, *333*, 333(t), *334*, *335*
     survival rate in, 334
     treatment of
       en bloc resection in, *333*, 333–334
       triple incision technique in, 334–335, *335*
   melanoma of, 336
   Paget's disease of, 332
Vulvectomy
   in anal cancer, 179

Whitmore-Jewett staging system
   in prostate cancer, 277–278, 278(t)